# Food Technology, Science and Marketing:

## EUROPEAN DIET IN THE TWENTIETH CENTURY

# Food Technology, Science and Marketing:

## EUROPEAN DIET
## IN THE TWENTIETH CENTURY

*Edited by*
*Adel P. den Hartog*

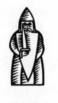

TUCKWELL PRESS

First published in 1995 by
Tuckwell Press Ltd
The Mill House
Phantassie
East Linton
East Lothian EH40 3DG
Scotland

British Library Cataloguing-in-Publication Data
A Catalogue record for this book
is available on request from the
British Library

The publisher acknowledges subsidy of
the Scotland Inheritance Fund; General Biscuits
Netherlands; the Foundation LEB Fonds; the
Department of Human Nutrition of the Wageningen
Agricultural University.

Typeset by Hewer Text Composition Services, Edinburgh
Printed and bound by
Cromwell Press, Broughton Gifford, Wiltshire

# CONTENTS

Contents

# CONTRIBUTORS

*Burnett, J.* Department of Government, Brunel The University of West London, Uxbridge, Middlesex UB8 3PH, United Kingdom.

*Chiapparino, F.* Instituto Universitario Europeo, Dipartimento di Storia, via dei Roccettini 9, 50016 S. Domenico di Fiesole, Italy.

*Crawford, E. M.* Department of Economic and Social History, The Queen's University of Belfast, Belfast BT7 1NN, Northern Ireland.

*De Knecht-van Eekelen, A.* Medical Faculty, Section Medical History, Free University of Amsterdam, van der Boechorststraat 7, 1081 BT Amsterdam, the Netherlands.

*Den Hartog, A. P.* Department of Human Nutrition, Wageningen Agricultural University, P.O. Box 8129, 6700 EV Wageningen, the Netherlands.

*Fenton, A.* European Ethnological Research Centre. c/o National Museums of Scotland, York Buildings, Queen Street, Edinburgh EH2 1JD, Scotland.

*Hietala, M.* University of Joensuu, Department of History, P.O. Box III, SF-80101 Joensuu, Finland.

*Horrocks, S. M.* Department of Economic and Social History, University of Leicester, Leicester, LE1 7RH, United Kingdom.

*Kisbán. E.* Magyar Tudományos Akadémia, Néprajzi Kutatóintézete [Institute of Ethnology of the Hungarian Academy of Sciences], Országház u 30, 1250 Pf-29, H-1250, Budapest, Hungary.

*Kjærnes, U.* SIFO, National Institute for Consumer Research, P.O. Box 173, N-1324 Lysaker, Norway.

*Oddy, D. J.* University of Westminster, Faculty Business, Management & Social Studies, 309 Regent Street, London W1R 8AL, United Kingdom.

*Pinard, J.* Faculté des Lettres et Sciences Humaines, Université de Limoges, 22, Avenue de la Libération, F-86000 Poitiers, France.

*Schärer, M. R.* Musée de l'Alimentation, Quai Perdonnet/Rue de Léman, BP 13, CH-1800 Vevey, Switzerland.

*Scholliers, P.* Centre for Contemporary Social History, Free University of Brussels, Pleinlaan 2, B-1050 Brussels, Belgium.

*Spiekermann, U.* Historisches Seminar, Westfälische Wilhelms-Universität, Domplatz 20–22, H 8143 Münster, Germany.

*Teuteberg, H. J.* Historisches Seminar, Westfälische Wilhelms-Universität, Domplatz 20–22, H 8143 Münster, Germany.

*Thouvenot, C.* Alimentation Cultures Espaces Sociétés, CNRS, Faculté de Médecine, Université de Nancy I, BP 184, F 54505 Vandoeuvre, France.

*Van Otterloo, A. H.* University of Amsterdam, Department of Sociology, Oude Hoogstraat 24, 1012 CE Amsterdam, the Netherlands.

*Weinhold, R.* Karl Marx Strasse 52F, o 1109 Dresden, Germany.

# I

# INTRODUCTION

## Adel P. den Hartog

This book is the outcome of the third symposium of the International Commission for Research into European Food History, held at the Wageningen Agricultural University, the Netherlands, in May 1993.[1] The International Commission for Research into European Food History is a multidisciplinary working group, organizing among others biennial symposia on substantive issues in food history, with emphasis on the 19th and 20th century. The first symposium was held in 1989 at the University of Münster, Germany, and dealt with research issues in European food history.[2] The second symposium, held in 1991 at Brunel University, West London, was devoted to the origins and development of food policies in Europe.[3] The symposium at the Wageningen Agricultural University brought together 20 contributors from 12 different countries, whose edited papers are contained in this volume. The Wageningen symposium addressed the role of food technology, science and marketing in the making of the European diet in the 20th century.

For a better understanding of present and future dietary developments in Europe it is of importance to make an analysis of factors which have shaped the modern diet. Based on discussions during the Symposium it became clear, as was expected, that a European diet as such does not exist. However, there is a very strong common denominator, marked by similarities in trends relating to how food technology, science and marketing have transformed the various diets in Europe. The process has led to an elimination of food shortages and hunger, and a change from a poor and monotonous diet to a highly diversified diet for nearly all segments of society.

Schumpeter in his classical study on economic development makes a distinction between invention and innovation.[4] He puts less emphasis on the inventor as such but more on the entrepreneur, thanks to whose leadership the invention may be put into practice as the actual innovation. In the food industry sciences have played a role in the invention of various methods of food processing, but the innovation, the product development and making of marketable products have been mainly the work of the entrepreneurs. The various papers in this volume indicate that the strength of the food industry in relation to the diet has been in the field of innovation. The food industry has not so much invented new foods, except for classical exceptions like margarine, chocolate bars and carbohydrated soft drinks. It has, however, made impressive progress in mass production of food with new alternations, standardization, distribution systems and marketing techniques. Sciences have been used to promote the quality of food and as a result the diet.

Taking Roger's theory on diffusion of invention into account, one may at country level distinguish early and late adopters of modern food technology and its related diet.[5] Countries such as Britain, followed by Germany, can be considered as early adopters. The question of which country adopts innovations earlier or later can be explained not only by the innovativeness of a society. It also depends on the geo-political situation and to what extent a country has room for making own decisions. Countries at the fringe of industrial Europe, such as Ireland, Finland and Hungary were relatively late adopters of modern food technology and the related diet. The papers on these countries indicate that the rate of diffusion was also influenced by periods of political dependency. The rate of adoption of modern foods in the diet depends also on the degree of access which people may have to resources such as income and formal education. This is what Amartya Sen calls entitlement to food, the command that people can exercise over resources to get sufficient food, both in quantity and quality.[6] The various papers in this volume demonstrate that in the course of the time food entitlement has become a self-evident phenomenon in the industrialized countries.

The first part of this book deals with food industry and food innovation. How the food industry is making use of nutritional sciences is presented by Horrocks. In the 1930s the British chocolate manufacturer Cadbury successfully introduced on nutritional and commercial grounds vitaminized cacao products. Not all nutritionally inspired food innovations were successful. An attempt by the Swiss food manufacturer Julius Maggi to introduce a protein-rich bean powder for improving the diet of the labouring classes failed. Schärer points out that this new food, based on nutritional concepts, was not accepted as it did not fit into the dietary habits and had the image of a poor man's food. The infant food industry is a classical example of the application of the nutritional and medical sciences in product development. Using the situation in the Netherlands as an illustration, de Knecht-van Eekelen analyses artificial versus breast feeding, changes from home-made preparations to proprietary infant formulas, and growing cooperation between the food industry and physicians.

The influence of innovations in the field of food preservation and food manufacturing is treated in the papers of Teuteberg, Burnett and Weinhold. Teuteberg shows the impact of the modern cooling and freezing techniques on society in Germany. The change from natural ice to a mechanical way of cooling and freezing took place in the second part of the 19th century. It allowed for mass transport of perishable foods from the production regions to the consumers. After the Second World War cooling and freezing techniques became widely available at household level. An interesting effect is the increase in taste for cooled beverages. The place of bread as a staple in the industrialized society is discussed for England by Burnett and in a former centralized economy by Weinhold for East Germany. England like other West European countries has shown a steady decline in bread consumption in the years 1950–1990. Burnett wonders whether bread can be considered any longer as a staple food of the contemporary diet. Its long-term decline can be seen as a casualty of the affluent society. The last decade of the 19th century marked a turning-point for the baking industry. The industrial technique of roller-milling produced fine white flour. Technology entered the baking industry with the introduction of flour-sifters, mechanical dough-kneaders, draw plate ovens and temperature-controlled gas or oil fired ovens. Two giant milling/baking combines now dominate the market, but master bakers still survive by offering speciality breads.

In the former German Democratic Republic, the authorities heavily subsidized the mass production of bread, a cheap staple food for the working class. Weinhold demonstrates how the communist authorities favoured large-scale bread baking by importing machines from East European countries and nearly destroyed the skills of the master bakers in Dresden. After the unification of the both Germanies, there is a revitalization of the master bakeries. Part one is concluded with a contribution by Fenton on the role of Milk Marketing Boards in Scotland. The introduction of modern dairy techniques combined with the consumer orientated activities of the Milk Marketing Boards caused a sharp increase in the consumption of milk during 1939–1952. This was due to cheap supplies for schools and social welfare, general increase in purchasing power and promotion to the general public of 'safe' milk. The promotion of milk as a healthy drink was much supported by nutrition experts. Because of requirements of the European Union and pressure within the UK, the Milk Marketing schemes will be revoked in 1994.

Part two is devoted to dietary patterns in relation to the food industry. The contribution of Kjærnes on how nutritional sciences promoted the dairy industry and milk consumption in Norway, is a diet orientated continuation of Fenton's paper on Scotland. It was not until the discovery of vitamins, mainly after World War I, that milk developed into a kind of nutritional 'miracle food' in Norway. For a long period the dairy industry found nutrition and health experts useful allies, and promotion of milk was successful. The situation changed gradually in the 1960s when the dietary fat-cardiovascular disease hypothesis gained acceptance. In Norway, as in other European countries, there is a decline in total milk consumption, and a shift from whole milk to low-fat milk and dairy products.

Pinard and Scholliers demonstrate by means of two entirely different products, cheese and chocolate, how industrial food processing has contributed to mass production and consumption. In France in the 19th century cheese was a major component of the rural poorer households. The 'fromage blanc' or cottage cheese was prepared at home, mainly from goat milk, by the house-wife. Cheese production at factory level and modern transportation contributed to the spread of a great variety of cottage cheeses among the urban consumers. In this process cheese has lost much of its locally based taste. In France cheese has changed from a food of poor families to a highly appreciated place as a dessert at a meal. Scholliers demonstrates how in Belgium chocolate as a luxury product at the turn of this century developed from an elite product to a product for the general consumer. Mechanization of the chocolate industry lead to a decrease in the price of chocolate. Intensive promotion campaigns and increase of income made it possible for the worker to buy a chocolate bar on special occasions. In the 1920s chocolate could be purchased on a daily basis.

Changes from a poor and monotonous diet and food shortage to the present affluent diet is given for Italy by Chiapparino and for Finland by Hietala. In Italy round 1900 meat was hardly to be found on the table. Pellagra, a nutrition deficiency disease, caused by a monotonous diet based on maize, was still common. After 1950 the diet improved because of a sharp increase of income and the rise of a modern large scale food industry. Regional differences, however, remain. In the less prosperous south and in central Italy the food system is still dominated by a small-scale food industry and food retailing. Finland experienced in 1867–1868 a widespread famine. Hietala explains how this famine has stimulated in Finland a drive towards a food policy based on self-sufficiency. In the interbellum the foundation was laid for a modern food industry. At present Finland is faced, like other European countries, with problems of an overproduction in food and an affluent diet. Dietary patterns in a centralised economy are discussed by Kisbán for Hungary for the period 1945–1990. The main target for the state owned industry was to produce in the first place quantity, and not variety of food products. From the late 1970s with more liberalisation food supply in shops improved considerably in quantity, variety and quality. Before the War, there were serious nutrition deficiencies amongst some groups of the working classes, but these problems disappeared after 1950. Although the food availability improved, there was limited room for food innovation. Kisbán argues that now Hungary is making up for a diet comparable to other industrialized countries.

Part three covers various aspects of food retail and marketing. The development of modern food retailing is analysed for the UK by Oddy and for Germany by Spiekermann. Both countries have experienced like other European countries the change from the corner shop to the food retail chain. There are, however, striking differences. Oddy demonstrates that in modern food retailing the UK was an early starter. In the interwar years the multiple shops became firmly established and introduced their own food labels. By the beginning of the 1990s the multiple shop retail chains have acquired a dominant position in food retailing. In Germany the food retail chain, both cooperative and private, gradually increased till the end of the 1920s. Spiekermann points out that this process was halted in the 1930s by the Nazi regime on ideological grounds. It was the aim of the government to establish a broad and decentralized network of independent single viable shops. After the 1950s the importance of the multiple shops increased rapidly.

For Ireland, Crawford points out the dual role of shopkeepers for the provision of food and also credit to low income customers, a phenomenon which was widespread in all other European countries. Despite the shift from low income families towards supermarkets, in present Dublin more than half of the poor families visit local cornershops when larder stocks run dry and credit is needed. Crawford is concerned that in the second half of the twentieth century food retailers provided an ever increasing variety of products, but have made a limited contribution to improved nutritional standards. Changes in food retailing for vast rural areas is discussed by Thouvenot in his paper on rural Lorraine in north-east France. It deals with food retailers travelling from one village to another, a phenomenon which also existed in other European countries such as Germany and Scandinavia. The intensification of the itinerant food trade in Lorraine started after the First World War. This was due to the introduction of the motor car and changes in rural life. In the 1960s the itinerant food trade started to decline. A major reason is the setting-up of large supermarkets at the outskirts of towns.

It is of interest to note that when food technology, science and marketing succeeded in providing an unprecedented food availability, both in quantitative and qualitative terms, to all layers of society, gradually in most European countries a public distrust of modern food technology emerged. The rise of distrust of modern food technology is dealt with by van Otterloo, taking the Netherlands Consumer's Union as an example. The growth of the Consumer's Union has been impressive during the last 40 years. The quality of food has been an important issue right from the start of its existence as an organization. The Consumer's Union became gradually professionalized by hiring experts in the field of food science and nutrition. The participation of consumers in food issues is an indication of a shift in the social structure of power between the different parties of the food system, such as industry, retailing and science.

Food advertising is a powerful factor in influencing the diet and in spreading nutritional knowledge among consumers. Advertising of food is closely linked with the development of a wider circulation of newspapers and magazines, the rise of the food industry and the emergence of brand names of food products in the latter part of the 19th century. All sorts of arguments are used in food advertising in order to persuade the consumer. In the early period of food advertising much reference was made to concepts of quality and hygiene. In the 1960s and 1970s there is a clear shift to 'natural' aspects of food and rural traditions. How the food industry tried to spread knowledge on nutrition among consumers as part of their food advertisements is presented by den Hartog. In the Netherlands, like other European countries, the food industry had an early interest in using nutrition and nutrition related items in their advertising activities. Nutritional terms and concepts from the nutritional sciences have frequently been used in food advertising over a long period. One may assume that the food industry in the course of time has contributed much to a greater familiarity with nutritional terms such as vitamins, proteins, calories, cholesterol, linoleic acid and problems of cardiovascular diseases. Advertisers make use of those parts of scientific information that may promote the sale of their products. This coincides often with current research themes.

## Notes

1   The editor in his role as Symposium organizer wishes to express his thanks to the Wageningen Agricultural University and the Rabo Bank for sponsoring the Symposium, which was held when the Agricultural University celebrated its 75th anniversary. Special mention must be made of the help received from Ms Sioe Kie Kroes and Ms Jaapje C.M.M. Nooij for organizing the conference and the editing of this book.

   Finally my thanks go to those who have generously supported this publication with a grant: the Scotland Inheritance Fund in Edinburgh, General Biscuits Netherlands, the Foundation LEB Fonds and the Department of Human Nutrition of the Wageningen Agricultural University.

2   Teuteberg, Hans J. (ed.), *European food history: a research review.* (London, Leicester University Press, 1992).

3   Burnett, John, Oddy, Derek J. (eds.), *The origins and development of food policies in Europe.* (London, Leicester University Press, 1994).

4   Schumpeter, Joseph A. *The theory of economic development, an inquiry into profits, capital, credit, interest and business cycle.* (Cambridge Ma, Harvard University Press, 1959).

5   Rogers, E.M. *Diffusion of innovations.* (New York, Free Press, 1983).

6   Sen, Amartya. *Poverty and famines: an essay on entitlement and deprivation.* (Oxford, Clarendon, 1987); Sen, Amartya, Muellbauer, J., Kanbur, R. *The standard of living.* (Cambridge, Cambridge University Press, 1988).

# 2

# NUTRITION SCIENCE AND THE FOOD INDUSTRY IN BRITAIN, 1920–1990

## Sally M. Horrocks

The history of nutrition science in 20th century Britain has generally been written in terms of its theoretical development, especially the emergence of the vitamin concept, and its relationship to public health and medicine.[1] The food manufacturing industry, another important means by which the findings of this discipline entered the public arena, has remained relatively neglected. From the 19th century onwards, however, nutrition science has been part of the range of scientific resources upon which the industry has drawn to both manufacture and promote its products. In the 1920s scientists working in industry learned to exploit the 'Newer Knowledge of Nutrition',[2] more systematically, in the process adapting it to suit their own specific needs. Since that time nutrition science has continued to play a role in the work of industrial food scientists, but it has never come to dominate their work, despite the criticism of several generations of health campaigners, who have sought to raise its profile. Instead nutrition science has remained as just one of a wide range of considerations to be taken into account by those working in the commercial sphere.[3] This paper, by considering the industrial exploitation of nutrition science in the context of the more general scientific activities of British food manufacturers, will suggest that manufacturers were able to draw on the resources of this new branch of science in a variety of ways, adapting it to their own ends, which did not necessarily conform to the expectations of nutrition scientists working in other institutional environments. This can be seen clearly when we examine the emergence of nutrition science as a significant element of the work of British industrial food scientists during the interwar period. After looking at the extent of interest across the industry as a whole this paper will turn to consider the variety of ways in which it was exploited by one firm, the cocoa and chocolate makers Cadbury. It will then go on to examine the involvement of industrial food scientists with the Nutrition Society in its early years before surveying some of the developments which took place in the postwar period.

**Science and the British Food Industry**

Prior to the 1920s the majority of large British food manufacturing concerns paid little attention to developments in the field of nutrition science. Several attempts, some highly successful such as that of Liebig, had been made by scientists to market foods based on scientific dietary principles, but there is no evidence to suggest that existing firms had undertaken any systematic research in this area.[4] These firms were, however, turning to trained scientists to provide skills they needed to expand their operations. Indeed, food manufacturing in Britain must be seen as a technologically sophisticated sector of industry by the interwar period. Despite the developments in the newer knowledge of nutrition which took place before World War I, it was not until the interwar period that these really began to be regarded as important by scientists working in the food industry. A number of events indicate the growing attention which was being paid to this field. Articles on the subject appeared with increasing frequency in the journals most often read by industrial food scientists, including *Food Manufacture*, *Chemistry and Industry*, and *The Analyst*. They began to be written by industrial food scientists and to include the results of their own investigations. Within firms themselves an increasing amount of time and resources were allocated to nutrition investigations, and its study was an important part of the only university course which specialised in the chemistry of foodstuffs which started in the mid-1920s.[5] When H.B. Cronshaw, the editor of *Food Manufacture*, presented his much debated paper on 'The Training of the Food Technologist' to the Food Group of the Society of the Chemical Industry in 1935, he suggested that the course should include nutrition. This raised little comment – by now it was an obvious requirement.[6] The formation of a separate Nutrition Panel within the Food Group, which was dominated by industrial food scientists, marked the coming of age of the subject as a specialism within industrial food science.

The rising prominence of nutrition in the practice of industrial food science was quickly reflected in both the products and promotional practices of firms. One indication of the extent of these activities is the concern they attracted from the Chief Medical Officer of Health, Sir George Newman, who condemned the 'sophistication' of foodstuffs in his 1932 report.[7] By the end of the 1930s 'vitaminised' foods were widely available, with products appearing in provisions stores and pharmacies throughout Britain. Vitamin supplements were also available in increasing numbers, and by 1939 they were even marketed for dogs. The construction by the Swiss chemical firm Roche of a plant to manufacture vitamins B1 and C in 1938 was hailed as a landmark in the 'era of re-adjustable foods'.[8]

Nutrition research was concentrated within those few companies which had a large enough research staff to enable specialisation, such as Lyons, Unilever and Cadbury, and in smaller firms which had been established

8

specifically to exploit the new knowledge, such as Vitamins Ltd. A number of pharmaceutical companies, notably British Drug Houses, carried out extensive research in the field, and the Pharmaceutical Society Laboratory provided support services to fee paying clients. Other enterprises were able to have access to this area of expertise through the services of consultants. In addition many food scientists already working in industry developed an interest in nutrition to add to their already wide range of skills. A number of firms began to employ trained biochemists where previously chemistry had been the standard requirement. Many of those in industry who worked on nutrition had, however, received no formal training in the subject, and their investigations were circumscribed both by this lack of expertise and by the immediate needs of their employers. Most industrial research laboratories had neither the facilities nor the inclination to emulate the types of experiments conducted by academic nutrition scientists. Instead they concentrated on determining the nutritive value of processed foods, on the effects of different processing techniques on this, and on how this could be controlled and altered on a large scale.[9]

The first two foods to be widely and successfully marketed with added vitamins were margarine and baby milk. Research into the possibility of adding a vitamin concentrate to margarine was initiated by Planters, a subsidiary of Lever Bros., later part of Unilever, in 1914 in an effort to bring its vitamin content into line with that of best butter. It took until 1927 to develop a margarine which was ready for commercial production, and which was sold under the brand name 'Viking' as a premium product at a price close to that of best butter. Early sales figures were disappointing, probably because of the high cost, and it was not until the quality of the concentrate had improved, and it was added to a variety of lines, that the concept of adding vitamins to margarine achieved commercial success.[10] As a result of the expertise gained from this project the company was able to market two vitamin supplements, 'Essogen' and 'Advita'. These were used extensively during a three year investigation undertaken by the research department into the effects of vitamin intake on sickness levels among the company's work force. These tests involved hundreds of employees, and led to the conclusion that vitamin supplements were responsible for improving general health levels and reduced absenteeism. Such a result had clear implications for the sale and promotion of the firm's products.[11]

In contrast to the difficulties experienced by margarine producers, Glaxo's efforts to produce babymilk with added vitamin D enjoyed rapid success. Joseph Nathan, the parent company, initiated the manufacture of milk powder in order to use the surplus skimmed milk from butter and cream production, and seems to have become involved with vitamins largely through the influence of Harry Jephcott, who rose from a position as quality control chemist to become the company's managing director. It was through its development of vitaminised food products that Glaxo began its move from food to pharmaceuticals, which accelerated during World War II. Prominent among Glaxo scientists who worked in this area was A.L. Bacharach, one of the most outspoken industrial experts on nutrition, who became the first Honorary Treasurer of the Nutrition Society. 'Sunshine Glaxo', their first product of this type, was launched in 1928, and a number of others were introduced soon afterwards. By 1938 the company was selling 22 different products in the British market, more than any other individual firm. Its growth in a number of countries throughout the world was closely linked to the success of these vitaminised products.[12]

Investigations in the field of nutrition science arose in some companies through the personal initiative of scientists themselves, but this did not prevent them benefiting the enterprise concerned. An example of this is the research into the vitamin C content of cooked food undertaken by M. Olliver of Chivers. This helped to fill a gap which had been left by the focus of academic work on raw foodstuffs, and led to the identification of blackcurrants as a potent source of vitamin C. Chivers became a major producer of blackcurrant concentrates during World War II.[13]

Both Unilever and Glaxo used nutrition science to advertise products as well as to develop new lines. The practice of advertising the nutritional benefits of food products, which had existed for a long time, and predated the emergence of the vitamin concept, was adapted to include claims based on the micronutrient content of foods. Heinz advertised the vitamin C in their tomato ketchup, Cadbury the vitamin D in milk chocolate, and many other firms followed suit. Scientists across the food industry were called upon by their employers to provide the material needed for the preparation of what was called 'medical propaganda' to promote products. While the requirements of advertising did not lead to fundamental advances in the science of nutrition, they did serve to raise public awareness that vitamins were an essential component of food, and contributed to the ways in which particular foods came to be regarded as good or bad.[14] In addition the range of foodstuffs whose nutritional composition had been analysed was extended.

*Cadbury*

Having looked at the food manufacturing industry in general our attention now turns to a more detailed study of the way in which one firm, Cadbury, used nutrition science for commercial purposes. The firm made extensive use of nutrition science in its advertising campaigns during the 1930s, as well as drawing upon these findings to find a profitable use for one of its waste products. Throughout, however, nutrition investigations were only one component of an extensive scientific organisation which served the entire company, and they remained firmly integrated into a general strategy which regarded all scientists within the firm as an important resource in the pursuit of profit. The firm first employed its own chemist in 1901 after a period of reliance on outside consultants. Initially N.P. Booth was involved in analysing raw materials and products, later extending his work to include the development of new lines. The staff of the Cadbury laboratory grew rapidly, and by World War I it had considerably extended its range of activities. Expansion continued during the interwar period, and scientists cooperated with staff from throughout the factory to ensure its efficient operation. At the same time they carried out fundamental investigations into the chemistry of production processes which ensured that the firm was able to draw upon a unique fund of technical information not accessible to its competitors.[15]

The earliest record of nutrition research by the firm was a series of rat feeding experiments carried out by H.W. Bywaters in 1919. Despite the indications that Cadbury's Dairy Milk Chocolate promoted vigorous growth, this line of enquiry was not pursued again until the late 1920s, when nutrition science became a regular pursuit. It did so in the context of a close relationship between the Advertising Office and the Chemists' Department, and began with a number of campaigns which focused on the nutritional composition of the firm's products after the attention of the Board had been alerted to the promotional possibilities of vitamins by the efforts of other manufacturers. The possibility of emulating Glaxo and taking out a licence to manufacture irradiated ergosterol under the Steenbock patents was discussed, but the firm was reluctant to pay for the use of this process.[16] This reluctance was compounded by the discovery that Cadbury's Dairy Milk Chocolate already contained vitamin D anyway. The opportunities that this offered for product promotion were rapidly seized, and A. Churchman, the chief biochemist, was instructed to prepare a pamphlet for the medical profession emphasising the nutritional advantages of chocolate consumption. This initiated a long period of collaboration between scientists and advertisers, which was particularly targeted at the medical professions. Throughout there was a concern to ensure that no claims were made which could not be backed up with scientific evidence. It was not until 1938, for example, that the Research Committee was satisfied that cocoa as well as chocolate contained vitamin D, and gave its permission to the Advertising Department to use this information in publicity material.

Throughout the 1930s Churchman devoted much of his time to work on vitamins for advertising purposes. He regularly attended medical exhibitions as a consultant, and gave conducted tours of the factory to local groups of the British Medical Association. A special pamphlet on the Bournville laboratories was prepared for doctors, and emphasised the hygienic conditions of production as well as the beneficial dietetic effects of the company's products. The Advertising Office even went so far as to suggest that, 'as far as our visitors are concerned the Chemists' Department is our principal concealed asset.' In 1934 a major advertising campaign for Cadbury's Dairy Milk promoting its food value was launched, and feeding tests were carried out. The emphasis of the advertising campaign was on the product as a food rather than as a snack, and great stress was given to the way in which the goodness of milk was complemented by the chocolate to provide a convenient source of essential nutrients. Other measures, including a publicity film for nurses, were planned. In 1936 it was decided that any recipe change would have to be examined for its effects on the nutritive value of the product, as well as for the familiar qualities of taste and texture, a move which indicates the growing importance which had come to be attached to nutrition within the firm. The launch of a diabetic chocolate in 1937 was viewed as establishing an important 'propaganda line', and the research facilities available to the company were emphasised in advertising material for the product.

Advertising was not the only area in which Cadbury were able to exploit this new area of science, as it proved to be of value in the continuing search for profitable uses for waste materials. The most significant left-over from the production process was cacao shell, which had a variety of outlets, none of which was particularly profitable. In his attempts to improve this situation A.W. Knapp analysed the product in meticulous detail and proposed a number of schemes for its use. In 1934 his analysis revealed that cacoa shell was the most potent vegetable source of vitamin D, and feeding trials were initiated to examine its use as cattle fodder.

These were carried out in collaboration with the National Institute for Research in Dairying, and indicated that cows fed on cacao shell had enhanced levels of vitamin D in the milk they produced. After widespread publicity for these findings the demand for cacao shell rose, as did its price. Later it was advocated as an excellent food for pit ponies.[17]

The uses to which nutrition science was put by Cadbury fit into the general pattern of scientific activities to be found within the firm, which involved maintaining a close watch on outside developments and then adapting and exploiting them to serve the needs of the company. The scope of research was strictly limited to these needs, and the widespread publication of results should be seen as part of this strategy, probably doing more to enhance the image of the firm than to further the discipline of nutrition science. In this they were typical of major food manufacturers in interwar Britain, whose interests in nutrition science were based primarily on the commercial possibilities which it offered.

## Industrial Scientists and the Foundation of the Nutrition Society

The divisions which existed between the practice of nutrition science in industry and its pursuit in other institutional settings are suggested by the reactions of industrial food scientists to the foundation of the Nutrition Society. Few of them would have identified themselves primarily as nutrition scientists, and they constituted a very different professional group from those researchers in the academic community who were interested in nutrition. The divide between these groups was clearly apparent during the foundation of the Society in 1941. Few scientists working in either the food or pharmaceutical industries were prominent in this process, and several leading research directors in industry declined to join when approached. These included Leslie Lampitt of Lyons, probably the most influential member of the industrial food science community, and E.B. Anderson of United Dairies, who was also a leading member of the Food Group. It is not clear exactly why they declined to join, but it is possible that both of these men felt that the Nutrition Panel of the Group already fulfilled the need for a forum for researchers interested in this area, and thus regarded another society as unnecessary. Despite his reservations over this duplication of effort, Lampitt was keen to ensure that there was cooperation between the two organisations. None of the instigators of the scheme to form the Society were from industry, although A.L. Bacharach of Glaxo, who became the first Honorary Treasurer, was involved from an early stage. Although a number of industrial scientists did eventually join, those members listed as coming from firms in the food and pharmaceutical industries combined constituted well under ten per cent of the membership of the Society in its early years.[18]

By 1945/46, however, 30 companies, including Kraft Cheese, Lever Bros, Reckitt & Colman, Marmite Food Extract Co., Macfarlane Lang, Spillers, Newforge, Ovaltine, and Chivers were represented among the membership.[19] These firms manufactured a wide range of foodstuffs, including food drinks, dairy products, biscuits, canned foods, pet foods, and condiments. The involvement of firms from such a variety of sectors within food manufacturing indicates the widespread acknowledgement within the industry of the importance of nutrition expertise. Staff from a number of large firms, including Lyons, were still conspicuous by their absence. Scientists from this firm did, however, attend meetings and presented papers which related to commercial food processing operations. The introduction of regulations which restricted membership of the Society to those who had 'contributed to the scientific knowledge of nutrition' may have discouraged some of those in industry who had an interest in the area and made extensive use of its findings, but whose responsibilities in other fields gave them little time or scope for original or publishable work. Industrial scientists may also have been reluctant to join an organisation which was so dominated by other interests when many found that the existing structures associated with the Society of the Chemical Industry fulfilled their needs. The lack of serious involvement in the Nutrition Society by industrial scientists in the early years thus reflects both the divisions to be found between the interests of academic and industrial scientists, and the position of nutrition science as just one of a range of skills possessed by scientists in the food industry.

**Postwar Developments**

In the years immediately following the end of World War II there were a number of major changes in the organisation of food research in Britain in both the academic and the industrial spheres.[20] Across British industry in general there was increasing emphasis on fundamental research, reflected in the movement of scientists from senior university posts into industry. Jack Drummond, for example, followed his stint as scientific advisor to the Ministry of Food during the war not by returning to his professorial position at University College London, but by taking up a post as research director for Boots, a major manufacturer of pharmaceuticals.[21] These changes affected the nature of the relationship between academic and industrial science across a number of fields, including nutrition science. Industry grew in relative importance as a source of finance for nutrition research as the lavish funding provided by the Medical Research Council in the interwar years dried up at the same time as nutrition was gaining acceptance as an independent academic subject at the undergraduate level. The pioneer in this was John Yudkin at Queen Elizabeth College (now part of King's College), whose department produced the first nutrition graduates in the mid 1950s.[22]

Food science and technology also began to receive recognition as academic subjects soon afterwards, although a number of courses existed prior to this which were related to the needs of the food industry. The subject was developed in response to the demands of industry, and included both undergraduate teaching and postgraduate conversion courses for those qualified in other disciplines. Many of the early pioneers had been trained in more traditional fields but were readily able to apply their knowledge to food. A good example was A.G. Ward, who headed the Leeds University Department of Food Science, and who was an expert in colloidal physics. By 1970 courses were offered by the universities of Leeds, Nottingham, Reading and Strathclyde, by Queen Elizabeth College and the Polytechnic of the South Bank in London. Their character reflected the tremendous diversity to be found in food science, and included attention to nutrition as part of a much broader range of interests. There was close collaboration between industry and university departments from the outset, and grants for research were increasingly derived from this source, both from individual firms and from trade organisations.[23] This led to concerns that the dietary advice which emerged from such studies was far from the kind of disinterested council which was necessary if the nutritional health of the nation was to be improved. These misgivings were intensified during the 1980s as increasing publicity was given to each new study which explored the relationship between diet and disease, and as foods came to be increasingly labelled as good or bad for health on the basis of this research. Scientists who failed to agree with the prevailing orthodoxy were loudly criticised, as D. Naismith of

Queen Elizabeth College discovered when he produced a report in the 1980s on potato crisps which included the observation that they contain, 'more fibre than wholemeal bread, six times as much vitamin C as an apple and less salt than cornflakes'.[24] Concerns about the quality of the British food supply came under the scrutiny of campaigning organisations such as the London Food Commission and Parents for Safe Food. These groups drew attention to what they regarded as a serious lack of concern with nutrition content by manufacturers, who, they argued, placed profits above long term health considerations. These criticisms, which often accused industrial food scientists of complicity in this process, were countered by drawing attention to the many other aspects of their work, and by stressing that nutrition was but one of a range of concerns which needed to be taken into account in the development and manufacture of food products.[25]

This emphasis on nutrition science as just one of many skills is even more evident if we examine the increasing technological capabilities of food retailers, an aspect of industrial food science where the postwar era stands in marked contrast to the interwar period. Investment in laboratory facilities has been used by retailers to increase their control over their suppliers, especially as own label supermarket products increased their share of the grocery market. J. Sainsbury, now one of the largest retail chains, first employed their own chemist in 1935, and by 1948 had expanded scientific services to the point where they needed to separate chemical and bacteriological laboratories. In 1956 the laboratories moved to new premises, and included laboratories for routine chemical and bacteriological work, along with research laboratories for bacteriology, biochemistry and physical chemistry, and a library. Laboratories were also maintained at factories in other locations. In the 1970s the laboratories moved yet again, and were brought together on one site for the first time since 1948. The extensive literature produced by the firm which discussed the functions of these laboratories up to the mid-1970s stressed their role in ensuring that products conformed to food safety legislation, in assessing customer complaints, and their crucial importance in the control of production and distribution. Little specific attention seems to have been devoted to nutrition, although it was clearly one of the many areas of interest which were included in laboratory activities.[26] While the mobilisation of nutrition science has undoubtedly played a part in the more widespread use of scientific expertise in the battle for market share which has been taking place in the British food retailing industry over the last decade, it would be foolish to place overdue emphasis on its significance. Instead it is important to view it as just one of a range of factors which have helped to determine the nature of the food products offered to consumers.[27]

**Conclusion**

The incorporation of nutrition science into the skills of industrial food scientists and its exploitation by the pharmaceutical industry during the interwar period brought onto the market a whole range of products which embodied a new understanding of the nature of good food, and led to changes in the way some existing products were marketed. A knowledge of nutrition joined the already extensive range of fields with which the industrial food scientist was required to be familiar, leading to the development of nutrition investigations shaped by the commercial environment from which they emerged. Profits not preventative medicine were the goal which motivated this research. After World War II, despite a number of changes in the organisation of food research, and the growth of both nutrition and food science as university subjects, this pattern remained basically unchanged.

**Notes**
1. Smith 'thesis', Petty (1989), Mayhew (1988).
2. This phrase is taken from the title of Elmer V. McCollum's book, and refers to nutrition science after the emergence of the vitamin concept.
3. For a more general account of this see Horrocks, 'thesis'.
4. Finlay (1992).
5. *Prospectus of university courses in the Municipal College of Technology, Manchester, session 1926/7* (Manchester, *1926*), pp. 158–60 and 230–1.
6. *Chemistry and Industry* 54 (1935), pp. 192–4. On the Food Group see Kay (1972).
7. Newman (1932).
8. *Chemist and Druggist*, supplement, 25/3/39, p. xxxi and *Food Manufacture* 13 (1938), p. 423.
9. Horrocks (1994).
10. Wilson (1954) vol. I, pp. 306–7 and 338.
11. 'Vitamins and sickness absence', *Pharmaceutical Journal*, 134 (1935), p. 642.
12. Davenport-Hines and Slinn (1992), pp. 5–132.
13. *Food Manufacture*, 10 (1935), p. 435.
14. Graves and Hodge (1940), pp. 189–90 claims that 'vitamins were all-weather favourites: . . . before the end of the Thirties they were lettered from A to E in the hearts of even the most backward villager.'
15. On the firm as a whole see Williams (1931) and Cadbury Bros (1946). The work of Cadbury scientists up to 1939 is covered in Horrocks, 'thesis', ch. 5. this account is based on the firm's archives, especially the Annual Reports of the Chemists' Department and the Minutes of the Research and Advertising Committees. I would like to thank Cadbury Bros for permission to use this material.

16. Apple (1989).
17. Knapp, Arthur W. and Coward, Katherine H., 'The vitamin D activity of cacao shell', *Biochemical Journal* 50 (1935), pp. 728–35.
18. Smith, 'thesis', ch. 4.
19. *The Nutrition Society: list of officers, committees, etc. 1945/46.*
20. DSIR (1948).
21. *Obituary Notices of Fellows of the Royal Society* 9 (1954), pp. 99–130.
22. Smith, 'thesis'. Yudkin received funding from at least 18 different firms and 3 food producing organisations between 1947 and 1973 (King's College Archives, QA5/GPF 3/1).
23. Ward, Alan G., 'The emergence of food science', *New Scientist*, 18 (1962), pp. 674–5 and 'Planning food research', *Chemistry and Industry*, 95 (1976), pp. 1011–8.
24. Quoted in Smith, 'thesis', p. 469, note 54.
25. Clutterbuck and Lang (1982) and Cannon (1987). The London Food Commission, now the Food Commission, produces its own magazine, *The Food Magazine*.
26. *JS Journal*, Feb 1951, July 1957, Aug/Sept 1968, Feb 1969, Sept 1975 and Quarmby, D.A., 'Food retailing: the challenge to food scientists and technologists', *Food Science and Technology Today*, 3 (1989), pp. 222–7.
27. Senker (1988).

## Literature

Apple, Rima, 'Patenting university research: Harry Steenbock and the Wisconsin Alumni Research Foundation', *Isis*, 80 (1989), pp. 375–94.

Cadbury Bros, *Industrial record: a review of the interwar years* (Bournville, 1947).

Cannon, Geoffrey, *The politics of food* (London, 1987).

*Chemistry and Industry.*

Clutterbuck, Charlie and Lang, Tim, *More than we can chew* (London, 1982).

Davenport-Hines, Richard P.T. and Slinn, Judy., *Glaxo: a history to 1962* (Cambridge, 1992).

Department of Scientific and Industrial Research, *Annual Reports 1939–48* (London, *1948*).

Finlay, Mark R., 'Quackery and cookery: Justus von Liebig's extract of meat and the theory of nutrition in the Victorian age', *Bulletin of the History of Medicine*, 66 (1992), pp. 404–18.

*Food Manufacture.*

Graves, Robert and Hodge, Alan, *The long weekend: a social history of Great Britain, 1918–1939* (London, *1940*, reprinted *1991*).

Horrocks, Sally M., 'Consuming science; science, technology and food in Britain, 1870–1939' (unpublished PhD thesis, University of Manchester, 1993).

Horrocks, Sally M., 'The business of vitamins: nutrition science and the food industry in interwar Britain', in H. Kamminga and A. Cunningham (eds), *The Science and Culture of Nutrition* (Amsterdam, 1994).

Kay, Herbert D., 'A short history of the Food Group', *Journal of the Science of Food and Agriculture*, 23 (1972), pp. 127–60.

Mayhew, Madelaine, 'The 1930s nutrition controversy', *Journal of Contemporary History*, 23 (1988), pp. 445–64.

McCollum, Elmer V., *The newer knowledge of nutrition: the use of food for the preservation of vitality and health* (2nd edition, New York, 1922).

Newman, George, *On the state of the nation's health* (London, 1932).

Petty, Celia, 'Primary research and public health: the prioritization of nutrition research in inter-war Britain' in J. Austoker and L. Bryder (eds), *Historical perspectives on the Medical Research Council* (Oxford, 1989), pp. 83–108.

Senker, Jacqueline, *A taste for innovation: British supermarkets' influence on food manufacturers* (Bradford, 1988).

Smith, David F., 'Nutrition in Britain in the 20th century' (unpublished PhD thesis, University of Edinburgh, 1986).

Williams, Iolo A., *The firm of Cadbury, 1831–1931* (London, 1931).

Wilson, Charles, *The history of Unilever: a study in economic growth and social change* (2 vols, London, 1954).

# 3

# ANALYSIS OF NUTRITIONAL STATUS, THE FOOD INDUSTRY AND PRODUCT INNOVATION IN THE LATE NINETEENTH CENTURY, WITH REFERENCE TO PREFABRICATED PULSE POWDER

## *Martin R. Schärer*

There are not many cases in the 19th century where it is possible to examine in detail the interplay between an analysis of the nutritional status of a defined section of the population, the philanthropic efforts of a welfare association, the intentions of a food manufacturer, and a resultant product innovation and its acceptance. One case in which these conditions do apply, thanks to the abundant source material available, relates to the pulse or legume powder (Leguminosenmehl) intended for the worker population, which was brought onto the market by Julius Maggi in 1884. The following presentation is based on the general nutritional situation of the time, in the context of a nonprofit social-service organization, the 'Schweizerische Gemeinnützige Gesellschaft' (SGG), and against the background of the nascent food industry.

### The nutritional status in Switzerland in the closing years of the nineteenth century

From the Middle Ages almost to the end of the 18th century, Switzerland – apart from a self-sufficient area in the heart of the Alps and a transition zone with a ley farming economy – was characterized essentially by two contrasting patterns of nutrition. The Alpine areas (pasture country) were dominated by cheese and other dairy products as well as meat (game and small farm animals), while on the plateau round the northern rim of the Alps (arable land) food consisted chiefly of cereal preparations and bread (plus, from the second half of the 18th century, potatoes), pulses (legumes) and vegetables.

These highly different zones increasingly converged since the very early onset of industrialization at the end of the 18th century, to such an extent that they were no longer a determining factor in the four decades leading up to the

First World War which are of interest to us here. The period is also characterized by another – social – convergence which was, however, less far-reaching: considerable social differences still existed on the eve of the war. After a period of movement, the use of new foodstuffs and an altered nutritional situation altogether were now consolidated: potatoes, coffee (very often surrogate coffee) and the bread-and-coffee breakfast were widely adopted; cooking became increasingly mechanized; some processing activities shifted from the home to specialized premises; private preserves' production diminished; hardly any households were able to cover their own needs any more, even in small towns, and what little self-sufficiency remained was restricted to small vegetable plots; numerous cookery books were published, including some aimed specifically at workers; an increasing general level of prosperity made better nutrition possible. Naturally, these changes did not take place in step and displayed typical variations from one region to another. Cereal and dairy products, potatoes, pulses, cabbage, root vegetables and local fruit provided the staples; they were augmented by meat, fish and fowl to varying degrees according to individual purchasing power. Quality and quantity depended on a household's economic situation, while choice and preparation were a matter of local tradition; a generalization of nutritional patterns was initially observable in fully market-dependent worker circles. Products of the slowly emerging food industry had yet to make any general impact; there can be no talk of mass consumption until the 20th century.[1])

Besides the numerous isolated works,[2] the two single nutritional balances covering the whole of Switzerland are of interest for the decades immediately preceding the First World War. The calculations of the chemist Rudolf Theodor Simler[3] referring to the year 1870 and specifically described as a 'contribution to the establishment of a chemistry in the interests of the state and the national economy', attempt to 'investigate the sources from which the population of a national territory derives the energy which it converts each day into the living power of physical and intellectual work'. He justified the basic interest in the question with the recognition that 'in the final analysis, this energy, in other words those foodstuffs which are the very basis of material existence . . . [influence] the petty politics of constituencies as they do the affairs of state'. However, as he in a sense puts the cart before the horse by calculating Swiss production from requirements (computed with the help of various nutritional factors), which he equates with consumption, and import surpluses, it is impossible to deduce real consumption figures from his work.

Infinitely more informative is the work by Salome Schneider,[4] even if it does refer to the later years 1908–12. With an average daily intake of 2,900 kcals (3,100 allowing for alcohol) – 2/3 of vegetable, 1/3 of animal origin – the Swiss can be considered to have been adequately nourished. To summarize the most important consumption figures (given in grams per capita per month, except where otherwise stated): bread 9,700, flour 2,000, maize (sweet corn) 1,600, rice 280, vegetables 2,900, potatoes 11,000, fruit 6,300 (of which apples 3,400), milk 26 litres, butter 410, cheese 920, eggs 8 units, meat 3,800, sausage 5 units, poultry 140, fish 110, coffee 250, surrogate coffee 120, sugar 2,000, wine 5.9 litres, cider 2.5 litres, beer 6 litres. A breakdown by nutrient reveals a decidedly well-balanced picture: 98 g proteins, 84 g fat and 440 g carbohydrates (all figures without alcohol). Naturally, these figures (like all calculations before the First World War) reflect utilization and not actual consumption, i.e. they do not take in account either waste or spoilage and as such are too high. Furthermore, the figures are Swiss averages; consumption among the worker population, particularly at its lower levels, was considerably less. The only significant difference from today in the percent share of nutrients of vegetable and animal origin is in fats: in 1908/12, 84% of fats were of animal origin (with milk and dairy products taking the lion's share with 52%), whereas they account for barely half today. Self-sufficiency calculations are also interesting (never in its history has Switzerland been self-supporting): self-sufficiency stood at 55% for vegetable and 99% for animal products. Schneider concludes by noting that nutrient consumption is high in comparison with other countries and that its composition had undergone a substantial shift in favour of fat and protein since Simler's survey.

As in other countries, budget calculations[5] for Switzerland are plentiful. An analysis of household expenditure for the year 1912[6] – i.e. at the end of the period we are interested in – allows some general conclusions to be drawn: the higher the income the greater the expenditure for the individual food-stuffs in absolute terms, with the exception of potatoes, flour, pasta and animal fat; more purchasing power is invested in protein-rich items as well as in fruit and vegetables. But – as is well-known – this is paralleled by a decline in the relative outlay for essentials: unskilled workers spend an average of 374 francs, skilled workers 406 francs, state employees and office workers 442 francs a year on food and drink. These outlays represent 52%, 48% and 40% of their respective total budgets. An extensive study of real wages among Swiss industrial workers between 1890 and 1921[7]) carried out by the University of Zürich comes to the following findings: 1890 54%, 1900 48%, 1910 53%, 1920 54%.

A major step in bringing about a reduction in spending on food is represented by the development of cooperative societies around the middle of the last century. They offered first a reduced, then an ever more extensive range of modestly priced good products. As the cooperatives were not all organized the same way it is difficult to make a global evaluation of their financial advantages, but actual savings over buying at other shops were probably in the region of 5–10% of expenditure on food.[8]

## Worker nutrition, Fridolin Schuler and the Schweizerische Gemeinnützige Gesellschaft (SGG)

A few examples of the extensive contemporary literature dealing with the situation of workers in the 19th century will be presented briefly here in order to put Schuler's analyses into better perspective. Bernhard Becker was a parson in Linthal in the canton of Glarus, which industrialized at a very early stage. In his monograph 'Ein Wort über die Fabrikindustrie',[9] published in 1858, he was already exercised by many questions which Schuler was to explore in more detail later. For example, he deplored the inadequate lunch breaks and the gulping down of meals in factories, putting the blame not just on the imposed organization of work but also on erroneous behaviour on the part of the workers, who preferred to stay at work over midday to earn more rather than go home. He pointed to the very high (34% in 1854) level of unfitness for military service as a sign of poor attention to health. Becker advises 'rather feeding the inner man' than decking oneself out with 'inane apparel'.[10] He calls upon societies and social organizations for concrete advice and assistance: 'I am of the opinion that there is always far too much theorizing and not enough cooking.'[11]

In 1868, the chemist J.F. Schneeberger brought out a prize-winning publication on food, in particular that of the 'working and lower classes', as a 'contribution to the improvement of our social and economic circumstances and principally in order to combat the demon drink'.[12] He comes to the conclusion that alcohol abuse is a result of poverty, deficiency and misery, and that these arise from wrong living and eating. Neither legal wage agreements nor public support promised a permanent improvement in the situation; 'the only possible solution [is] to be sought and found in self-help, and this in turn in the moral fibre of the individual and in the education of the rising generation.'[13] He sees food in context, asserting that reforming diet also means reforming habits, customs, way of life, prejudices and sloth(!), and has no illusions as to the difficulty of the task. Schneeberger sees success as depending largely on the existence of a prospering economy, protected by tariffs, in a stable and liberal political order based on self-responsibility (hence the stress placed on the importance of education). One of his detailed criticisms is aimed at the cheese industry for taking milk out of circulation for consumption. Even at this early stage, he also sees the high nutritional value of pulses.

In his report on worker and factory conditions in Switzerland[14] published on behalf of the Swiss general committee for the Vienna World Fair, Karl Victor Böhmert, professor of political economy and statistics at the University of Zürich, is concerned less with describing the state of nutritional conditions – although he does give some annual price comparisons and budgets – than with presenting existing 'measures' designed to improve them, such as the sale of cheaper food by the manufacturers, the setting up of factory canteens and public soup kitchens as well as hostels with both eating and sleeping facilities for single workers. The importance attached to milk is interesting: it is described as the healthiest and cheapest food, 'which will most effectively displace alcoholic liquor and in particularly promote the development of a stronger breed of men'.[15] This explains the propagation of farm and factory links. The cooperative associations are above all cited as stemming from workers' own initiatives.

The Glarus doctor and federal factory inspector Fridolin Schuler (1832–1903), in whom we are particularly interested here, is therefore part of a considerable tradition of sociopolitical analysis; he draws on earlier studies from Switzerland and other countries and presents a detailed picture of factory workers' living and working conditions in various publications. His work is central to an assessment of worker nutrition in the late 19th century. He deals with nutritional questions extensively in several publications, particularly in the years 1882 to 1889; from as early as 1878 till 1902, he was one of the first three factory inspectors, together with the former teacher and politician Wilhelm Klein and Edmund Nüsperli, owner of an engineering works, to be appointed under the new 1877 Factories Act.[16])

As Schuler recounts in his memoirs,[17] he became interested in worker nutrition and housing conditions very early on. So when, in 1882, he was asked to talk at the annual meeting of the SGG[18] in his native canton of Glarus, where he had previously been cantonal factory inspector, he could think of 'nothing better to do'[19] than to speak 'On the nutritional status of factory workers and its deficiencies'.[20] He observes in workers a considerable proneness to disease as well as nutritional deficiency (above all in proteins and fats) and is the first to attempt to define a worker-specific food specification. He said that workers' food must be easier to digest than peasants' food and contain more animal proteins; good bread should be preferred to potatoes and vegetables; Schuler also realized the importance of semiluxuries in the monotonous daily round. On the question of whether workers could afford more protein-rich and hence more expensive food in the first place, he found on the basis of – admittedly isolated – statistical studies that, though the rising cost of living in recent decades had certainly made this more difficult, malnutrition was in most cases not due to inadequate income. He ascribes much more blame to the time factor, asserting that the strict timetable of factory work precludes the time-consuming preparation of meals, resulting in digestive problems and a loss of nutrients which take a particularly high toll on children; furthermore as there is not enough time to eat, workers all too often turn to unhealthy snacks between meals at work. Overindulgence in alcohol is also implicated: 'Many a once-fit and industrious worker has turned to spending his days in taverns in anger at the pitiful food his wife serves up for him because she does not know how to buy or cook. Certainly, she knows something about the old, traditional dishes, many of which would suit the stomach of a field labourer well enough, but which would would represent an indigestible burden to that of the factory worker.'[21] Even when Schuler tries to understand the worker in the transition from the agricultural to the industrial age with its new nutritional demands and to explain the nutritional deficiencies in structural terms, he does not quite exonerate him from blame: he did after all have the possibility of feeding himself better by frittering away less money on unhealthy pastries and other luxuries, for example. There is no lack of suggestions on how to improve the situation: establish cooperative societies; fight food misrepresentation; propagate underconsumed foodstuffs such as milk and dairy products, oats, barley and pulses; introduce new and appropriate foods such as pulse powder; make breaks long enough for cooking and eating; introduce a good milk coffee in work breaks; sell modestly priced light wine or cider or beer to combat the consumption of spirits; establish cooking schools, inexpensive restaurants and day nurseries with good-quality meals; create cookbooks for workers.

Just two years later, in 1884, he returns to the subject – on behalf of the Ministry of the Interior – this time in relation to alcoholism.[22] He reviews the different regions of Switzerland and picks up much from his first publication such as the link between poor nutrition and the liquor problem, and comes to the conclusion that the necessary measures in association with an increase in the price (and also an improvement in the quality) of distilled spirits would help to bring about a reduction in alcohol consumption. Switzerland's first Alcohol Act – it came into force in 1887 – saw some important innovations: the introduction of a state liquor monopoly, a licensing system for the sale of spirits, a tax on distilleries, and allocation of 10% of the proceeds of the monopoly to the fight against alcoholism.[23]

Following a report on pulses published in 1885 – i.e. one year after their introduction – to which I revert in part 4 of this paper, and numerous essays on other topics, Schuler in 1889 published 'A short word to the people. Healthy food'[24] in which, as in an earlier family magazine,[25] he set out his ideas in broadly understandable terms and with concrete, price-related meal suggestions. Among other things, he propagated – as he had done back in 1881 – not only pulses but above all the increased use of low-fat cheese, a product he devoted efforts to improving, though without success.[26]

Schuler's data, which are both highly summary and disconnected, provide an insufficient foundation for a detailed and class-specific account of worker nutrition. Additional sources of information are necessary, sources which are rarer in Switzerland than for instance in Germany. Erich Gruner has given an account of worker nutrition in a socio- and historico-economic context.[27] The lower working classes in particular suffered from malnutrition, most especially with respect to proteins, less so as regards fat, and hardly at all in terms of carbohydrates. The mainstays of the diet were surrogate coffee and milk, bread, potatoes, flour dishes and pasta preparations, with occasional cheap meat and rarely vegetables; distilled spirits provided extremely important stimulants.

Since its foundation in 1810, the Schweizerische Gemeinnützige Gesellschaft repeatedly addressed itself in meetings and publications to, among many other things, agricultural problems (not mentioned here) and nutritional questions, in the process generating countless new suggestions for improvement:[28] 1817 public soup kitchens, 1837 cereal stockpiles, 1881, 1888, 1890 and 1899 alcoholism, 1882 the feeding of the factory population, 1888 food as payment in kind for needy itinerants, 1889 healthy food, 1892 a food inspectorate, 1903 compulsory cooking schools. Permanent commissions were devoted to cooking schools and alcohol addiction.

The widespread food misrepresentation of the times and the insecurity of the population with regard to many new industrial products prompted Schuler in an 1885 lecture to the Central Association of Physicians to plead for the establishment of a Chair of Hygiene at the Federal Technical High School (ETH), founded in Zürich in 1855[29] – a proposal that was implemented some ten years later.[30] The production of healthy, cheap food for the people represented a major challenge to the young food industry, whose products were much less in evidence in Swiss homes towards the end of the 19th century than Schuler's expositions might lead one to believe.

## The food industry in the 1880s

The food industry, a relative latecomer to the industrialization process, got off to an even later start in Switzerland than in other European countries, despite the fact that the Alpine confederation was one of the earliest nations to industrialize. The reason presumably lies in the lack of large-scale urbanization, the ability of smaller centres to maintain (partial) self-sufficiency to a later date, and the fact that the supply of fresh products in the larger towns presented no serious difficulties.

It is hardly possible to speak of a food industry before 1850; mechanization only began to gain momentum after 1870. By the end of the 'eighties the following products were being produced in Switzerland, exclusively in tiny, small and medium-sized enterprises: mineral water (from 1789), chocolate (1819), pasta products (1839), malt extract (1865), condensed milk (1866), infant cereal (1867), canned products (1868), surrogate coffee (1870s), pulse and powder soups (1884) and margarine (1889). Chocolate and condensed milk, together with cheese, represented the principal food exports.[31]

Swiss factory statistics[32] from 1882 (the first ever),[33] 1888[34] and 1895[35] give a rough idea of the importance of the food industry, which experienced substantive growth above all from the 'nineties onwards – 'rough' because the statistics cover only establishments subject to the 1877 Factories Act. Furthermore, as the definition of a 'factory' was changing all the time, all cross-comparisons must be qualified.[36] The 1882 statistics indicated a total of 47 firms in the pasta, condensed milk, infant cereal, chocolate and surrogate coffee sectors, with 1,631 workers (i.e. 1.8% of all factories and 1.2% of all factory workers). By 1888 their numbers had grown to 68 firms with 2,183 workers, corresponding to 1.8% of firms and 1.4% of workers. Finally, in 1895, the figures show 95 factories with 3,711 workers (1.9% and 1.8%, respectively, of the totals). For soup preparations, there were no factories in 1882, 2 in 1888 and 5 in 1895.

It is against this background of the general nutritional status, its analysis, above all by Fridolin Schuler, and the development of the food industry that the launch of a – for the time – completely novel product will now be presented.

### The launch and distribution of a new product: Maggi pulse preparations

In his report on pulses as food for the people[37] published in 1885 following the introduction of the new product and designed for propaganda purposes, Schuler goes into considerable detail about the nutritional aspects of pulses, praising them as a cheap source of protein. However, he cautions that they must be properly cooked in order to provide an easily digestible, palatable meal. He also notes that the powders and soup bars[38] on sale for some time were generally too expensive; thus he recognized price, in addition to taste, as a decisive factor in a food designed for widespread consumption. This publication was the end-result of an extensive train of events which began three years before.

After his pivotal lecture at the 1882 meeting of the Schweizerische Gemeinnützige Gesellschaft, the decision had, as stated, been taken to follow up the project.[39] The appropriate partner was found in the person of Michael Johann Julius Maggi (1846–1912).[40] His father had fled to Switzerland from Monza as a political refugee in 1834 and had bought mills in Frauenfeld and Kemptthal. After a commercial apprenticeship in Basle and some two years spent with a Budapest milling company, Julius took over the Kemptthal mill in 1869 and acquired others in Zürich and Schaffhausen. He was a widely known and respected businessman as well as a member of the Zürich cantonal government. Maggi's eagerness to diversify his operations, after his father's death in 1881, must be understood against the background of the milling industry crisis of the 'eighties (the switch to the roller system, powerful foreign competition). It was for this reason that he took up the SGG's challenge and started experimenting.

The technical problems to be solved for the manufacture of pulse powder were considerable and required the design of new equipment.[41] It seems unlikely that Maggi was influenced by direct contacts with other manufacturers of similar products. He developed a powerful cleaning system for his supplies of peas, broad beans and lentils and designed a roasting vessel, because fresh pulses are difficult to grind. The roasting process converted the starch partly into dextrin and sugar but retained the solubility of the protein, thereby achieving a better flavour, increasing the digestibility of the product, improving the level of nutrient absorption by the body, reducing the bloating properties of the pulses and eliminating toxicity. In addition, keeping capacity was extended, and – a matter of prime importance – subsequent cooking time was cut to just 20–30 minutes, as against about 45 minutes for a competing product of similar high quality. (Fresh pulses had to be soaked the night before and even then cooked for hours.) Only now, and with both the mills and the screens suitably modified, was it possible to grind the peas, beans and lentils – with the addition of cereal grain. These innovations cannot be fully appreciated without realizing the great risk represented by the use of water (the traditional enemy of every miller) and fire in an all-timber building. During the almost two-year experimental phase, Maggi was in permanent contact with Schuler, Ernst Schulze, professor of agricultural chemistry and farming technology, and the chemist Dr Johannes Barbieri, both of the ETH in Zürich, as well as with the physiologist, Prof. Johann Friedrich Miescher, in Basle, who repeatedly analysed the products and made suggestions for improvements. In addition, practical trials were carried out in hospitals, poorhouses and prisons, in the army and private homes. In a shrewd strategic move, Maggi had sent 5 kg of the new product to each member of the SGG central commission for them to try out themselves.[42] Breakthrough therefore seemed assured – some products, such as another Maggi powder product consisting partly of pulses, had already been put on the market – and Schuler could state with satisfaction that 'the Maggi preparations leave hardly anything to be desired with regard to nutritional value and digestibility.'[43] They were also attested as being distinctly superior to all competing products. The only problem remaining was the question of taste. Further countless experiments and trials finally led to the production of no less than nine varieties with different flavours: A, B, C (low fat), AA, BB, CC (medium fat) and AAA, BBB, CCC (high fat). As stated on the packaging and in the publicity, the A types always contained the most protein and fat and the least carbohydrates. Applications of the new manmade product were virtually unlimited – soups, puree, flour dishes, cakes, etc. – though the wide range of varieties and relatively complicated letter-based coding system cannot have helped.

Now that the new product had been developed to the complete satisfaction of all concerned, Schuler proposed that the SGG should take an official position on it,[44] whereupon the central commission decided on 10 November 1884 to hold a joint session with the cooking commission in the presence of Schuler and Maggi. The fact that this meeting took place a good week later, on 19 November 1884, and that there was already a draft contract with a manufacturer on the table, shows how important the whole affair was. This meeting, held in the Zunfthaus zur Schmieden, an old guild hall, in Zürich, was attended by a total of ten people including no less than four clergymen.[45]

The drawing up of a contract between the SGG and Julius Maggi[46] was a serious business. Maggi undertook to respect the prices agreed for Switzerland.

Price rises were only allowed with the approval of the central commission and in the event of increases in raw-material prices. Furthermore, Maggi was required to produce quarterly sales statistics. The agreement says nothing about any reciprocal services to be rendered by the SGG. Only the preamble mentions the prior history of the undertaking and the decisions made by the SGG, including the one concerning dissemination of the Schuler report. The contract,[47] dated 19 November 1884, was probably only signed by the association's president Spyri, its secretary Denzler and Julius Maggi a few days later, as the astute Kemptthal businessman wanted to raise the agreed prices at the last moment.[48] This is shown by the fact that the old prices were crossed out in the draft contract and raised by 10 Rappen (centimes). Moreover, Maggi also wanted to include two cheaper varieties in the contract. The central commission approved both changes. The contract, together with a summary of the events leading up to it, was published in the features section of the Neue Zürcher Zeitung and in the appendix to the Schuler pulse brochure. The profit margins can be calculated because the wholesale, dealer and retail prices are all known. The resale margin was 10% to 12.5%, according to the variety. Maggi pulse products were a bargain compared to competing products.[49]

As soon as the contract was signed, Maggi must have lobbied the SGG with the bold request to formally declare that it would not patronize any pulse products but his, justifying this demand by his 100,000-franc investments and the high business risk he bore, because the minutes of the 16 December 1884 meeting of the central commission[50] already mention 'quite extensive correspondence' on this subject. Maggi was very highly thought of, and although people were aware of the danger of tying themselves down it was decided to give exclusive support to Maggi products for three years, a decision which invited the wrath of other manufacturers. The resultant general downward pressure on the prices of competing products can be counted as a gain for the consumers.[51] The SGG could not avoid at least performing expert surveys on other products (the results of which were also communicated to Maggi, incidentally) or carrying out detailed examinations of unsolicited samples and recognition requests, though the findings were not published so as not to prejudice anybody.[52]

Besides the new-product promotion based mainly on widespread distribution of Schuler's publications by the SGG, Maggi also did some advertising of his own for his pulse products. This included, indirectly, packaging design. This was 'simple, unassuming, because it should above all not add to the cost of the product'.[53] Maggi used simple printed paper bags, lined with parchment paper for the fattier varieties, marked: 'Manufactured on behalf and under the price control of the Schweizerische Gemeinnützige Gesellschaft.'[54] 'Those who desire more elegance, greater convenience, can purchase the pulse preparation in metal cans at a slightly higher price.'[55] Maggi placed his first advertisement in the Winterthur 'Landbote' on 10 September 1884, that is to say two months before the signing of the contract with the SGG. Like

28

many others after it, it was simply a list of stockists.[56] Finally, a first insertion couched in advertising language appeared on 7 November 1885: 'The best, healthiest foods, at prices unequalled by any competitor, are the soup powders recommended to the Swiss people by the Schweizerische Gemein-nützige Gesellschaft. More nourishing than meat, just as easy to digest, very cheap, and quickly prepared. Distinction at the Swiss Cookery Exhibition in Zürich, 1885. First-Class Diploma.'[57] In the memoir published for the International Congress on Hygiene and Demography held at Vienna in 1887, Maggi's publicity for his meat extract as a condiment and invalid food was accompanied by promotion of his cheap and protein-rich pulse pre-parations, which were also suitable for military rations; it also mentioned, for Austria, the 'Imperial and Royal Ministerial Councillor and Central Trade Inspector, Dr Migerka' as a proponent of the new products.[58]

The sales statistics to be drawn up by Maggi were furnished until early 1890, even though SGG's patronage came to an end in 1887.[59] Sales first fell from 212 tonnes (1885) to 110 t (1886), then increased again to 133 t (1887) followed by a much steeper rise to 470 t (1889) – a remarkable achievement for a completely new product. Sales were understandably higher in the cold half of the year. Of the different tastes, peas and lentils proved more popular than beans, oats and barley. Fat and low-fat pulses were roughly on a par. In the peak year (1889), consumption in Switzerland was 13 g per month, or just about one bowl of soup per head of the population. As there were various other similar products on the market for which statistics are lacking, overall consumption of pulse powder must have been higher. The statistics, orga-nized as they are according to canton, do not reveal any clear correlation between degree of industrialization and pulse consumption, only a tendency.

The relatively modest consumption figures tally with contemporary observations concerning the acceptance of the new product.[60] The expected breakthrough failed to materialize, and precisely in those sections of society the pulse products were aimed at – among the workers. If it were merely a matter of the introduction of a commercial speciality, the results of this introductory year could be seen as highly gratifying. Rarely, according to the Maggi Pulse Products sales points, has a product become established and spread so quickly as this. But where the new food has really caught on is among the upper classes of the population and the more affluent workers. Among the peasantry, as well as in the lower classes of the population, who live more from hand to mouth, that is to say where coffee and possibly even stronger stimulants represent actual food, the initial impact had very little effect. [Maggi was aware of the acceptance difficulties in worker circles: see his remarks on these findings in a letter to President Spyri with the observation: '. . . ought we to say "unfortunately" or "naturally"?'[61]] If one thinks how long it took for potatoes to become a real part of everyday diet, there is hope that the new food, too, will gradually filter down from top to bottom. It offers the greatest prospects of success in the form of soup powder; it would, however, be highly desirable if it were to catch on in the more solid form of pasta products. (Maggi incorporated these in his product range; they were manufactured by Weilenmann Bros. of Veltheim near Winterthur.[62]) Of these, pea pasta proved to have the most appeal, and after various trials production was for the time being limited to this.[63] In view of the slender cash resources in peasant circles as well as the general disinclination to buy food, it was proposed, in the light of these findings, to encourage people to grow legumes and to trade in the crop for pulse powders.

What was the reason for the disappointing results of pulse product sales, particularly in the specific target group? It can hardly have been due to the price, as there was nothing cheaper on the market in this line. Or can it? Were the Maggi pulse products in their unattractive paper bags 'wrongly positioned' as popular and (though not put in so many words) poor-people's food, and therefore inferior to more expensive products in glossy packaging? It is impossible to answer this question, as we do not have statistics for other brands. It is also doubtful whether the newspaper and magazine advertising had any impact at all in worker circles. Deeper reasons surely lie in food habits themselves. It is understandable that sons and daughters of the land would be sceptical about a wishy-washy factory product with a strange-sounding name and a complicated letter-based designation system. But what about factory workers? Would not people with no land of their own, people who were entirely dependent on the market and generally did their shopping on a day-to-day basis be expected to welcome a ready-made, ready-packed food with open arms? Did it not require, on the other hand, considerable insight to integrate into one's personal diet a food with a decidedly abstract, professedly healthful image which afforded little pleasure to the palate? However this may be, these resistance factors seem to have far outweighed the time-savings, appreciated more in lower middle-class households without maids, to be expected from the convenience aspect. Even the new product's promoters had to concede that its unfamiliar taste could be an important reason for the lack of acceptance: 'What did them [the Maggi powders] the most harm was immoderate use, leading to satiety and digestion problems. This was particularly the case in our difficult-to-please population, whereas in other countries the original simple preparations are still consumed in great quantities.'[64] Or, put in a nutshell: '. . . it [the pulse powder] is making only slow progress in general consumption and, to boot, only among educated people, and altogether there can be few people who place a Maggi soup on a level with a juicy roast in terms of taste.'[65]

For all these reasons it is understandable that Maggi himself, as the main party concerned, sought to remedy the situation. His first step was to refine his product by further increasing the solubility of the protein and improving the taste – twin aims which were difficult to achieve because greater solubility and better taste are not necessary compatible.[66] He worked in association with the Institute of Hygiene of the University of Munich.[67] As a result of these improvements, he was able to announce in a newspaper advertisement in 1887: 'Maggi Pulse Products, the only products with fully burst cells.'[68] He subsequently developed the pulse powders into soup powders (from 1886), with the addition of spices, herbs and other ingredients, as the basis of a more appetizing meal. The soup powders very soon ousted their precursors; they paved the way for the Swiss soup industry, whose products have a permanent place in the modern, time-saving kitchen. The Schweizerische Gemeinnützige Gesellschaft, like Schuler, also lost their interest in pulses and turned their attentions to propagating other foodstuffs, particularly milk and cheese.

A handful of people and institutions with very varied backgrounds and interests came together to develop a new product in several years of intensive collaboration: the factory inspector Fridolin Schuler who triggered the whole process in the first place with his analysis of worker malnutrition and his urge to find a solution; the Schweizerische Gemeinnützige Gesellschaft, which took up such causes in its dedication to matters of general welfare; and the shrewd and innovative businessman Julius Maggi, eager to restructure his milling operations. The reason why success did not measure up to the high hopes and great goals of all concerned has little to do with the concrete manner in which the project was prosecuted but lies rather in a failure by all the actors involved to take sufficiently into account some basic phenomena of human eating habits.

## Notes

1  For a survey on Swiss food history and the literature, see Schärer (1991; 1992a; 1992b).
2  Strahlmann (1975).
3  Simler (1873–5).
4  Schneider (1917). I refer to to the rectified figures in Howald (1924), pp. 244–246.
5  Schärer (1992a), p. 273.
6  Gruner and Wiedmer (1987), pp. 362ff.; see also Gruner (1968), p. 124.
7  *Reallöhne* (1981), vol. 2, Der NFRL-Preisindex 'Nahrungsmittel, Getränke, Heizung und Beleuchtung', ed. Urs Kern, pp. 112ff.
8  Gruner (1968), pp. 1048ff.
9  Becker (1858).
10  Ibid., p. 92.
11  Ibid., pp. 103f.
12  Schneeberger (1867–9).
13  Ibid., vol. 1, p. x. [ = page ten]
14  Böhmert (1873), in particular vol. 1, pp. 300–381.
15  Ibid., p. 320.
16  Eichholzer (1952).
17  Schuler (1903), pp. 66ff.

18 Proceedings in SZG, 21(1882), pp. 509–521.
19 Schuler (1882), p. 67.
20 Schuler (1882).
21 Ibid., p. 24.
22 Schuler (1884).
23 Wunderlin (1986), in particular p. 116.
24 Schuler (1888).
25 List of his publications in Schuler (1903), pp. 155ff.
26 Ibid., p. 70.
27 Gruner (1968), pp. 133ff.; Gruner and Wiedmer (1987), pp. 362ff.
28 Rickenbach (1960), quotes also the preceding commemorative publications.
29 Schuler (1885b).
30 The first professor of hygiene of labour, nutrition and bacteriology was Otto Roth, *Eidgenössische Technische Hochschule* (1955), p. 344.
31 Schärer (1991), p. 28.
32 Gruner and Wiedmer (1987), pp. 107ff and 118f.
33 *Schweizerische Fabrikstatistik* (1883).
34 Ibid. (1889).
35 Ibid. (1896).
36 *Das Bundesgesetz* (1900), pp. 9–63.
37 Schuler (1885a).
38 For the history of prefabricated soup see *'Die sehr bekannte'* (1989), p. 73ff.; Teuteberg (1990), pp. 51ff; Stoffel (1957).
39 *Protokoll*, Nov. 19th, 1884; also quoted in Schuler (1885a), p. 15.
40 Schmid (1946); Pfister (1942); *Frank* (1992), pp. 169–253; Schmidt (1987); Frei and Schmidt (1990).
41 Schuler (1885a), pp. 10ff; writings of Karl Schleich and Eugen Hefti, Alimentarium Food Museum, Vevey, Switzerland.
42 *Protokoll*, Nov. 10th, 1884.
43 Schuler (1885a), pp. 11f.
44 See ref. 49.
45 See ref. 46.
46 Draft of the contract in *Protokoll*, Nov. 19th, 1884.
47 ASGG, A1880–89 Y 4; also quoted in Schuler (1885a), p. 16. In the published annual report of the Central Commission of the SGG, the non rectified version is given in error, SZG 24(1885), p. 383.
48 *Protokoll*, Nov. 22nd, 1884, addendum.
49 Schuler (1885a), pp. 8 and 13f.
50 *Protokoll*, Dec. 16th, 1884.
51 'Berichterstattung' (1886), p. 102.
52 *Protokoll*, Dec. 1st, 1885, Jan. 7th and May 6th, 1886; see also SZG 25(1886), p. 219.
53 Schuler (1885a), p. 13.

54 Collection of the Alimentarium Food Museum, Vevey, Switzerland.
55 See ref. 65.
56 Müller (1961), appendices 12 and 22.
57 Müller (1961), appendix 25.
58 *Denkschrift* (1887).
59 SZG 25(1886), pp. 104f.; 27(1888), p. 96; 29(1890), pp. 120 and 222 the figures for 1888 are not to be found.
60 SZG 24(1885), p. 383; 'Berichterstattung' (1886), pp. 101ff.; Schuler (1889), p. 7; Schuler (1903), pp. 68ff; Pfister (1942), p. 11.
61 See ref. 63.
62 Müller (1961), appendix 24.
63 'Berichterstattung' (1886), p. 101.
64 Schuler (1903), p. 68.
65 Schuler (1889), p. 7.
66 See ref. 63.
67 *Frank* (1992), pp. 134f.
68 Landbote Winterthur, Sept. 4th, 1887.

**Literature**

ASGG = Archives of the Schweizerische Gemeinnützige Gesellschaft in Zürich
SZG = Schweizerische Zeitschrift für Gemeinnützigkeit.

Becker, Bernhard, *Ein Wort über die Fabrikindustrie, Mit besonderer Hinsicht auf den Canton Glarus* (Basel, 1858), ed. Hans-Ulrich Schiedt (Bern, 1990).
'Berichterstattung über die Einführung der Leguminosen als schweizerische Volksnahrung pro 1985', *SZG*, 25(1886), pp. 101–103.
Böhmert, Victor, *Arbeiterverhältnisse und Fabrikeinrichtungen der Schweiz, Bericht, erstattet im Auftrage der eidgenössischen Generalcommission für die Wiener Weltausstellung*, 2 vols. (Zürich, 1873).
*Das Bundesgesetz betreffend die Arbeit in den Fabriken vom 23. März 1877, Kommentiert durch seine Ausführung in den Jahren 1878–1899* (Bern, 1900).
*Denkschrift der Firma Julius Maggi & Co. in Kemptthal (Schweiz) und Bregenz (Vorarlberg) für den VI. Internationalen Congress für Hygiene und Demographie in Wien, September 1887* (Kemptthal, 1887).
Eichholzer, Eduard, 'Die drei ersten Fabrikinspektoren', *Industrielle Organisation, Schweizerische Zeitschrift für Betriebswissenschaft*, 21(1952), pp. 42–44.
*Eidgenössische Technische Hochschule 1855–1955* (Zürich, 1955).
*Frank Wedekinds Maggi-Zeit, Reklamen/Reiseberichte/Briefe*, ed. Hartmut Vinçon (Darmstadt, 1992, Pharus, 4).
Frei, Alfred G. and Susanne B. Schmidt, 'Julius Maggi (1846–1912) – von der

Mühle zur Lebensmittelfabrik', in Herbert Berner (ed), *Singener Stadt-geschichte, vol.* 2, Singen, Dorf und Herrschaft (Konstanz, 1990, Beiträge zur Singener Stadtgeschichte, 15; Hegau-Bibliothek, 55), pp. 543–556.

Gruner, Erich, *Die Arbeiter in der Schweiz im 19. Jahrhundert, Soziale Lage. Organisation, Verhältnis zu Arbeitgeber und Staat* (Bern, 1968, Helvetica politica, A3).

Gruner, Erich and Hans-Rudolf Wiedmer, *Arbeiterschaft und Wirtschaft in der Schweiz 1880–1914, Soziale Lage. Organisation und Kämpfe von Arbeitern und Unternehmern, politische Organisation und Sozialpolitik, vol. 1, Demographische, wirtschaftliche und soziale Basis und Arbeitsbedin-gungen (Zurich, 1987).*

Howald, Oskar, 'Die Ernährung der schweizerischen Bevölkerung in den Jahren 1920/22', *Zeitschrift für schweizerische Statistik und Volks-wirtschaft,* 60(1924), pp. 237–251.

Müller, Fritz, *Maggi-Chronik, vol.* 2. 1. Juli 1912–31. Dezember 1947, manu-script (Winterthur, 1961).

Pfister, G., *Maggi-Chronik, vol.* 1, 1832–30. Juni 1912, manuscript (Kempt-thal, 1942).

*Protokoll der Zentralkommission der Schweizerischen gemeinnütz. Ge-sellschaft, vol.* 3, Jan. 14th, 1873 – May 6TH, 1886, in ASGG, C1g.

*Reallöhne schweizerischer Industriearbeiter von* 1890 bis 1921, 5 vols., ed. Hansjörg Siegenthaler, manuscript (Zürich, 1981).

Rickenbach, Walter, *Geschichte der Schweizerischen Gemeinnützigen Ge-sellschaft* 1810–1860 (Zürich, 1960).

Schärer, Martin R., *700 Jahre auf dem Tisch, Oder: Die 7 ausgestellten Ausstellungen, Ernährung in der Schweiz vom Spätmittelalter bis zur Gegenwart und Möglichkeiten, Ernährungsgeschichte im Museum auszus-tellen* (Vevey, 1991).

Schärer, Martin R., 'Ernährung und Essgewohnheiten', in Paul Hugger (ed), *Handbuch der schweizerischen Volkskultur* (Zürich, 1992a), pp. 253–288.

Schärer, Martin R., 'Food History in Switzerland: A Survey of the Litera-ture', in Hans J.Teuteberg (ed), *European Food History* (Leicester, 1992b), pp. 168–198.

Schmid, Hans Rudolf, *Julius Maggi 9. Oktober 1856 bis 19. Oktober 1912, Zu seinem hundertsten Geburtstag* (Kemptthal, 1946)

Schmidt, Susanne B., 'Julius Maggi, Singens würziger Weg zur Industries-tadt', in Alfred G. Frei (ed), *Habermus und Suppenwürze, Singens Weg vom Bauerndorf zur Industriestadt* (Konstanz, 1987), pp. 110–143.

Schneeberger, J.F., *Die Ernährung des Volkes mit besonderer Berücksichti-gung der arbeitenden und niedern Klassen* . . ., 2 vols. (Bern, 1867–9).

Schneider, Salome, 'Die Erzeugung und der Verbrauch von Nährwerten in der Schweiz', *Zeitschrift für schweizerische Statistik und Volkswirtschaft,* 53(1917), pp. 275–335.

Schuler, Fridolin, 'Über die Ernährung der Fabrikbevölkerung und ihre

Mängel, Erstes Referat für die Jahresversammlung der Schweiz. gemeinnützigen Gesellschaft den 19. September 1882 in Glarus', *SZG*, 21(1882),
pp. 365–418 (and Zürich, 1882).

Schuler, Fridolin, *Zur Alkoholfrage, Die Ernährungsweise der arbeitenden
Klassen in der Schweiz und ihr Einfluss auf die Ausbreitung des Alkoholismus*
(Bern, 1884).

Schuler, Fridolin, *Leguminosen als Volksnahrung, Gutachten herausgegeben
im Auftrage der schweiz. gemeinnützigen Gesellschaft* (Zürich, 1885a).

Schuler, Fridolin, 'Soziale Aufgaben der Lebensmittelchemie', *Correspon-
denz-Blatt für Schweizer Aerzte*, 15(1885b), pp. 567–571.

Schuler, Fridolin, 'Gesunde Nahrung, Ein kurzes Wort an das Volks von der
Schweiz. gemeinnützigen Gesellschaft', *SZG*, 27(1888), pp. 328–336 (and
Zürich, 1889).

Schuler, Fridolin, *Erinnerungen eines Siebenzigjährigen* (Frauenfeld, 1903).

*Schweizerische Fabrikstatistik* (Bern, 1882ff.).

*'Die sehr bekannte dienliche Löffelspeise', Mus, Brei und Suppe – kultur-
geschichtlich betrachtet*, ed. Fritz Hug (Velbert-Neviges, 1989).

Simler, Theodor, 'Versuch einer Ernährungsbilanz der Schweizer Bevölkerung', *Zeitschrift für schweizerische Statistik*, 9(1873), pp. 158–169;
10(1874), pp. 15–26; 11(1875), pp. 1–22.

Stoffel, Alexander Eric, *Die Absatzprobleme der schweizerischen Suppenindustrie* (Zürich, 1957).

Strahlmann, Berend, 'Erhebungen über den Lebensmittelverbrauch der
schweizerischen Bevölkerung in historischer Sicht', in Georg Brubacher
and Günther Ritzel (eds), *Zur Ernährungssituation der schweizerischen
Bevölkerung, Erster schweizerischer Ernährungsbericht* (Bern, Stuttgart,
Wien, 1975), pp. 42–56.

Teuteberg, Hans-Jürgen, *Die Rolle des Fleischextrakts für die Ernährungs-
wissenschaften und den Aufstieg der Suppenindustrie, Kleine Geschichte der
Fleischbrühe* (Stuttgart, 1990, Zeitschrift für Unternehmensgeschichte,
Beiheft 70).

*Über die Ernährungsweise der arbeitenden Klasse im Kanton Zug, Beleuchtung
der bezüglichen offiziellen Darlegung von Hrn. Dr Schuler, eidgen. Fabri-
kinspektor*, Regierungsrath des Kantons Zug (Zug, 1884).

Wunderlin, Dominik, 'Die Antialkoholbewegung in der Schweiz', *Hessische
Blätter für Volks- und Kulturforschung* NF20(1986), pp. 113–128.

# 4

# THE BEST SUBSTITUTE FOR MOTHER'S MILK: PROPRIETARY PREPARATIONS BETWEEN THE RISE OF PAEDIATRICS AND THE SCIENCE OF NUTRITION IN THE NETHERLANDS DURING THE TWENTIETH CENTURY

## Annemarie de Knecht-van Eekelen

*Bottle-feeding is a prime example of the application of an artificial technology to a natural biological function.*
(Gallagher (1978) p. 79)

## Introduction

On the one hand opinions on infant feeding today are the same as one hundred years ago. At that time physicians considered mother's milk the best food for infants and today this view has again gained an unassailable position in their minds. On the other hand the practice of artificial infant feeding has radically changed during the past century and this change will be the subject of this paper. Three main aspects concerning the developments in artificial infant feeding can be distinguished: 1 the frequency of artificial feeding versus breast-feeding, 2 the shift from home made preparations to proprietary infant formulas, 3 the growing cooperation between food-industry and physicians or the medicalisation of infant feeding.

These days in the Netherlands a mother can choose only between breast-feeding and bottle-feeding with a proprietary food for infants. Since 1990 home made preparations are advised against by all official institutions. This advice is based on a literature study published by the 'Studiegroep Zuige-lingenvoeding' [Study Group Infant Nutrition] in 1985.[1] With this advice the food industry achieved a strong position which became even more conso-lidated as in the following years proprietary formulas were recommended not only for the first half but also for the second half of the first year of life. In contrast to the 1985 report the Public Health Authorities stated in 1991 that cow's milk is inappropriate for infants and proprietary formulas should be used for: 1 young infants when breast-milk is unavailable and 2 for all infants between ½ and 1 year old. The arguments for this advice were taken from the nutritionists' views that the composition of formulas are in better agreement with the physiological needs of the infant.[2]

This shows the decisive influence of scientific opinions on the introduction of formulas to the public. The same procedures can be noticed during the past hundred years. In my view – as I also described in my thesis – the developments in the science of nutrition have been the main directive forces that influenced the industrial preparation of artificial infant feeding.[3] The recent industrial monopolisation of the production of foods for infants has only been made possible by the use of the scientific knowledge on nutrients and the nutritional needs of the infant. The close collaboration between industry, nutritionists and physicians resulted in proprietary infant formulas that guarantee an optimal development of the infant.

## Infant feeding and the development of the science of nutrition

Infant feeding can be divided into two main topics: breast-feeding and artificial feeding. Some words must be said about breast-feeding before I can go into the changes in artificial feeding that took place during the last hundred years. From the nineteenth century no precise figures on the use of breast-feeding versus artificial infant feeding are available. Dutch physicians unanimously held the view that mothers should breast-feed their children. Their arguments were several. In this period the position of the woman as the centre of the household performing all motherly tasks was strongly advocated and breast-feeding should be the foremost duty of a good mother.[4] As life-chances of artificially fed infants were notably worse this also was a strong argument against bottle-feeding.

However, all nineteenth century literature indicates the widespread use of pap-feeding in the Netherlands. Usually infants were exclusively breast-fed during the first two weeks of life and then supplementary pap was given in combination with breast-feeding. Pap was made of a mixture of water with sugar and some kind of farinaceous food such as arrowroot, rice-flour, wheat-flour, barley, rusk or breadcrumbs. In combination with breast-feeding no other milk was used as this was thought to interfere with the substances in mother's milk.[5] Mothers stuck to the idea – and that is a widespread opinion even nowadays – that their milk is not nourishing enough for an infant. So they reached out for nourishing supplementary foodstuffs in order to rear a heavy chubby baby that in their opinion was supposed to be a healthy baby. This belief has always been the most important motivation when choosing artificial infant feeding and the producers of proprietary infant foods intensified this belief in their advertisements. The impact of the advertising campaigns of infant-food companies around the turn of the century on the move to bottle-feeding can be seen all over Europe and in the United States.[6]

As long as mother's milk was the main food for the young infant his life chances were reasonable. Overfeeding with the additional pap was a frequent cause of indigestion which could end in severe dehydration and consequent death. Even worse was the situation for infants who had to be reared on artificial feeding only. For them diluted cow's milk – or when available goat's, sheep's or ass's milk – was the main nourishment. Ass's milk was thought to have the closest similarity to women's milk as regards its contents of protein, carbohydrate, fat and minerals.[7] For the young infant sugar was added and for the older ones also some of the already mentioned farinaceous nutrients.

During the nineteenth century the kind of milk, the dilution of the milk and the sorts of sugar and farina to be used according to the age of the infant were passionately discussed by physicians. Also the preparation of the artificial infant feeding – should milk be boiled or not? –, the way of providing the food – by spoon or in a bottle – and the hygienic preparation were important topics in their discussions. Their aim was to provide a food with the same properties as mother's milk, a starting-point of most research on infant food during the past century.[8]

Views on the composition of artificial infant feeding were based on chemical analyses of the different sorts of milk. As the insights into the chemical structure of proteins, carbohydrates and fats increased and the analytical methods improved the differences between mother's milk and the various animal milks became obvious. One has to remember that for instance the structure of proteins was unknown during the nineteenth century, while figures on minerals were also scarce and vitamins were not known at all.

During the second half of the nineteenth century some important discoveries were made which greatly influenced the practice of artificial infant feeding. The impact of the rise of bacteriology on the ideas about the preparation of artificial infant feeding has been immense. All forces were recruited to fight bacteria, the invisible enemies. Milk was found to be an important carrier of all kinds of bacteria so sterilisation of milk was thought inevitable. However, negative results from the use of highly sterilised artificial infant food were reported from the middle of the eighties on. Rachitis and scorbut were often observed in infants using these foods. In reaction to the sterilising mania physicians looked for an opportunity to prescribe clean germ free milk that could be used raw.

Important for infant feeding was the discovery of enzymes in the gastrointestinal tract that activate the breakdown of carbohydrate, fat and protein. By then former worries on the impossibility of the digestion of these nutrients were over, but of course other problems arose. There remained differences in the digestibility of mother's milk and cow's milk that could not be accounted for. Very fundamental research on the energy balance of infants was executed in 1898 by the German paediatrician Otto Heubner (1843–1926) and his colleague, the physiologist Max Rubner (1854–1932). According to their findings more physiological quantities of food could be prescribed so total or partial over- or underfeeding could be prevented.[9]

The solution for many unanswered questions was provided in the twentieth century when the vitamins were discovered as vital substances essential to life. During the 1920s and 1930s nutrition research all over Europe was directed towards the elucidation of the chemical composition of the different vitamins and their role in human physiology. Analyses were made of the quantities of vitamins in mother's milk and advice was given on the necessary daily intake of vitamins by infants at different ages. Artificial infant feeding was fortified with vitamins and supplementary vitamin A and D were prescribed for breast-fed infants. The discussion on the infant's needs for vitamins has been continued to the present day and now vitamin K is a subject of discussion.[10]

## Physicians take an interest in infant feeding

Before 1919 all activities to improve the conditions for infants came from private persons, often physicians and upper class ladies. Physicians with a special interest in paediatrics had joined in the 'Nederlandsche Vereeniging voor Paediatrie' [Dutch Society of Paediatricians] that was founded in 1892. One of their goals was 'to improve the fate of the children in the Netherlands'.[11] They all held the view that artificial infant feeding was the cause of the untimely death of a large number of children. The first reliable data on infant feeding were obtained by a large scale inquiry in the Hague and the neighbouring village of Scheveningen in the year 1908. Results from this study were published in 1913 in the well known 'Haagsche Rapport' [Report from the Hague].[12] Data relating to 6989 infants born in 1908 were compiled under the supervision of Hendrik W. Methorst (1868–1955), the director of the 'Centraal Bureau voor de Statistiek' [Central Bureau of Statistics] in the Hague which had been founded in 1899. At birth 18.8 per cent of the newborn were bottle-fed and 7.2 per cent got a combination of breast and bottle. Figure 1 shows the situation at 13 weeks with less than 50 per cent of the infants still breast-fed.[13] Very interesting is the fact that mothers from the lower social classes used less artificial infant feeding than those in the higher social levels. Death during the first year of life was among breast-fed infants 7.0 per cent and among artificially fed infants 17.8 per cent. This striking difference led to the conclusion that on the one hand breast-feeding should be encouraged, while on the other hand young women in all social levels should be educated on the nursing and feeding of infants. This education became one of the tasks of the infant welfare centres that were established in the Netherlands from 1901 on.[14] However, it took until the 1970s before 95 per cent of all infants were taken to an infant welfare centre: The 'Nederlandsche

Bond tot Bescherming van Zuigelingen' [Dutch Association for the Protection of Infants] founded in 1908 promoted infant welfare centres, but as this association depended on private initiative it had a slow start. In 1927 the local activities came under supervision of the Public Health department and from that time on the number of infant welfare centres increased from 47 in 1926 to 387 in 1930 and to around 3000 in 1976. By that time the 'Bond' did not exist any more, as the lack of new goals brought an end to the organisation in 1971.[15]

During the 1920s and 1930s the number of bottle-fed infants decreased considerably (see figure 1). Infant welfare centres are supposed to have been one of the main factors in this process. However, during the 1950s and 1960s a reverse effect can be noted (see figures 1 and 2). Some authors doubt if infant welfare centres really promoted breast-feeding like they stated.[16] The increase in the number of mothers visiting the centre surely improved the health of the infants and decreased mortality, but this seems more due to the instructions on preparing and feeding artificial infant food than to the augmentation of breast-feeding. During the decline in the numbers of breast-fed infants in the 1960s, as is shown in figures 1 and 2, the number of infants seen in a welfare centre increased. As the choice to breast-feed is made before the delivery, the first visit to the welfare centre will be too late to change this decision. Figure 2 shows the negative attitude of mothers towards breast-feeding up to 1975. The change in their opinion has been largely due to campaigns of women's organisations promoting breast-feeding.

## Proprietary farinaceous foods for infants

From the preceding remarks on the wide-spread use of artificial infant feeding in the Netherlands it will be clear that there was a market for infant food. Indeed, as soon as the food industry developed, proprietary foods for infants were introduced to the public. One should consider two different branches occupied with foods for infants: the flour-mills and the dairy industry.

At the end of last century the more than 2000 flour-mills operating in our country reorganised and concentrated milling in a much smaller number of large enterprises.[17] Rival industries tried to enter the market by producing proprietary brands. As to a proprietary flour for infants the flour-mills had a fairly easy task in introducing a fine quality of rice-flour, wheat-flour or other flour as especially apt for infants. Mothers had always used such products and a reliable standard quality had its advantages as long as the difference in price from the similar regular product was not too high.

'Molenaar's kindermeel', produced by the flour-mill of P. Molenaar & Comp. in Westzaan (North-Holland), became one of the leading Dutch farinaceous products for the preparation of artificial infant feeding. Today it is still marketed under the same name though the firm has long been taken over by a large syndicate of flour producers. Molenaar, as well as other producers, advertised his products on a large scale. They spread leaflets for mothers showing letters from happy users and photographs of their chubby children.[18] Molenaar got a high reputation among physicians by going along with their advice. For example Molenaar adapted his advertisement according to the ideas of one of the leading Dutch paediatricians, Evert Gorter (1881–1954), professor in paediatrics at Leiden university.[19]

Another trade mark for farinaceous baby-food that is still on the market is 'Liga'. In the 1920s Liga, a biscuit special for children, was marketed by a biscuit-factory in Roosendaal (North-Brabant). The biscuit was used as a supplementary food for weaning infants and it was said to contain almost all necessary nutrients. Liga boomed in 1950s and 1960s when the birth-rate was high and the standard of life increased. However, circumstances were different in 1970s when the 'sellers'-market' changed into a 'buyers'-market' and Liga seemed to lose its share. Moreover, the growing attention to dental caries banished cookies from the nursery.[20]

In the 1980s General Biscuits, nowadays the producer of Liga, took the opportunity to put the ideas of the Study Group Infant Nutrition into practice. They employed one of the members of the Study Group Infant Nutrition and developed a new series of biscuits for infants and toddlers. 'Liga Baby-food' became a biscuit without gluten, with little sugar and no salt and fortified with calcium and iron. Liga is one of the most striking examples of the influence of the science of nutrition on the production of a food for infants.

## The first milk based proprietary foods for infants

The history of the production of proprietary milk for infants must be seen in the context of the development of the dairy industry in the Netherlands.[21] When in 1871 the first creamery in the Netherlands was founded, there already was marketed a canned infant food consisting of condensed milk and dextrinated wheat-flour. The first proprietary food for infants on a milk basis was 'Farine Lactée' prepared by the Swiss Company Nestlé. The founder Henri Nestlé (1814–1890) started the production in 1867. Dutch physicians were concerned about the aggressive advertisements of Nestlé, that in their opinion, withheld mothers from breast-feeding. Nevertheless Nestlé obtained a distinct position in the Dutch market for proprietary infant food. In 1912 the company started a factory in Rotterdam by the name of 'Galak' where various Nestlé products were manufactured.

However, at that time some factories of Dutch origin had already started their own proprietary foods. The leader had been the 'Hollandsche Fabriek van Melkproducten Hollandia' [Dutch Factory of Dairy Products Hollandia] an enterprise under the direction of a former army officer Constant

H. Wagenaar Hummelinck (1843–1914). He opened his factory for the production of condensed milk in Vlaardingen [South-Holland] in 1882. In those days physicians were not unanimous about the usefulness of condensed milk as infant food, but Hummelinck assured his consumers that 'Hollandia's infant food becomes by the day more and more the infant food par excellence'.[22]

In fact the rise of bacteriology and the fear of bacteria played into the hands of Hummelinck. He could offer a clean and germ free product that became rather popular around the turn of the century. Hummelinck opened two more factories and the export of his products to England boomed. Four types of condensed milk were produced: full cream milk with or without sugar and skimmed milk with or without sugar. The advantages of a standardised composition and an easy way of preparing infant food with condensed milk surely tempted mothers to buy the 'bussenmelk' [canned milk]. Even physicians gave in to condensed milk for infants on the condition that full cream milk was used and supplementary fruit-juice was provided. In 1912 3.5 per cent of the Dutch milk-production was canned and mainly exported to England and to the Dutch colonies.[23] For ordinary daily use in the Netherlands fresh milk was available for each household. In the twentieth century the improved milk distribution and quality control ensured fresh milk for everyone at a fairly low price. So what need was there for proprietary infant food?

## Patent food for weak infants

As long as the bottle-fed infant was healthy usually a home-made mixture of cow's milk, water, sugar and flour was used. However, the problems started when the infant had trouble with this food. Around the turn of the century a large variety of mixtures was composed based on different opinions of paediatricians, chemists and other interested parties. One of these prescriptions – an idea of the German professor in agriculture Alexander Backhaus (1865–1927) – was bought by Martinus D.M. van der Hagen (1861–1928), owner of a creamery in Zoetermeer [South-Holland] where butter, cream and other diary products were produced. His brother Johannes C.I. van der Hagen (1857–1918) was a physician who saw possibilities for this new product after he had heard of Backhaus's preparation at a meeting in Germany in 1895. Van der Hagen started with the production of Backhaus milk in 1901. Backhaus milk was made of skimmed fermented cow's milk with cream and sugar added after filtration of the coagulated protein. The composition resembled women's milk as it had a low protein and a high sugar content. Backhaus used the name 'Nutricia' for his enterprises and Van der Hagen, who had bought this name too, changed his factories name into 'Nutricia' in 1901.[24] Already in the same year Dutch Backhaus-milk was available in special Nutricia shops in cities of North- and South-Holland in four varieties in sterilised bottles of 125, 200 or 300 grammes. The expansion of a network of own shops and retailers was one of the strategies to make this name known to the public. In the 1920s their products were sold by almost 300 retail-dealers.

Of course Nutricia was not the only dairy factory trying to obtain a place in the market for infant food, but this company is the only one that survived from the nineteenth century on till today. Already in a few years time Nutricia broadened the assortment of its products. In 1904 the production of condensed buttermilk for infants was started. Buttermilk had always had a good reputation in the Netherlands for the feeding of infants with a little stomach trouble and in some parts of the country (especially Friesland) buttermilk with sugar and starch was the ordinary artificial food for infants. Round 1900 several Dutch physicians propagated mixtures with buttermilk so Nutricia made haste to follow these insights. This has always been Nutricia's strategy. They closely followed the medical opinions and tried to apply them in an industrial product. When in 1910 the German paediatrician Heinrich Finkelstein (1865–1942) introduced his famous 'Eiweissmilch' for infants with indigestion, Nutricia started production in 1911. Some decades later in 1933 Nutricia joined in the vitamin offensive and produced the first buttermilk fortified with vitamin D. Supplementary vitamin C was added to all infant foods in 1937. From 1946, optimal doses of vitamin A, C and D based on nutritionist views were added.[25]

A real innovation was Nutricia's introduction of the first humanised milk [Almiron-A] for ailing infants in 1954. It had a low protein content and the concentrations of minerals were low and adapted to those of mother's milk. At first it was in liquid form but in 1961 the breakthrough to powdered infant food came with 'Almiron-B'. At that time one of the advantages of powdered milk was the possibility of fortifying with iron (Fe); however, powder was more expensive. From 1964, Almiron was marketed as an artificial infant feeding for healthy children who are not breast-fed.[26]

## Proprietary food for healthy infants

During the 1920s and 1930s most artificial infant food for healthy infants was prepared at home. Special sugar, mostly dextrin-maltose, for home made infant food was produced by several factories. Also the acidified whole milk – according to the principle of the American physician William Marriot (1885–1936) – which became popular in the Netherlands in the thirties was made at home. So it is characteristic for those days that the industries did not produce canned acidified milk, but a mixture of sugar and acid to mix with cow's milk and water when preparing the infant food at home. It was the professor in paediatrics in Groningen, Jan van Lookeren Campagne (1895–1978), who strongly advocated acidified whole milk for healthy infants. According to his prescription W.A. Scholten prepared 'Citrotrinose', a mixture of dextrin-maltose and citric acid. Just as the producers of food for infants, Scholten promoted his product with a brochure even written by a paediatrician.[27] Of course in due time Nutricia came with 'Citromalt' based on the same principle.

After the Second World War a rapid increase in the production of proprietary infant foods took place. In 1945 Nutricia marketed several new products such as condensed and powdered whole acid milk and powdered protein-milk. The following year Nutricia introduced 'Olvarit', canned vegetables for babies, in accordance with the medical advice that early supplementation with minerals was desirable. Their medical advisor was the paediatrician J.H.P. Jonxis, the successor of van Lookeren Campagne in Groningen. The paediatricians from Groningen have always taken a strong interest in nutrition problems. During the next decades Nutricia expanded the production of these non-milk foods with fruit and meat for babies (1958) and whole meals for toddlers (1961). Moreover Nutricia's farinaceous products increased in popularity. At the same time the 'Friesche Vlag' dairy factory in Leeuwarden introduced an assortment of milk-foods for infants that became popular in the northern provinces. Just as Nutricia, the Friesche Vlag had paediatricians as medical advisors. Professor Gorter, for instance, wrote a brochure for them.

During the sixties more powdered humanised milks such as Almiron-M2 (Nutricia), S.M.A. (Wijeth Laboratories) and Similac (M & R Laboratories) were marketed. Paediatricians, however, were not awaiting these products and one of the leading textbooks read at that time: 'They are useful products no doubt, but as to the current application of ready for use nutrition (Nutricia, Friesche Vlag) I haven't felt the need for these new preparations until now.'[28] Nevertheless powder formulas have conquered the market after a long period in which liquid and powder both were available. The composition underwent changes according to the changing medical opinions. For instance in 1975 Almiron was produced without saccharose because of the attention to dental caries in those years. In the 1980s the fatty acids and cholesterol were brought into vogue, so this had its impact on the Almiron formula. The latest changes have been the addition of taurine and/or carnitine, and the decrease of the protein concentration according to recent studies on protein metabolism of infants.[29] Moreover there is a strong tendency towards a smaller assortment of well-balanced foods; the days of elaborate adjustments for each individual infant are over.

## Concluding remarks

The possibility of satisfactory artificial feeding of the normal newborn became a realistic goal in the middle to late nineteenth century, when chemical techniques were developed for determining the constituents of human and animal milk. The success of the proprietary preparations, due largely to private entrepreneurship and integrity, supported much of the research responsible for progress in nutrition. The statement from the 1920s, that the first year of life is dominated by nutrition and nutrition problems, lost its threat as the quality of artificial infant feeding improved.[30]

However, in the Netherlands it took till after the Second World War before the preparation of formulas had moved from the kitchen to the factory. Before 1940 Dutch paediatricians supported the home-made preparation, because 'all proprietary products are no better for healthy children and often worse', as Gorter stated.[31] After 1945 things changed. Van Lookeren Campagne mentioned that the ones who could afford it, bought proprietary infant food. But in the 1950s even Gorter had to admit that 'the advantage of proprietary infant food is the supplementation with enough vitamin D'.[32] The increasingly sophisticated, ready-made and convenient products designed to meet all the individual food requirements of infants were more and more recommended by health workers as bottle-feeding affords an objective measure of the amount of milk consumed by the infant at each feeding. As the American physician Gallagher states: 'Although many contemporary pediatric authorities recommend breast-feeding over bottle-feeding, their recommendation does not extend to the providing of breast milk from other than the infant's own mother. The breast-milk bank and the wet-nurse are extinct social institutions . . . This suggests that the advantage attributed to breast-feeding is regarded as a relative advantage, not an absolute to be achieved at all costs.'[33]

The increased use of artificial infant feeding in the 1960s was accompanied by a sharp decline in breast-feeding practices. This was a concern to Dutch physicians, one of them complaining that 'The physician's general lack of training in this field may explain why, despite the many studies already done on this subject, so little progress has been made.'[34] During the 1970s, however, breast-feeding gained popularity among 'back to nature' movements, in whose philosophy of a more natural life-style breast-feeding in the traditional way was given an important place.[35] This renewed conscience led to a critical evaluation of the activities of industrial producers of infant food. In May 1974, the Twenty-seventh World Health Assembly also took a clear stand on breast-feeding and formulated its resolution WHA27.43 as follows: 'Urges Member countries to review sales' promotion activities on baby foods and to introduce appropriate remedial measures, including advertisement codes and legislation where necessary.'[36]

The advice on infant feeding formulated by the Study Group in 1985 offered the possibility of a balanced relation between breast-feeding and bottle-feeding. An increase in breast-feeding during the first six weeks and the prolonging of the use of proprietary food till one year could satisfy all parties. Medicalisation of the feeding of infants has been made possible by a close cooperation between physicians and food-industry.

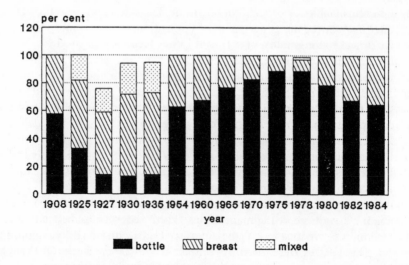

*Figure 1.* Infant feeding in the Netherlands at *13* weeks (1900–1978) and at 4 months (1980, 1982, 1984); compiled from Hennink (1966), Swaak (1975), Voorhoeve and Booy (1975), Swaak (1979), Van der Klaauw et al. (1979), Schilpzand and Uithof (1980), De Knecht-van Eekelen (1984), Obermann-de Boer and Kromhout (1985).

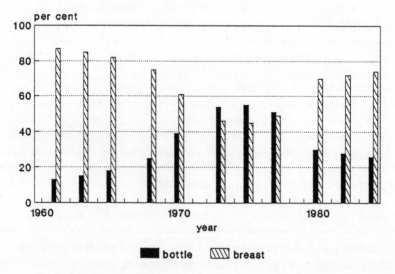

*Figure 2.* Infant feeding in the Netherlands at day *1–10* (*1960–1985*); compiled from Hennink (*1966*), Swaak (*1975*), Voorhoeve and Booy (*1975*), Swaak (*1979*), Van der Klaauw et al. (*1979*), Schilpzand and Uithof (*1980*), De Knecht-van Eekelen (*1984*), Obermann-der Boer and Kromhout (*1985*).

## Notes

1  Uitentuis (1985).
2  *GHI bulletin* (1991), p. 32; see also Wharton (1990).
3  De Knecht-van Eekelen (1984).
4  De Knecht-van Eekelen (1984), pp. 214–220.
5  De Knecht-van Eekelen (1984), pp. 245–248.
6  Apple (1980), pp. 404–406; Apple (1986), p. 4.
7  De Knecht-van Eekelen (1984), pp. 180–183; see for modern biochemical considerations of milk Jelliffe and Jelliffe (1978).
8  De Knecht-van Eekelen (1984), pp. 175–179, 188–197, 249–293.
9  De Knecht-van Eekelen (1984), pp. 108–118.
10  Fernandes (1990), p. 210.
11  De Knecht-van Eekelen (1984), p. 81.
12  At the First European Sanitarian Congress held in Brussels in 1876 infant mortality was one of the main topics. The relation with artificial infant feeding was obvious to all participants; De Knecht-van Eekelen (1984), pp. 234–236; see *Gezondheidscommissie 's-Gravenhage* (1911–1912).
13  Hennink (1966), pp. 56–61; Swaak (1975), pp. 27–28; Voorhoeve and Booy (1975), p. 338; Swaak (1979), pp. 162–163; Van der Klaauw et al. (1979), pp. 12–18; Schilpzand and Uithof (1980), pp. 42–50; De Knecht-van Eekelen (1984), p. 234; Obermann-de Boer and Kromhout (1985), p. 123.
14  Voorhoeve (1976); De Knecht-van Eekelen (1984), pp. 75–79; Marland (1992).
15  *Overzicht* (1932), pp. 45–46; Voorhoeve (1976), p. 34.
16  Hennink (1966), p. 92; the same remarks have been made for Great Britain: Ellis (1960), p. 169.
17  De Jonge (1976), pp. 217–222.
18  Molenaar (1936).
19  Gorter (1922).
20  Van Kasteren (1991).
21  Mol (1980).
22  De Knecht-van Eekelen (1984), pp. 251–255; Apple (1986), p. 5.
23  For more information on the Dutch East Indies see: Den Hartog (1986), pp. 158–163.
24  Wennekes (1991), pp. 9–24; Jelgersma (1991).
25  *Nutricia Kroniek* (s.a.).
26  Beck (1988); Almiron-A was intended for infants with a kidney or heart disease, disorders of unknown origin and vomiting children. In 1964 'Almiron M2' was provided for premature and small underweight infants, but in 1974 Nenatal was marketed for this purpose.
27  Van Lookeren Campagne (1938/39); Keyzer (1941); Van Lookeren Campagne (1947), pp. 31–32. Citrotrinose was an alternative for the more aggressive lactic acid in Marriot's mixture.
28  Verboom (1964), 81; the meagre enthusiasm for milk-powder is in

contrast to the situation in Great Britain where the public already got to know this product in the Second World War by the issue of fortified National Dried Milk: Ellis (1960), p. 170.

29  Beck (1988); *Nutricia Memo* (1989); see also Bindels (1992).
30  De Lange (1921), p. 6.
31  Gorter (1929), p. 41.
32  Van Lookeren Campagne (1947), p. 3; Gorter (1954), p. 164.
33  Gallagher (1978), p. 80.
34  Hennink (1966), p. 93.
35  Jonxis (1980), p. 386.
36  *Contempory patterns* (1981), p. 7.


## Literature

Apple, Rima D., ' "To be used only under the direction of a physician": Commercial infant feeding and medical practice, 1870–1940', *Bulletin of the History of Medicine*, 54 (1980), pp. 402–417.

Apple, Rima D., ' "Advertised by our loving friends": The infant formula industry and the creation of new pharmaceutical markets, 1870–1910', *The Journal of the History of Medicine and Allied Sciences*, 41 (1986), pp. 3–23.

Beck, I., *Memo Nutricia. Overzicht Almiron-ontwikkeling* [Review of Almiron-development] (Zoetermeer, 1988).

Bindels, J.G., 'Artificial feeds for infants – human milk substitutes: current composition and future trends', *Current Paediatrics*, (1992), pp. 163–167.

*Contemporary patterns of breast-feeding. Report on the WHO collaborative study on breast-feeding* (World Health Organization Geneva, 1981).

De Jonge, Jan A., *De industrialisatie in Nederland tussen 1850 en 1914* [The industrialisation in the Netherlands between 1850 and 1914] (Nijmegen, 1976).

De Knecht-van Eekelen, Annemarie, *Naar een rationele zuigelingenvoeding. Voedingsleer en kindergeneeskunde in Nederland 1840–1914* [Towards a rational infant feeding. The science of nutrition and paediatrics in the Netherlands 1840–1914], Thesis Nijmegen (Nijmegen, 1984).

De Lange, Cornelia C., *De geestelijke en lichamelijke opvoeding van het kind, in vrije navolging van Prof. Biedert 'Das Kind'* [The mental and physical education of the child etc.] (Amsterdam, 1921).

Den Hartog, Adel P., *Diffusion of milk as a new food to tropical regions: The example of Indonesia 1880–1942*, Netherlands Nutrition Foundation Wageningen (Wageningen, 1986).

Ellis, R.W.B., *Health in Childhood* (Harmondsworth, 1960).

Fernandes, J., 'Ontwikkelingen in de voeding van zuigelingen [Developments in infant nutrition]', *Voeding 51*, (1990), pp. 206–210.

Gallagher, E.B., *Infants, mothers, and doctors* (Lexington (Mass.)/Toronto, 1978).

Gezondheidscommissie 's-Gravenhage, *Sterfte in verband met voedingswijze en sociale omstandigheden, onder de kinderen beneden het jaar in 1908 geboren te 's-Gravenhage en Scheveningen* [Mortality related to nutrition and social circumstances among the children younger than one year old born in 1908 in the Hague and Scheveningen], Part 1, (The Hague, 1911–1912).

*GHI bulletin, Zuigelingenvoeding. Uitgangspunten en praktische aanbevelingen* [Infant nutrition. Premises and practical recommendations] (Rijswijk, 1991).

Gorter, Evert, *Over kindermeel* [On farina for infants] (Leiden, 1922).

Gorter, Evert, *De voeding van gezonde en zieke zuigelingen* [The nutrition of healthy and sick infants] (Leiden 1929, 1954).

Hennink, Marius P., *Borstvoeding. Een onderzoek te Leiden naar enkele sociaal-geneeskundige aspecten met betrekking tot borstvoeding* [Breast-feeding. A research into some social medical aspects concerning breast-feeding in Leiden], Thesis Leiden (Leiden, 1966).

Jelgersma, B., *Memo Nutricia. Aanvangsdatum onderneming* [Date of establishment of Nutricia] (Zoetermeer, 1991).

Jelliffe, Derrick B. and E.F. Patricia Jelliffe, *Human milk in the modern world. Psychological, nutritional, and economic significance (Oxford/New York/Toronto, 1978)*.

Jonxis, J.H.P., 'Borstvoeding' [Breast-feeding], *Voeding* 41, (1980), pp. 386–389.

Keyzer, J.L., *Over de voeding van gezonde en zieke zuigelingen met volle zure melk* [On the feeding of healthy and ailing infants with acidified whole milk] (Foxhol/Groningen, 1941).

Lookeren Campagne, Jan van, 'Citrotrinosemelk [Citrotrinose-milk]', *Maandschrift voor Kindergeneeskunde* 8, (1938/1939), pp. 85–86.

Lookeren Campagne, Jan van, *Voeding en voedingsstoornissen bij zuigelingen* [Nutrition and nutrition disorders of infants] (Amsterdam, 1947).

Marland, Hilary, 'The medicalization of motherhood: doctors and infant welfare in the Netherlands, 1901–1930', in Valery Fildes, Laura Marks and Hilary Marland (eds), *Women and children first. International infant welfare, 1870–1945* (London/New York, 1992), pp. 74–96.

Mol, J., 'Van melkinrichting tot levensmiddelenfabriek [From dairy-shop to food-factory]', *Voeding* 41, (1980), pp. 166–172.

Molenaar & Co.'s Meelfabrieken, *Het eerste levensjaar* [The first year of life] (Westzaan, 1936).

*Nutricia, Kroniek* [Chronicle], typescript (s.l., s.a.).

*Nutricia, Memo. Achtergrondinformatie eiwitverlaging Almiron m2 en a–b* [Background information on decrease of protein Almiron m2 and a–b] (1989).

Obermann-de Boer, G.L. and D. Kromhout, 'Voedselconsumptie van zuigelingen (het Leidse zuigelingenen peuteronderzoek) [Nutrient intake of infants (the Leiden Pre-School Children Study)', in B.C. Breedveld et al. (eds), *Voeding tijdens zwangerschap en lactatie* [Nutrition during pregnancy and lactation] (Alphen aan den Rijn/Bruxelles, 1985), pp. 120–131.

*Overzicht over het sociaal hygienisch werk in Nederland op het gebied van den Dienst der Volksgezondheid* [Survey of the social sanitarian work in the Netherlands in the field of the Public Health Service] (The Hague, 1932).

Schilpzand, Rutger and Wiebe Uithof, *Ontwikkeling van de zuigelingenvoeding in Nederland vanaf 1900* [Development of infant nutrition in the Netherlands from 1900], Department of Human Nutrition publication nr 80–15 (Wageningen, 1980).

Swaak, A.J., *Bouwstenen voor een sociale kinderhygiëne* [Materials for a social children's welfare] (Nijmegen, 1975).

Swaak, A.J., 'Een oriënterend onderzoek naar de voeding van zuigelingen in de eerste zes levensmaanden in de provincie Noord-Brabant [A preliminary research into the nutrition of infants during the first six months of life in the province of North-Brabant]', *Voeding* 40 (1979), pp. 157–165.

Uitentuis, J., *Zuigelingenvoeding. De huidige inzichten* [Infant nutrition. The present insights] (Utrecht/Antwerp, 1985).

Van der Klaauw, M.M., Th.H.M. de Beer and G.A. de Jonge, *Borstvoeding in Terneuzen* [Breast-feeding in Terneuzen], research year 1977, Part 1, (Leiden, 1979).

Van Kasteren, J., 'General Biscuits vertaalt Richtlijnen in produkt [General Biscuits translates Guidelines in product]', *Voeding* 52, (1991), pp. 231–233.

Verboom, C.H., *Zieke zuigelingen. Een handleiding bij de herkenning en behandeling van de belangrijkste ziekten op de zuigelingen- en kleuterleeftijd* [Sick infants. A manual etc.] (Assen, 1964).

Voorhoeve, H.W.A. and R.W. Booy, 'Epidemiologie van borstvoeding [Epidemiology of breast-feeding]', *Voeding* 36, (1975), pp. 338–345.

Voorhoeve, H.W.A. (ed), *75 jaar Kinderhygiëne in Nederland. Van zuigelingenzorg tot jeugdgezondheidszorg* [75 years Children's Welfare. From infant welfare to youth health care] (Assen/Amsterdam, 1977).

Wennekes, Wim, *De vaders van Nutricia 'De Min van Nederland'* [The fathers of Nutricia 'The wet-nurse of the Netherlands'] (Abcoude, 1991).

Wharton, Brian, 'Milk for babies and children. No ordinary cows' milk before 1 year', *British Medical Journal* 301, (1990), pp. 774–775.

# 5

# HISTORY OF COOLING AND FREEZING TECHNIQUES AND THEIR IMPACT ON NUTRITION IN TWENTIETH-CENTURY GERMANY

*Hans Jürgen Teuteberg*

The Seventh International Ethnological Food Research Conference, which took place in Bergen (Norway), dealt for the first time exclusively with the development of the preservation of human foodstuffs and examined this topic from the most various points of view.[1] Strangely enough none of the 25 speeches dealt with freezing techniques, although they belong to the great innovations of the industrial age. This innovation has not only extended the millennium-old provision economy, but has also reshaped the nutritional culture essentially. The great divide in the history of human nutrition seems remarkable: only forty years ago not even one per cent of German households owned an electric refrigerator, which is why the Federal Minister of Finance even wanted to impose a luxury tax upon it. In Germany today it belongs to the most essential need which is considered not to be done without. Even public assistance recipients as the poorest of the poor receive an allowance for the acquisition of a refrigerator. Therefore almost every household is equipped with such a refrigerator. Other industrial nations cannot imagine the daily food supply without this modern cooling technique, either. As we lack a scientific comprehensive presentation of food-cooling and the significance of the industrial freezing techniques for the change in nutritional habits this contribution aims at a summary of the current research.[2]

## Early practices of cooling foodstuffs

Like most techniques this one has a longer previous history. From mere observation one already knew in the early days that the perishability of most foodstuffs has something to do with the water content, which can rise in meat according to fat content to 55–75%, in raw milk to 88% and in some fruits and vegetables even to 95%. This shows the truth of the old alchemist wisdom, 'corpora non agunt nisi fluid', i.e. bodies, more precisely decomposing substances, can only be effective at a sufficient liquidity level. Grain, which can be stored almost indefinitely at a water content of 13%, showed the importance of the process of drying. By means of drying, smoking and salting the water was drawn from the foodstuffs and thereby the pathogenous putrefactive bacteria lost their basis. Olive oil, wood- and wine-vinegar, high-proof alcohol- and sugar solutions as well as heating to achieve the exclusion of air, which was recommended by the Frenchman Denis Pain in the late 17th century, tried out by the Italian Lazarro Spalanzi in the 18th century and first successfully and permanently put into practice by the French cook Nicolas-François Appert in the early 19th century, have extended the possibilities of preservation.

Ancient authors as well as literary sources from the Chinese, Indian and Arabian cultures also repeatedly reported experiments on the cooling of drinks, fruits and meat with the help of natural snow and ice. Contrary to other preservation techniques this remained an extremely expensive luxury which even royal sovereigns could only occasionally afford.[3] While the preparation of ice-cream and frozen fruit juices gradually increased on the noble tables of Italy, France and then also Germany from the late 17th century, the use of ice in the daily food storage was altogether only of minor importance until the beginning of the 19th century.[4]

### The rise of natural ice manufacturing

At first a new development was in the offing in the English colonies of North-America, because an increased erection of 'ice-houses' took place in the second half of the 18th century. In these houses the valuable meat could best be protected from putrefaction in the long and humid summers. The growing demand for cooling possibilities, which also made itself felt in other tropical colonies of the Europeans, stimulated a wish to produce, store and even transport natural ice on a larger scale. After the Bostonian shipowner Frederick Tudor had brought ice from New England to the island of Martinique in the Caribbean, where plantation owners were willing to pay a lot of money for such a cooling system at the beginning of the 19th century, the natural ice industry experienced a quick boom. Fast-sailing American 'clippers' brought the ice-blocks not only to South America, but also to South Africa and after the inauguration of the Suez Canal even to India as well as Australia. A whole new branch of trade now dealt with the cutting of regular ice-blocks, which made the development of specific tools necessary.[5] The natural ice also served for the cooling of milk and dairy products in the American towns, where flying ice-traders and especially 'Ice cars' appeared in the streets. On the first US railways at that time foodstuffs often had to be shifted. Since 1857 one therefore tried to freight the extremely expensive meat of deer and poultry with the help of cooling-carriages running on rails. Nathan B. Sutherland from Detroit was the first to take out a patent for such cooling-carriages. While Cincinnati as the first big centre of industrial meat processing had been able to slaughter and salt as well as transport the meat southwards on the Ohio-river only in winter, the slaughtering business with the help of ice-cooling was now possible even in summer. Chicago also profited from this innovation. Large amounts of meat were now taken easily from the meat factories to the markets of the American East coast with the help of cooling-carriages.[6] Compared to the live delivery of cattle the freight charges were diminished by two thirds. Thereby the ice had made the erection of a totally new meat and packaging industry possible. It turned into a real promotor of the new frozen food. The banana, which first came to New York from Cuba in 1804, also conquered the whole of North-America with the help of 'Ice boxes on wheels'.[7] The new cooling-carriages transported meat, vegetables and fruit from far-away manufacturing areas into the big towns and made them more independent of the supply from the surrounding areas. The urbanisation of North America, which grew more and more quickly, would hardly have been possible without these cool-storage transports. The cooling of foodstuffs turned out to be a profitable business which employed thousands of people and triggered off capital investments to the extent of millions of dollars.

Economic-technical encyclopedias and magazines of the 18th century prove that in Europe there were already 'ice-farms' with 'ice-pits' and 'ice-houses', but all this took place in the normal course of conventional housekeeping.[8] A first commercialisation could be observed in the fishery business. In 1786 one already sent the invaluable Scottish salmon to London in ice-boxes. The necessary natural ice was hacked from the numerous Scottish lakes and was stored in humid soil-huts in summer. Since 1800 the herring-fishery also made use of preservation with ice. With the extension of the railway fresh seafish managed to gain ground all over the country for the first time. From the middle of the 19th century a fishmonger called Hewett began to preserve the salted herrings while he was still in the open sea. The fishermen from Grimsby and Hull, who got their ice from Norway, were now able to extend their journeys to Greenland and the fish-processing industry experienced a great boom. The farmers in the surrounding areas of London considered the hacking-off of ice-blocks in the Thames marshes a profitable business. These blocks were then carted off to the central fish market at Billingsgate. In 1902 Great Britain already imported fresh seafish for 4 millions.[9] The 'fish and chips' shops opening everywhere prove that fresh seafish became a cheap national popular dish through the cooling principle.[10]

Since 1886 and after the completion of the railway system the German fishery, which for centuries had only been pursued as in-shore fishing, was extended after the English model to become an efficient deep-sea fishery with the help of the state. Steam trawlers, mechanical net winches, cutting boards and wireless telegraphy raised the catch results immensely. Some kinds of commercial fish, like e.g. redfish, were put on the home market for the first time. From 1890 all larger German harbours had their own ice-works.[11] Special 'fish trains' ran directly from the fish auctions to the great towns. Corresponding to this new offer the demànd for natural ice and domestic refrigerators also increased. The suburbs of Berlin became the first centres of the ice trade. The Havel and Spree formed numerous lakes which were suitable for an 'ice harvest'. In 1840 the Berlin butcher Louis Thater, then the trader Eduard Murack and finally the bricklayer Carl Bolle in 1863 began to erect ice-houses after the American model. Later on the 'North German Ice-works' owned 18 such ice-houses on 1400 square metres of the Rummels-burger Lake. They had steam-engines, shops and a refrigerator production, which was also joined by branches in Köpenick, Hannover, Frankfurt Main and Vienna. After the First World War this enterprise employed 1200 people. Almost 200 ice traders with 400 horse-drawn vehicles, whose coachmen wore a standardized uniform, were united in the 'Artificial Ice Society', founded 1915. This society supplied dairies, hotels, refreshment kiosks, butchers, slaughter-houses and breweries. In 1935 the Berlin classified directory still listed 93 ice traders. In Frankfurt Main the ice trade was dominated by the company Günther & Co, which had 30 coaches driving through the streets of the town in 1925. The consumption of natural ice in German private house-holds was far below that of the American per-capita consumption, though the offer of all sorts of ice-creams nevertheless seems to have been larger.[12]

Even though the domestic 'ice-cellars', 'ice-pitches' and 'ice-farms', in which the meat and milk could be stored in small rooms, continued to dominate especially in the rural areas in the mansion-houses near the Eastern part of the Elbe, the demand for small refrigerators for the urban-bourgeois households increased simultaneously with the growing urbanisation since 1860. At the world exhibition in Vienna in 1873 one could already see a large number of models of such 'portable ice-cellars'. The growing dependence on the food trade, the decreasing possibilities to store larger provisions as well as the growing demands on quality and freshness, interplayed. Apart from farmers, hospitals and pubs, especially larger aristocratic households were interested in such an acquisition. The industry offered simple ice-boxes as well as repre-sentative cabinets with neo-gothic carved work, marble arrangements and crystal glass as well as an unleaded enamel varnish inside the refrigerator.[13] Because of the continually melting ice the humidity content could not be avoided, which led to malodorous oxidation and mildew. Therefore the refrigerator had to be scoured with tin-sand, washed and dried once a week. The continuous cleaning and replacing of ice was very time-consuming and the task of the servants. It is therefore no surprise that contrary to the USA these refrigerators were only temporarily used during the summer heat and could still not replace the old pantry. The natural ice was also sometimes polluted so that carcinogens could easily be transmitted.[14]

### First ideas and experiments with artificial cold

The defects and relatively high costs of a cooling system with natural ice had led to pre-occupation with the question of how one could achieve an artificial cooling system for foodstuffs at a very early stage. One had already realized in early advanced civilizations that evaporating water emits cold and that through the solution of salt this process could even be intensified, but only since the middle of the 16th century did there appear systematic descriptions about cooling drinks made this way.[15] The new natural sciences became the actual pacemaker for the artificial deep-freezing techniques. The English chemical engineer Robert Boyle, who had found the law for the compression of gases, found out in test series between 1665 and 1668 that the mixture of sulphuric acid, hydrochloric and especially nitric acid with snow produces an 'artificial cold'. He explained this with the thesis that the salts had obviously changed the aggregate state of the snow. He had correctly realized that cold is released while ice or snow melts or evaporates.[16] From the point of view of science in the 17th century cold had a material character. Especially in nitric acid one assumed a cold-producing character, the 'prinium frigidum'. The French natural philosopher Pierre Gassendi even maintained that the water particles also attach themselves to the nitric acid sediment and then turn themselves into a spinous-firm body of ice. At the beginning of the 18th century research dealt more intensively with the circulation process of the physical sciences and their practical applicability. The conditions under which gas turns into liquid and liquids turn into material were particularly discussed. A large number of experiments in this field as well as on pressure and vacuum, heating and cooling down were done in England, France and Germany and the Netherlands, but did not lead to practical use. The observation of the English physicist Michael Faraday turned out to be the most important one. During the liquefaction of gas he discovered that the ammonia gas, which he produced through heating in a U-tube, condensed into a coolant at the other end of the tube. If one leaves the ammonia to itself, it evaporates and produces artificial cold. In 1788 his colleague Charles Blagden, who like the physicist Gabriel Fahrenheit from Danzig had occupied himself with the freezing of mercury, reported about all kinds of experiments on the cooling of water below freezing point. By means of various admixtures he tried out different mixtures of cold.[17] Thereby further basic theoretical insights were gained, but the practical application still turned out to be extraordinarily difficult. The first patents for the production of artificial cold were granted, but did not lead to an economically profitable solution.[18]

**Founding fathers of the modern freezing techniques**

The first breakthrough was achieved by the French civil engineer Fernand Philippe Edouard Carre who constructed an ammonia-absorption-machine in 1857, in which the water was made to freeze through the quick evaporation of condensed ammonia. His 'ice-machine' already managed to produce a few thousand pounds of artificial ice and achieved a small sensation at the world exhibition in Paris, the more so because he also presented a refrigerator for the kitchen. His 'appareil refrigerant pour la production de la glace' was made of a cauldron filled with ammonia, a freezer as well as a reservoir. It needed two hours to produce 1 kilogram of artificial ice. It is not surprising that his ice-machine was not appropriate for the normal household. At this time another series of 'refrigerators' was put on the market, most of them based upon the 'ether ice-machine' of the American Jacob Perkins, who lived in England and had developed this machine for the first time in 1834. In Darlington Harbour near Sidney the first factory for frozen meat was erected by Thomas Sutcliffe Mort after he had made experiments together with the French navy engineer Eugene Dominique Nicolle. The 'New South Wales Fresh Food and Ice Company' founded by Mort, like Carre applied the ammonia-compression-principle. This company worked technically in a faultless way as did a slaughter-house erected in 1875 with cold rooms, but could not prevail on the market against the cheaper natural ice.

In 1877 the French refrigerator ship 'S.S. Frigorifique' transported for the first time Argentinian meat to France with the help of a mechanical cooling system after the Carre principle and under the direction of the French engineer Charles Tellier, but after a journey of 104 days the meat was spoilt. During a second journey with the cold-storage steamer 'Paraguay' in the same year, 80 tons of mutton at 30 degrees Celsius were taken from Buenos Aires to Le Havre and still came up to all demands on quality.[19] At the first international congress on cooling in 1908 Charles Tellier was appointed 'Père de froid' on application of Argentina for his great feat. All over the world this great success stimulated experiments to arrange the shipment of frozen meat. Apart from Argentina, Australia and also New Zealand, became great exporters of meat.

In Europe at this time the realisation came that it would be more economic to switch over to the production of artificial cold. Meanwhile physical science had proved that there were three ways of lowering temperature and producing ice: 1. through liquefaction of firm bodies (e.g. salts), 2. through evaporation of fluids, and 3. through the extension of gases. The first method seemed most suitable for the continuous production of small amounts of ice, the other two seemed to be applicable for the fabrication of ice with the help of complicated machines. Understandably one turned to the cheapest method first, but the small cooling machines introduced by the Italian Toselli and the technical Professor Heinrich Meidinger could not be converted into an economically realizable form despite the correct physical specifications.[20]

The actual pioneering success in the field of artificial cooling techniques was achieved by the engineer Carl Linde (1842–1934).[21] The Professor for mechanical engineering, who had already been called to the Polytechnikum at the age of 26, presented a paper in 1870 with the title 'Wärmeentziehung bei niedrigen Temperaturen durch mechanische Mittel' and a year later his epoch-making treatise 'Verbesserte Eis- und Kühlmaschinen' was published and made the 'beer town' Munich sit up and listen. The great brewery owner Georg

Sedlmayr was immediately willing to have such a machine constructed at his own expense. Contrary to other scientists Linde was not concerned to replace natural ice, but particularly wanted to find other means of transmitting artificial cold. At the world exhibition in Vienna in 1873 he presented a totally new programme. His central idea was to integrate the cooling machines into the economically highly advanced natural ice technique and to connect coolants and atmosphere consistently to reduce the cooling costs drastically. He thereby wanted to help the artificial cold to a broad industrial application. With this approach Linde immediately caused an international sensation. In 1875 he already constructed a completely new ammonia-ice-machine, in which the vapours of the liquid ammonia, which was contained in a tube appliance, were primed by a pump and then led back to the capacitor. With the co-operation of the coolants flowing around the tube helix the vapours were condensed to a liquid again and then returned the evaporator. Based upon the experiences concerning cold-storage plants in breweries and slaughter-houses he later constructed a handy household appliance which was equivalent on the whole to today's compressor refrigerators. After several experiments his new cooling-machine had a very much higher degree of efficiency than all other competing models. Like nobody before him Linde had brought scientific insights and industrial realizations together optimally.

After two machine factories had built and distributed his cooling-machines successfully in Europe, he founded his own company in Wiesbaden in 1879, which first concentrated on the supply for breweries. After a mild winter in 1883/4, when the natural ice harvest turned out to be small, he was hit by a 'downpour of orders'. In the meantime the breweries had noticed that through the new artificial ice they could achieve complete independence from the seasonal variations in temperature. Production, storage and distribution could do without natural ice. Similar to the fruit, fish and meat trade they could be extended supra-regionally and even internationally for the first time. The artificial cold paved the way for the transition to an efficient mass production. While the 'Linde's Ice-machine Society' had delivered only 10 machines in 1877, they already delivered 429 in 1896. At this time there were 2,756 cooling-machines worldwide, 900 of them in breweries, 297 in meat processing factories, 122 in ice factories, 109 on sea-going vessels and 80 in dairies. Most cooling-machines were to be found in Germany, England, the U.S.A. and Austria; but Linde also had some customers in South-America, China and Egypt. As far as he himself was concerned, he fell back upon research into low temperatures in his experiment station at the University of Munich, but without completely breaking away from his company. In 1895 he achieved together with William Thompson and James Prescott Joule a first liquefaction of air. This resulted in a totally new physical science of low temperatures and first examinations of the high vacuum. Linde's inventions accelerated the construction of slaughter-houses, cold-storage depots, refrigerator ships and refrigerator vans everywhere; between 1887 and 1891 alone his company produced 60 cold-storage plants. The quaity of meat, whose consumption rapidly grew in Germany at this time, was thereby decisively improved, but also fishmongers and butter and cheese traders, mushroom growers, wineries as well as chocolate producers, the chemical industry and the gum and sugar manufacturers discovered the profit of artificial cold.

Linde's success did not let the designing engineers who constructed household fridges rest. In the first decades after the turn of the century engineers and machine-producing factories everywhere busied themselves with the problem of replacing natural ice in the household by artificial cold. US companies took charge in this field. The automobile managers Arnold Goss and Edmond Copeland from Detroit developed a household fridge which was called 'Kelvintor' by the New York advertising agency Thompson in memory of the physicist Lord Kelvin. In 1918 67 fridges were sold under this name. When the big automobile combine General Motors took over a small company called 'Guardian Frigidair', which had been founded in Fort Wayne in 1915, they helped them to a fast sale of their fridge with the same name. The name 'Frigidaire' became the synonym for the fridge in the USA. More than fifty companies tried to convince the customer of the quality of their household refrigerators. While production in the USA in the year 1910 comprised only 100 fridges, it rose to 5000 in 1921 and to 850.000 in 1930. This meant about ten per cent of all fridges sold, but we should not forget that the wide rural areas in the USA had still not been connected to electricity. The sale of refrigerators turned more and more into a mass business in North-America. This had something to do with the quickly falling prices and the large-scale series production which had been taken over by the automobile construction. At the beginning of the 1930s the chain-store Sears, Roebuck & Co already included refrigerators in their supply. In 1934 they could already sell 59,000 pieces, i.e. 5 per cent of the total fridge turnover; in 1939 the sales figures rose to 285,000 or 15 per cent of the total turnover in the United States. The success was also promoted by the circumstance that e.g. the new Colspot-model had received a streamlined look which had been approved by aviation.[22] In 1936 already 9 million fridges were standing in American households, and 850,000 pieces were sold yearly.

### The birth of the deep-cooling age in Germany

The breakthrough to the modern deep freezing age happened in Germany, as in other European countries, with a delay of twenty years. Certainly the food departments of the new department stores, delicatessen shops, bakeries, ice-cream parlours, breweries and landlords were interested in the new artificial 'small cold' long before the First World War, but household cooling-machines were not in high demand. The 'Allgemeine Elektrizitätsgesellschaft' (AEG) in Berlin did offer a first model of an automatic ice and cooling machine for the households in 1912, but the model cost 1500

Goldmarks or the average income for two years of work. The small compact fridges which were put on the market by the companies Ahlborn (Hildesheim), the Bayer Brothers (Augsburg) and the 'Bergedorfer Eisenwerke' near Hamburg aimed only at the industrial customer. In 1930 the AEG offered the model 'Santo', the Siemens AG (in later times working with the Linde company) offered their model 'Protos Frigor' and the enterprises Bosch and 'Eisfink' offered small refrigerators which were partly based upon US patents. Even these fridges were relatively expensive and consisted of sheet iron, copper pipes as well as visibly rotating axles and driving belts. The cooling case and cooling apparatus did not form an integrated whole as yet, and one could recognize the model of the old natural ice box. Furthermore the models had leaks and the mechanical parts wore out after a while. The fact that until well into the 1930s and 1940s the natural ice industry still dominated is therefore not surprising. Attempts to introduce a 'popular refrigerator' with the help of the 'Reichsinstitut für Lebensmittelfrischhaltung' in 1936 to provide every household with a cheap fridge proved, unlike the similar projects 'Volkswagen' and 'Volksrundfunkempfänger' to be a complete failure. The acquisition of the electric refrigerators remained four times more expensive than the natural ice cabinets and the monthly operating costs were also 25 per cent higher. Until 1930 only 30,000 compression fridges had been sold, i.e. only 0.6–0.8 per cent of all households owned such an electric cooling unit, for which one had to go to the great expense of two monthly salaries of an industrial worker.[23] Contrary to the other electric appliances the fridge was not yet listed in the instructions for a modern efficient household.[24] The market was almost completely dominated by the American models. The US company General Electric for example managed to offer a model called 'Monitor Top', which fused the cabinet with the engine unit in a white varnished steel case to an aesthetic unity. The AEG, who had given up their first absorption model, now distributed this American top product under their own trade mark name 'Santo'.

The deep freezing economy also developed in a different field. The Danish fishmonger A.J.A. Ottesen (1860–1936) had initiated the artificial deep freezing of fish. In Denmark, which concentrated on the export of fish, one had closely observed the attempts to improve cooling techniques. Experiments on the improvement of ice farming at the agricultural school in Copenhagen illustrate this.[25] Since the invention of the profitable cold compression machine by Linde Ottesen it was realized that one did not need ice to preserve fish, but that one only had to cool a salt solution to protect the highly perishable fish. A useful solution failed because the fresh fish took in too much salt when dipped into the brine and therefore became uneatable. After several experiments the Danish fishmonger found out that every sodium chloride solution has a freezing point corresponding to its degree of concentration, at which ice is exuded instead of salt. A fish dipped into this solution no longer took in salt, but only cold. Now Ottesen chose a salt content of 28,9 per cent which freezes at a temperature of minus 21,2 degrees Celsius. Thereby the fish could now be frozen within 1–3 hours to about minus 20 degrees according to size and be preserved almost indefinitely. In 1912 the Danish machine-producing factory Saboe constructed a first deep freezer and in 1915 the first production was started in the harbour of Esbjerg. Based on Ottesen's patent Rudolf Plank, professor for thermo-dynamics at the Technical University of Danzig, presented a memoir 'Die Konservierung von Fischen durch Gefrierverfahren'. This memoir furnished proof that low temperatures employed as a shock treatment could best preserve the frozen products and the muscle and cellular tissue would only be changed slightly.[26] The fishery expert Walter Schlienz, who changed from the Prussian Ministry of Agriculture to the management of the 'Nordsee' enterprise founded in 1896, became the most enthusiastic advocate for the new deep freezing techniques and also played leading role in the foundation of a new frozen fish-stock corporation. The large-scale production at the production line, the mechanical filleting of fish and the first automatic fried-fish shop, and also the equipment of a first deep freezer ship, which fillets and deep-freezes the fish straight after the catch, as well as the establishment of the 'Gefriertechnische Gesellschaft deutscher Hochseefischerei' are on the whole owing to his work.

As a further development of the Ottesen brine-freezing technique the American fishery biologist Clarence Birdseye (1886–1956) presented a new plate freezer which led the frozen food through two metal strips sprayed with cooled brine. Birdseye also made first experiments on the freezing of carton-packed vegetables and fruit and turned the older American ice-cream boxes into handy deep freezers which helped the retail traders to offer deep-freeze household packages. Rudolf Planck observed these innovations closely and reported them immediately.[27] Since the middle of the 1930s this breakthrough was also achieved and 'Quick Frozen Food' celebrated its first triumphant successes in the USA. In the USA the total production of deep-freeze foods climbed to 170 000 tons per year, whereby fruit, vegetables and fish were at the top.

The 'four-year plan' proclaimed in Germany in 1936 and in particular the Second World War provoked a strong promotion of the deep freezing technique, because the regime of the National Socialists wanted to close the protein gap of the popular nutrition and wanted by all means to avoid famines like those during the First World War. Especially the German Armed Forces at the fronts were supplied increasingly. The industrial production of carton-packed fish fillets, the deep freezing of fruit and vegetables with the co-operation of the tinning industry, the construction of special flat-bed trailers for vans as well as the fish processing ships and the foundation of numerous enterprises and trade associations are the results of massive governmental financial support. The quick boom of the German deep freezing economy after 1945 was a logical consequence of these activities.

Unfortunately only little is known of the development and differentiation of the German retail trade with its turnovers of deep-freeze food, the motivations of the shopping housewives and the actual domestic consumption of frozen foods in the past decades. The data reveal that in 1960 only 3 per cent of all West German households owned a deep freezer, in 1969 at least about 18 per cent, whereby the rural households dominated by far. In 1965 52,6 per cent of all households were equipped with a fridge, in 1969 already 86 per cent, but in 1970 only 10 per cent of these households owned a three-stars-freezer compartment to store the frozen foods for a longer period of time. The consumption of frozen foods increased between 1960 and 1970 from 22,100 tons to 218,992 tons, which signified a tenfold increase. Through new forms of trade, especially the transition to the supermarket, the modernization of canteens and private kitchens and new offers concerning prefabricated food, frozen food continued its boom until today, whereby more and more deep freezers made their appearance in the urban households. Today special mobile home-services bring the frozen foods straight from the producer to the customers after they have ordered the products through a catalogue. The cold-chains which secured a high food quality have thereby become much closer. Looking back it seems that the years around 1860 and 1960 have been the most decisive years for the history of modern frozen foods and deep freezing but only new comparative studies can clarify whether this division into periods is actually correct.

## Notes

1  Riddervold/Ropeid (1988)
2  Preliminary studies are: Wirkner (1897); Anderson (1953); Plank (1954); Woolrich (1957); Thévenot/Fiedler (1978); Hilck/Auf dem Hövel (1979); Hellmann (1990).
3  Lippmann (1898); Hellmann (1990), pp. 27–40.
4  Wiegelmann (1964); Marperger (1716); Fincke (1958).
5  Giedeon (1948); Eltzner (1882); Cummings (1948); Jones (1982).
6  Cummings (1940), p. 60ff.; Critchell/Raymond (1912); Clemens (1923); Armour (1906).
7  Root/de Rochemond (1976), pp. 150–55; Levenstein (1988), pp. 30–43.
8  Concerning the spreading of ice-cellars in Germany see Künitz (1777); Menzel (1848); Harzer (1853); Nöthling (1896).
9  Burnett (1966), p. 135.
10  Walton (1992).
11  Rudolph (1946), p. 47; Wiegelmann/Maus (1986), pp. 75–92; Hitzbleck (1917); Stahmer (1913).
12  Hengsbach (1970); Kaufmann (1923); Heinel (1908); Rohrbeck (1928); Eiswerke (1906).
13  Swoboda (1868); Swoboda (1874), Meidinger (1888).

14 Heyroth (1888); Fritzsche (1895).
15 The many experiments on artificial cooling of foodstuffs and luxury foods in previous centuries for the purpose of preservation cannot be considered here. Compare the older literature in Beckmann (1799), pp. 197 ff. See Villafranca (1550); Bartholinus (1661).
16 Boyle (1744).
17 Blagden (1788).
18 See a detailed list of the early experiments with still imperfect 'ice-machines' in Figuier (1876), pp. 591-623. Compare Singer (1958).
19 Feldhaus (1970), p. 549; Tellier (1910); see Thévenot/Fiedler (1978).
20 Toselli (1868); Meidinger (1872), Meidinger (1875), Habermann (1888).
21 Linde (1984); Matschoss (1954); Gesellschaft (1896); Gesellschaft (1929).
22 Taubeneck (1936); Wallance (1956); Bush (1975); Meikle (1979).
23 Hellmann (1990); Mosolff (1941); Heiß (1939).
24 Meyer (1926).
25 Fjord (1877); Hilck/Auf dem Hövel (1979), pp. 11–18.
26 Plank (1915); Plank (1928).
27 Plank (1929); Plank (1937); Reader (1963).

## Literature

Anderson, Oscar E., *Refrigation in America. A History of a new Technology and its Impact* (Cincinnati, 1953).
Armour, Ogden, *The Packers, the Private Car Lines and the People* (Chicago, 1906).
Bartholinus, Thomas, *De nivis usus medico observationis variae* (Copenhagen, 1661).
Blagden, Charles, *Die Gesetze der Überkaltung und Gefriererniedrigung. Zwei Abhandlungen* (1788). Ed. by A.J. von Oettingen (Leipzig, 1894).
Beckmann, Johann, *Beyträge zur Geschichte der Erfindungen*, vol.4 (Leipzig, 1799).
Boyle, Robert, Philosophical Transactions; giving some Accompt of the Present Untertakings, Studies and Labours of the Ingenious in many Considerable Parts of the World, vol.1, London 1655, pp. 8–9.- An Experimental History of Cold, pp. 46–52. A Further Experiment of Mr Boyle as Experimental History of Cold, pp. 344–52. -Promiscuous Inquieries, chiefly about Cold, vol.1, London 1666, pp. 256–62.- An Frigorifick Experiment shewing, how a considerable Degree of Cold may be suddenly produced without Help of Snow, Ice, Haile, Wind or Niter and that any Time of the Year. In: *The Whole Works*, ed. by Thomas Bird, vol.2, London 1744, pp. 200, 266, 300.
Burnett, John, *Plenty and Want. A Social History of Diet in England from 1815 to the Present Day* (London, 1966).
Bush, Donald J., *The Streamline Decade* (New York, 1975).

Clemen, Rudolph A., *American Livestock and Meat Industry* (New York, 1923).

Critchell, James Troubridge and Joseph Raymond, *The History of Frozen Meat Trade*, 2nd ed. (London, 1912).

Cummings, Richard Osborne, *The American and His Food* (Chicago, 1944).

Cummings, Richard Osborne, *The American Ice Harvest: A History in Technology, 1880–1918* (Berkely/Los Angeles, 1949).

*Eiswerke J.H. Günther & Co* (Frankfurt a.M., 1906).

Eltzner, R.W., 'Eis-Gewinnung in den Vereinigten Staaten', *Deutsche Bauzeitung*, vol.16 (1882).

Farrer, K.T.H., *A Settlement Amply Supplied: Food Technology in Nineteenth-Century Australia* (Melbourne, 1980).

Feldhaus, Franz Maria, *Die Technik. Ein Lexikon der Vorzeit, der geschichtlichen Zeit und der Naturvölker ( 1914)*, 2nd ed. (München, 1970).

Figuier, Louis–Guilleaume, *Les merveilles d'industrie, ou description des principles industries modernes*, vol.3 (Paris, 1876).

Fincke, Heinrich, 'Beitrag zur Geschichte eisgekühlter und gefrorener Lebensmittel', *Süsswaren* vol.2 (*1958*), pp. 8–10.

Fjord, U.J., *Bericht über einen Versuch auf dem Gebiet der Eismeierei, ausgeführt auf der Landbauschule zu Kopenhagen und den Gütern Durupgaard und Gjedfergaard* (Hildesheim-Danzig, 1877).

Fritzsche, Anton, *Untersuchungen über die Qualität des Würzburger Natur- und Kunsteises* (Würzburg, 1895).

*Gesellschaft für Linde's Eismaschinen Wiesbaden* (Prospect), (Wiesbaden 1896).

Gesellschaft für Linde's Eismaschinen (ed.), *Künstliche Kälte für Fleischereien, Delikatess, Wild- und Geflügelhandlungen* (Wiesbaden 1925).

Giedeon, Siegfried, *Mechanization takes Command* (New York, 1948).

German: *Herrschaft der Mechanisierung*, (Frankfurt a.M., 1982).

Habermann, R., 'Die Eis- und Kälteerzeugungsmaschinen' *Verhandlungen des Vereins zur Beförderung des Gewerbefleisses* (Berlin, 1888).

Harzer, Friedrich, *Vorschriften und Regeln zur Anlegung von Eiskellern nebst vorausgehender Theorie und Praxis über die Abkühlung der Körper zu wirtschaftlichen und technischen Zwecken. Für herrschaftliche und landwirtschaftliche Haushaltungen, Konditoreien, Schlächter etc.* (Weimar, 1855).

Heinel, C., *Die wirtschaftliche Bedeutung der deutschen Kälte-Industrie im Jahre 1908* (München, 1908).

Heiß, Rudolf, *Die Aufgaben der Kältetechnik in der Bewirtschaftung Deutschlands mit Lebensmitteln*. Schriften des Reichskuratoriums für die Technik in der Landwirtschaft Nr. 77 A: Die Kühlkette, Das Gefrieren von Lebensmitteln (Berlin, 1939).

Hellmann, Ullrich, *Künstliche Kälte: Die Geschichte der Kühlung im Haushalt* (Giessen, 1990).

Hengsbach, Arne, 'Natureiswerke im Umkreis von Berlin'. *Jahrbuch für brandenburgische Landesgeschichte*, vol. 21 (Berlin, 1970).

Heyroth, Anton, *Über den Reinlichkeitszustand des natürlichen und künstlichen Eises*. Arbeiten aus dem kaiserlichen Gesundheitsamt (Berlin, 1888).

Hilck, Erwin/Rudolf Auf dem Hövel, *Jenseits von minus Null: Die Geschichte der deutschen Tiefkühlwirtschaft* (Köln, 1979).

Hitzbleck, H., *Die Bedeutung des Fisches für die Ernährungswirtschaft Mitteleuropas in vorindustrieller Zeit*, Diss. rer.pol. (Göttingen, 1971).

Jones, Joseph C., *America's Icemen*, (Humble, 1982).

Kaufmann, A., 'Der Eishandel in Berlin', *Zeitschrift für die gesamte Kälte-Industrie*, vol. 10 (Berlin, 1977).

Levenstein, Harvey A., *Revolution at the Table: Transformations of the American Diet* (New York-Oxford, 1988).

Linde, Carl von, *Aus meinem Leben und meiner Arbeit. Erinnerungen des Pioniers der Kältetechnik* (1916), Reprint, (Düsseldorf, 1984).

Lippmann, Edmund O. (Freiherr) von, 'Zur Geschichte der Kältemischungen', *Zeitschrift für angewandte Chemie*, vol. 11 (1898), No. 33 pp. 739–45.

Marperger, Johann Jacob, *Vollständiges Küchen und Keller-Dictionarium*, (Hamburg, 1716).

Matschoss, Conrad, *Grosse Ingenieure*, 4th rev.ed. (München, 1954).

Meidinger, Heinrich, 'Eismachen zur Bereitung von Gefrorenem', *Dingler's Polytechnisches Journal*, vol.204, (1872), pp. 409–14.

Meidinger, Heinrich, 'Die Fortschritte in der künstlichen Erzeugung von Kälte und Eis,' *Dingler's Polytechnisches Journal*, vol. 218, (1875), pp. 471–78.

Meidinger, Heinrich, 'Eismaschinen', *Badische Gewerbezeitung*, vol.12, (1868), No. 5, 7, 10, 11.

Meikle, Jeffrey, *Twentieth Century Limited: Industrial Design in America, 1925–1939* (Philadelphia, Pa.1979).

Menzel, Carl August, *Der Bau des Eis-Kellers* (Halle, 1848).

Meyer, Erna, *Der Haushalt* (Stuttgart 1926).

Mosolff, Hans, *Der Aufbau der deutschen Gefrierindustrie* (Hamburg, 1941).

Nöthling, Ernst, *Die Eiskeller, Eishäuser und Eisschränke. Ihre Konstruktion und Benutzung*, 5th rev.ed. (Weimar, 1896).

Plank, Rudolf/E.Ehrenbaum/K.Reuter, *Die Konservierung von Fischen durch Gefrierverfahren* (Berlin, 1915).

Plank, Rudolf, *Haushalts-Kältemaschinen* (Berlin, 1928).

Plank, Rudolf, *Amerikanische Kältetechnik* (Berlin, 1929).

Plank, Rudolf, Vorkühlungsanlagen für Obst. *Zeitschrift für die gesamte Kälteindustrie*, Beiheft 38(1937).

Plank, Rudolf, *Die Frischerhaltung von Lebensmitteln durch Kälte* (München 1940).

Plank, Rudolf (ed.), *Handbuch der Kältetechnik*, 5 vols. (Berlin, Göttingen, Heidelberg, 1954).

Reader, W., *Birdseye: The Early Years* (Walton-on Thames, Surrey, 1963).

Riddervold, Astri/Andreas Ropeid (eds.), *Food Conservation: Ethnological Studies* (London, 1988).

Rohrbach, Wilhelm, 'Die Bedeutung der deutschen Eisindustrie,' *Die Kälteindustrie* vol. 1928, No. 7.

Root, Waverley/Richard de Rochemond, *Eating in America* (New York, 1976).

Rudolph, W., *Nahrung und Rohstoffe aus dem Meer* (Stuttgart, 1946).

Singer, Charles et al. (eds.), *A History of Technology*, 5 vols. (Oxford, 1958).

Stahmer, Max, *Fischindustrie und Fischhandel* (Hamburg, 1913).

Swoboda, Karl, *Die Eisapparate der Neuzeit* (Weimar, 1868).

Swoboda, Karl, *Anlegung und Benutzung der Eiskeller transportabler und stabiler Eiskeller oder Eisschränke, Eisreservoire und amerikanischer Eishäuser* (Weimar, 1874).

Taubeneck, George F., The Development of American Household Refrigation Industry, *II. Internationaler Kältekongress*, s.l. (Netherland) s.a. (1936).

Tellier, Charles, *Histoire d'une invention: le Frigorique* (Paris 1910).

Thévenot, Roger/J.C.Fiedler, *Essai pour une histoire du froid artificiel dans le monde* (Paris, 1978).

'Toselli's Verfahren, um Eis von bedeutender Dicke zu fabricieren', *Dingler's Polytechnisches Journal* vol. 190(1868), p. 126.

Villafranca, Blasius, *Methodus refrigandi ex vocatu salenitro vinum, aquamque de potus quodiis aliud genu, cui accedunt varia naturalia rerum problemato, non minus iucunda lectu, quam necessaria cognitu* (Rome 1550).

Wallance, Don, *Shaping America's Products* (New York, 1956).

Walton, John K., *Fish and Ships and the British Working Class*, 1870–1940 (Leicester, London/New York 1992).

Wiegelmann, Günther,/Annette Maus, 'Fischversorgung und Fischspeisen im 19. und 20. Jahrhundert. Versuch einer quantitativen Analyse', in Hans J. Teuteberg/Günther Wiegelmann. *Unsere tägliche Kost, Geschichte und regionale Prägung*, 2nd ed. (Münster, 1986), pp.75–92.

Wiegelmann, Günther, 'Speiseeis in volkstümlichen Festmahlzeiten', *Deutsche Lebensmittel-Rundschau* vol.60 (1964), pp.201–224. Reprint: Hans J. Teuteberg/Günther Wiegelmann. *Unsere tägliche Kost.* 2nd. ed. (Münster, 1986), pp.217–224.

Wirkner, C.G.von, *Geschichte und Theorie der Kälteerzeugung* (Hamburg, 1897).

Wolrich, William R., *The Men who created Cold: A History of Refrigeration* (New York, 1967).

# 6

# THE DECLINE OF A STAPLE FOOD: BREAD AND THE BAKING INDUSTRY IN BRITAIN, 1890–1990

## John Burnett

### Introduction

Bread was a traditional food of the British people, eaten by all classes, and by the poor as the principal article of diet: its description as 'the staple food' and 'the staff of life' indicates the symbolic importance which was attached to it. Commercial baking of white and brown bread was already established in London by the twelfth century, and although mixtures of grains continued to be used in the countryside into the early nineteenth century, white, wheaten bread had by then become the normal, preferred form of the great majority of people.[1]

The nineteenth-century history of bread and baking has been previously described.[2] This paper outlines the changing place of bread over the last hundred years, during which there has been a marked secular fall in consumption interrupted by two World Wars when food shortages temporarily restored it to a major constituent of the nation's diet. The question is posed whether bread can any longer be considered as a staple of contemporary diet.

### 1890–1914

In economic terminology bread is an 'inferior good' – less of it is purchased by consumers with higher incomes, and this generalisation holds true both over time and at a particular point in time. Total U.K. flour consumption grew after the 1840s, peaking in the early 1880s at around 280 lbs per head per annum[3] under the impact of cheap, mass imports from North America, but then began a gradual fall as living standards for the majority improved. By 1909–13 total flour consumption stood at an estimated 211 lbs per head[4] implying a major decline in what was by now a cheap energy source and a shift towards more expensive foods such as meat, fish and dairy products. In 1880 English bread was made almost equally of home and imported grain, but by 1914 British farms contributed less than a quarter of total needs:

meanwhile, the average price of the quartern loaf (4 lbs) had fallen from 7d. in 1800 to 5.8d. in 1914.[5]

The 'average', however, included wide variations in the consumption levels of different social classes. As income declined the proportion devoted to bread increased and that to more expensive foods fell: in poor families bread became the staple – in some, almost the only – food, eaten at every meal, while in wealthier households it merely accompanied other, more palatable, foods or was used to carry tasty spreads and 'relishes'. For most working-class families in this period food took between 60% and 70% of income: within this total food budget it was estimated in 1881 that wage-earners spent on average 1.4d. on bread (the same amount as on beer) out of a total daily expenditure on food and drink of 9.6d.[6], a fraction of 14.6%. But in his study of the poor in East London in 1886–7, Charles Booth calculated that 22% of *total* income went on bread[7], and the budgets collected by Mrs Pember Reeves in a poor area of South London in 1911–12 showed as much as 36% of the food budget spent on bread: in some of these households there was less than 3d. per person per day for food[8]. The lowest of all regular wage-earners, agricultural labourers, in 1913 spent as much as 40% of their food budget on bread and flour for home baking[9] because of the need to meet their high energy requirements as cheaply as possible. By contrast, for better-off skilled and semi-skilled workers earning £1.5s. – £1.10s. a week in 1904, bread took 19% of the weekly food budget,[10] suggesting that despite its lower price by this time, bread had continued to hold a broadly similar share of working-class food expenditure since the 1880s.

One of the few enquiries into middle-class diet was included in Seebohm Rowntree's study of York in 1900, when he examined budgets from the 'servant-keeping class'. These families spent 15.99d. per person per day on food, providing 4039 calories and 126 grams of protein.[11] Home baking still continued strongly in Yorkshire, and all classes bought flour for this purpose as well as some bakers' bread: when computed into bread, working-class families consumed 6.3 lbs per head per week compared with 4.8 lbs by the servant-keeping class.

Grouping the budget survey data of 1887–1900, Oddy has estimated that in the poorest working-class families with incomes less than 18s.0d. a week, bread consumption averaged 5.5 lbs per head per week: it rose to 7.3 lbs with incomes over £1.10s., before falling back in the servant-keeping class[12]: as people moved out of extreme poverty they first consumed more bread, but having reached the level of satisfaction the effect of further income was to reduce consumption.

In middle- and upper-class households bread was merely an adjunct to a meal, mainly eaten at breakfast in the form of toast or rolls and at afternoon tea in the shape of thinly-cut bread and butter or sandwiches: it was important at the 'nursery tea', where children were encouraged to eat it with jam or honey before proceeding to the more popular cakes, jellies and blancmanges. At the substantial luncheons and dinners of adults, where meat, game and fish predominated, bread scarcely appeared, though it found a place in the form of variously-filled sandwiches at outdoor events such as picnics and shooting-parties. Its role in working-class meal patterns was much more fundamental. Men normally took a packed midday meal to work, in which bread was the main item, enlivened with whatever 'relish' of meat, bacon, cheese or dripping fat was available; they expected a cooked meal on their return in the evening, the assumption being that the chief 'breadwinner' had a right to whatever meat the household could afford. The consequence in many poorer families was that women and children practically existed on bread and tea with scrapings of butter, margarine or jam, occasionally varied by soups, stews or flour-based puddings and pies: the Sunday dinner was often the only occasion for a family meal of meat and vegetables. In poor families with many children bread was the staple food, sometimes even rationed to an 'allowance' of two slices per child per meal. As Mrs Reeves noted of South London children in 1913 –

'Bread . . . is their chief food. It is cheap. They like it; it comes into the house ready-cooked: it is always at hand, and needs no plate and spoon. Spread with a scraping of butter, jam or margarine, according to the length of purse of the mother, they never tire of it as long as they are in their ordinary state of health. It makes the sole article in the menu for two meals in the day'[13]

And in Salford, Lancashire, Robert Roberts recalled that –

A treat consisted of a round of bread lightly sprinkled with sugar – the 'sugar butty'. But such was the craving for sweetness among the most deprived, some children I have known would take leaves from the bottom of their father's pot and spread them over bread to make the 'sweet tea-leaf sandwich'[14]

The baking industry which supplied this large demand was still mainly small-scale and unrevolutionised in 1890, consisting of some 30,000 independent bakers. Around a third of these worked single-handed, but the rest generally employed 2–4 assistants, the Census of 1891 giving totals of 84,200 employed in the baking trade and a further 46,600 engaged as confectioners and pastry-cooks. The small capital outlay on premises and the ability to bake without machinery made it an easy trade to enter, but some of the worst practices of the mid-nineteenth century – widespread adulteration and the use of insanitary cellar bakeries – were by now under public control[15] and the scale of output was beginning to grow from the former average of 10 sacks of flour a week towards 20–25 sacks. The last decade of the century marked a turning-point for the trade in several respects. Bakers were now mainly using roller-milled flour from imported wheat instead of stone-ground as in the past. Roller-milling by steam power, invented in Switzerland in 1834, had been developed in Hungary in the next three decades and particularly in the United States in the 1870s and 1880s: it was then rapidly established in Britain, mainly at ports and on waterways, and between 1880 and 1910 three-quarters of English windmills and watermills were either destroyed or converted[16]. Roller-milling produced fine, white flour by removing the bran and germ which stone-grinding had been unable to do: it was specially suitable for the hard North American wheats which were mixed with a small quantity of 'soft' English wheat. Second, at the end of the century 'scientific baking' was being urged by men like William Jago and John Blandy who were well versed in chemistry and anxious to raise standards of knowledge in the trade: a National School of Baking was opened at the Borough Polytechnic in 1899, endowed by the Association of Master Bakers. Third, technology was beginning to enter the baking trade, stimulated by an International Exhibition of Flour Mill Machinery in London in 1881[17]: by the end of the century, larger bakeries were using flour-sifters, mechanical dough-kneaders which reduced the time of kneading from an hour to 15 minutes, draw-plate ovens and temperature-controlled gas or oil-fired ovens.

At last, the hope expressed as far back as 1815 that 'persons with capital' would gradually be drawn into the trade[18] was beginning to be fulfilled. By 1900 a handful of factory or 'plant' bakeries had been established in London as well as a few large Co-operative Society bakeries. Plant bakeries handling 100 or more sacks of flour a week sold either to grocers or directly to the public in their own retail bread shops and teashops such as J. Lyons and Co. The number of these multiple-shop bread firms grew from 11 in 1900, with 265 branches, to 25 in 1910 with 782 branches[19]: although their share of total bread sales scarcely reached 5%, they were an important presage of future trends.

## World War One

It has often been claimed that as a major food-importing country, Britain was ill-prepared for the conflict of 1914–1918, that serious food shortages and social unrest were allowed to develop until only in January, 1918, a limited scheme of rationing was hesitantly introduced. This is a somewhat harsh criticism. Britain's dependence on food imports, particularly on imported cereals, had long been recognised: British farmers produced only one-fifth of wheat requirements in 1914, yet bread was still the staple of national diet, contributing 31% of calories and 35% of protein. Patriotic pride in the power of the British Navy to safeguard the seaways tended to obscure the vulnerability of the Atlantic passage to German submarine attacks, but as early as 1903 the government had appointed a Royal Commission on the Supply of Food and Raw Materials in Time of War which had begun to consider strategic implications.

The immediate effect of the outbreak of war was to raise food prices sharply in anticipation of shortages: by May, 1915, imported wheat had almost doubled from the previous price of 36s.0d. a quarter to 70s.0d. and the price of bread had increased by more than 40%. In 1916 a Royal Commission was established to take responsibility for purchasing and holding wheat stocks, the first significant intervention into the free market. As losses of shipping increased and food supplies worsened, the Food Controller, Lord Devonport, introduced a plan for 'voluntary' rationing in February, 1917, in which consumers were urged to limit their bread consumption to 4 lbs per head per week, a proposal strongly criticised by nutritionists in The Royal Society, who pointed out that some men engaged in heavy work were eating between 10 and 14 lbs a week and needed as much to maintain their output. In place of the failure of self-denial, the government gradually raised the extraction rate of wheat from the pre-war level of 70–72% to 76% in November, 1916, 81% in March, 1917, and ultimately, to 92% in the spring of 1918: additionally, admixtures of up to 30% of maize, barley, oats, beans and potatoes were required.

The 'War Bread' which bakers had to produce from 1917 onwards, though strongly defended by most nutritionists for its higher proportion of bran and germ, was generally very unpopular with the public. Dark in colour, it had an unfamiliar flavour, was difficult to bake and tended to produce a moist, soggy and unpalatable crumb. Meanwhile, government control over the milling and baking industries was greatly increased. In 1917 government took over financial control of the mills, fixed flour prices and guaranteed millers a standard profit based on pre-war margins: in the face of serious industrial unrest over rising prices, bread was subsidised to reduce the average price of the 4 lb loaf from 1s. 0d. to 9d. and bakers' profit margins were also fixed at a level which proved generous to the large 'plant' bakers. Not until September, 1920, were the bread subsidy and price controls abolished, and only in 1921 were millers allowed to sell flour of varying qualities at competitive prices[20].

When rationing cautiously began in January, 1918, first of sugar and, later in the year of meat, bacon, butter, margarine, jam and tea, bread was deliberately left unrationed in order that individual energy needs could always be met. Despite its unpopularity after 1917, bread and flour consumption increased as other foods became scarcer, the average intake rising from 4.28 lbs per head per week in 1910–14 to 4.69 lbs in 1917 and 4.80 lbs in 1918[21]. Due largely to the continued availability of bread, the civilian population suffered only a negligible reduction in the calorific value of its diet, even in 1918 probably no more than 2½%. The advances in real wages meant that some people were actually able to eat better than in pre-war days. At the end of the war bread and flour took an average of 14.4% of family expenditure on food, excluding drink and tobacco[22].

A more optimistic view of British food control than that presented by Sir William Beveridge in 1928 has recently been argued by Dr Margaret Barnett[23]. She states that as early as January, 1915, five ad hoc committees had been appointed which successfully built up stocks of grain and sugar. The strong prejudice against compulsory rationing, which was having bad effects in Germany, could only gradually be overcome, while the price controls and bread subsidy in the latter half of the war worked well. Finally, after a slow start, British agricultural output was greatly expanded – in the case of wheat by 59% over 1914. Britain survived a dangerous period without serious threat of social revolution and with generally improved standards of civilian health[24].

## The Inter-War Years

These years present a paradox – on one hand rising standards of consumption for the majority, on the other, images of dole queues, Hunger Marches and derelict industrial areas where two-thirds or more of men were unemployed. Nationally, at the worst point of the depression in 1932/3, 22% of the insured population were out of work, but on the credit side, these were years of cheap food imports and, for those in work, a rise in real wages of c.30% between 1920 and 1939. In these circumstances average consumption of flour and bread fell from the wartime peak of 250 lbs per head per year in 1918 to 196 lbs in 1938, or, in terms of weekly consumption, from 4.80 lbs to 3.77 lbs[25]. Consumers who now had more choice in their food budgets increased their consumption of meat, fruit, vegetables, sugar, butter, cheese and eggs, demanding more variety and palatability than in the pre-war diet, coupled with the fact that the growth in sedentary occupations reduced the energy needs of the workforce.

Between the Wars bread and flour took rather less than 9% of national food expenditure (compared with 32% spent on meat and fish) at a weekly cost of 8.1d. per person[26]. In their study of the nation's diet in 1936 Crawford and Broadley found that the wealthiest class in the population (AA) consumed 48 ozs of bread per person a week while the poorest (D) ate 62.4 ozs, though the latter had to devote 12.4% of their weekly food bill to this item compared with only 3.4% by the wealthiest class:[27] this was despite the fact that the wealthiest class ate considerably more of the costlier proprietary brown breads such as Hovis which were strongly recommended by many nutritionists, purchasing 10.1 ozs per head per week compared with only 2.1 ozs in Class D.[28] This was an interesting inversion of the nineteenth-century pattern, when white bread carried the social *cachet* and brown bread was associated with poverty. The working-class consumer now almost always bought the cheaper, standard white loaf, and home baking of bread continued to decline except in a few strongholds like Yorkshire, the North-East and Wales, the quantity of flour sold for home baking falling from 85 lbs per head per year in 1920–24 to 59 lbs in 1935–8.

Bread was still the staple diet of the poorer social strata, especially of the unemployed existing on low levels of public relief which often involved a reduction of up to 50% on normal wages. Here, bread, tea, margarine and cheap jam were the mainstays of family diet, with whatever meat, fish or other savouries mainly reserved for the man. In his second social survey of York conducted in 1936, Rowntree described the diet of an unemployed man with a wife and 4 children living on unemployment benefit of 36s.0d. a week: they bought 21 lbs of flour a week, equivalent to c.28 lbs of bread, or nearly 5 lbs per head: bread was the principal item at breakfast and tea, usually spread with dripping or jam. By contrast, a skilled plasterer earning 72s.0d. a week with a wife and three children bought only 10 lbs of white bread but also 2 ½ lbs of brown bread and 2 lbs of malt fruit bread.[29] One unemployed man wrote –

'Bread, bread, bread! I hate the very word! The sight of bread makes me feel sick . . . If you want to vary it, you change from marg[arine] to lard, and when you're tired of that you go back to jam, if there's any left . . .'[30]

The baking industry itself began to undergo a major transformation in this period towards larger-scale firms employing more advanced technology and distributing bread over wide areas made possible by motor transport. In the large plant bakeries automated processes now controlled production from mechanical mixing and weighing to baking in travelling ovens to wrapping and even slicing the finished product: plants capable of baking up to 70,000 loaves a day were in use by the 1930s. Technical progress was much slower among the small master bakers, who typically employed a couple of assistants and baked around 750 loaves a day.

With a declining demand for bread and the increased capacity of plant bakeries strong price competition developed which amounted to something approaching a 'price war' in the early 1930s, with undercutting and the use of low-quality flours by some of the trade. The 4lb loaf which had sold for 9d. at the end of the War reached 12d. during the inflation of 1920 but subsequently fell back to 8½–9½d, in the 1920s and to as little as 7½d. in 1934;[31] some multiple grocers sold at even lower prices as 'loss leaders' to attract custom. Price competition continued despite the establishment of the Food Council which was set up by a Royal Commission on Food Prices in 1924: its duty was to recommend and publicise prices for bread, but it lacked compulsory powers and was largely ignored by plant bakers and non-baking retailers.[32]

In 1938 there were still 24,000 bakers and confectioners in the country, but the trade was increasingly concentrated in the larger units: plant bakers accounted for 24–26% of consumers' expenditure on bread, co-operative societies, which also included many plant bakeries, for 19–21%, while master bakers now produced only 53–57% of the bread bought.[33] Particularly significant for future developments was the establishment in 1935 of Allied Bakeries Limited by a Canadian, Garfield Weston, the first firm with a national distribution of bread. By buying up existing bakeries with their established shops and van networks, Allied Bakeries claimed by 1938 to have 17 modern factories, 86 shops and 494 delivery routes.[34] This development paralleled even greater concentration in the milling industry, where by 1939 the 'Big Three' millers controlled c.66% of flour production – the largest, Joseph Rank Limited 24–30%, Spillers Limited 17–20% and the Co-operative Wholesale Society 17%: this was achieved by the merger of small country mills, trustification and the rationalisation of production at vast new port premises.

## World War Two and Post-War Control, 1939–1956

In 1939 British agriculture supplied only 12% of wheat requirements, but the vulnerability of this dependence on imports had led to the appointment of a Food (Defence Plans) Department in 1936 and a Cereals Control Board in

February, 1939, which began to build up stocks in anticipation of the outbreak of War in September. With the rationing of many other foods, the pre-war decline in bread consumption was to be reversed: it was again regarded as the nation's principal source of energy, and remained unrationed and price-controlled throughout the War years. By 1940 average consumption stood at 3.8lbs per head per week, c.10% up on pre-war levels, and total calories in the diet remained at or above the standard of 3,000 a day.

The main problem of wheat supplies was shipping space in competition with military needs and the losses from U-Boat attacks. Partly to save shipping space and partly on the advice of nutritionists in the Ministry of Food, the extraction rate of flour was raised from 70–73% to 85% in March, 1942, and the darker-coloured National Wheatmeal Flour became compulsory; during the next year admixtures of barley, oats and rye were also required. From 1941 the price of bread was fixed at 2d. a pound and bakers were granted a subsidy of 4s.0d. a sack (280 lbs) of flour, an allowance which favoured the large efficient plant producers to the detriment of small master bakers. The result was further to concentrate production in large firms which could take advantage of economies of scale and automated processes, and to reduce the number of small independent firms: the total number of bakers in the U.K. claiming subsidy therefore dwindled from 20,600 in 1942 to 18,200 in 1945 and, more dramatically, to 12,500 in 1955.[35] The growth of plant baking was particularly rapid in the decade after 1945 when prices were still controlled and plant bakers were able to corner a larger share of the market by supplying bread shops and grocery chains.

Any hopes of a rapid return to a free market at the end of the war were dispelled by the poor world harvests of 1945 and the urgent need to relieve hunger in formerly occupied countries. In May, 1946, the Labour government raised the extraction rate to 90% and in July took the highly unpopular step of rationing bread for the first time on a coupon basis exchangeable at any retailer. It was a virtually inoperable scheme which many bakers ignored while some Ministry of Food offices found themselves deluged with sackfuls of uncounted coupons. It had a very modest effect in reducing consumption in the first six months (probably because of previous hoarding), but in retrospect it seems that bread rationing was largely a political bluff to persuade the United States of Britain's serious food shortage (potatoes were also briefly rationed at the end of 1947) and her continuing need for large supplies. Bread rationing formally ended in 1948: with improved supplies and strong pressure in the Conservative government for decontrol, the baking of white bread was permitted in 1953 provided it was fortified with vitamin B1, nicotinic acid, calcium and iron, and three years later freedom was restored to millers and bakers with the ending of the subsidy and the National Loaf.

By the time of decontrol, 4 out of every 10 loaves sold in England and Wales were baked by large plant bakeries. Garfield Weston's bakery empire, Allied Bakeries, expanded rapidly after the War, buying up country bakeries and the London chain of ABC teashops. After disagreements over price with the two largest millers, Ranks and Spillers, Weston began to import his own flour direct from Canada, so integrating his business backwards: in order to protect their markets, Ranks and Spillers retaliated by integrating forwards into baking, acquiring existing firms and respectively establishing British Bakeries Limited and United Bakeries Limited. The Co-operative Wholesale Society was already an integrated milling/baking business, so that by 1956 both branches of the industry were becoming highly rationalised and concentrated.

## 1956–1991

The Annual Reports of the National Food Survey chart the steep decline in the home consumption of bread since 1950

*Table 1:*  Domestic Consumption of Bread, 1950–1991

|  | Consumption (ozs per person/week) | | | | Expenditure (p. per person/week) |
|---|---|---|---|---|---|
|  | 1950 | 1960 | 1985 | 1991 | 1991 |
| White Bread | 50.91 | 36.63 | 19.37 | 13.71 | 27.27 |
| Wholemeal and Brown | 2.55 | 3.335 | 7.33 | 7.31 | 18.42 |
| Other Bread (inc. rolls) | 4.29 | 5.49 | 4.29 | 5.51 | 22.94 [36] |

**Source:**  Domestic Food Consumption and Expenditure: Annual reports of the National Food Survey Committee for 1950, 1960, 1985, 1991 (HMSO)

Total bread consumption, at 26.53 ounces per person per week, is now equivalent to less than one large loaf (1 ¼ lbs) and less than half that of 1950. The fall in the standard white loaf has been especially dramatic, only partially compensated by a trebling in the consumption of brown breads which have grown, particularly in the last decade when their higher fibre content has been promoted for health reasons. There are still considerable variations in bread consumption between different socio-economic classes, age groups and regions. Consumption is lowest in the wealthiest A1 class (household income more than £730/week) at 19.53 ounces per person, rising steadily to 28.77 ounces in Class D (income less than £140/week). The highest consumption is among Old Age Pensioners at 30.5 ounces per person per week[37], probably reflecting the relative poverty of some in this group and the fact of more meals being consumed at home. Bread consumption also increases steadily with increasing age up to the 65–74 age group, at which point it is a third higher than for those aged under 25. The consumption of brown and wholemeal breads, which are more expensive than the standard white loaf, has an unusual pattern, being highest in pensioner households and next highest in the wealthiest A1 class: whether health-consciousness or taste preferences determine this pattern is not possible to say.

Any explanation of the overall decline in bread consumption must take account of changes in meal patterns in Britain since the end of rationing. In the

1950s meal occasions were still traditional – a cooked breakfast plus bread or toast, a midday meal, which often consisted of sandwiches for those unable to return home, and an evening meal or 'high tea' in which bread and 'spreads' also played a significant part[38]. Today, British people eat less food in total, particularly of energy-supplying sources, and have fewer formal mealtimes; the principal cooked family meal has become the evening meal, in which bread often has a minor rôle. Several trends have militated against consumption – the generally lighter meals, the increased employment of married women away from home, the growing use of breakfast cereals, pasta and rice dishes as alternatives to bread and the popularity of 'eating out' in restaurants where bread is not an important constituent. For many people the standard white loaf, sliced and wrapped, which now accounts for over 50% of all bread sales, is convenient but unexciting and lacking in flavour: in a period of generally rising standards of living, it has a boring image which commands little affection despite the use by major bakery companies of emotionally-charged brand names such as 'Wonderloaf', 'Sunblest' and 'Mother's Pride'.

Concentration of the baking industry proceeded rapidly after the ending of control in 1956. The number of small master bakers has now declined to c.4,000 from 10,000 in 1964: on the other hand, two giant milling/baking combines, Rank Hovis McDougall and Associated British Foods (formerly Allied Bakeries) now dominate the market, having absorbed the baking activities of Spillers and the Co-operative Wholesale Society. By 1985 ABF held 30% of the British bread market, RHM 23%, master bakers 31% and independent plant bakers 7%: the remainder is composed mainly of 'in-store' bakeries in supermarkets and 'hot bread-shops', developments since the 1970s which are having some success by the attraction of freshness. Master bakers survive by offering speciality breads at premium prices and by sidelines in cakes and confectionery, but cannot compete in price with the large plant combines which can subsidise their baking activity from their milling profits and offer large discounts on bread to supermarket chains where it is sometimes sold as a 'loss leader'. From the 1960s onwards the larger plant bakeries had fully automated processes and the advantages of economies of scale and nationwide distribution networks. The most important technical development was the Chorleywood Bread Process, invented in 1961 at the Baking Industries Research Centre, which by very high-speed mixing of the dough reduced fermentation time from 3 hours to 3–4 minutes and allowed other economies in the use of flour: by 1980 75% of bread was made by this process.

Whether bread can any longer be regarded as a major staple of the British diet must be open to question. It now takes an average of only 1/18th of food expenditure and provides 10% of energy needs, the same amount as milk or vegetables and considerably less than meat or fats[39]. However, its importance rises considerably in low-income and pensioner households, where consumption is half as much again as in the wealthiest social class. As in the past, bread remains the cheapest and most convenient way of satisfying hunger, and a recent study of the diets of the unemployed showed that when money was short spending went largely on bread, sandwiches, chips and beans while that on meat, fresh fruit and vegetables was cut[40]. The current recession may well have slowed the decline in bread consumption: ironically, it would seem that with economic recovery bread would resume its long-term decline as a casualty of affluence.

**Notes:**
1  Ashley (1928), pp. 1–8
2  (a) Burnett (1963), pp. 98–108.
    (b) Burnett (1966), pp. 61–76.
3  Reekie (1978), p. 22.
4  Orr (1936), Table II, p. 18
5  Kirkland (1917)
6  British Association for the Advancement of Science. Report of the 51st Meeting (1881), p. 276 et seq.
7  Booth (1969), p. 138
8  Reeves (1979), pp. 133–143
9  Rowntree & Kendall (1913), Ch. 3
10  Board of Trade. Memoranda, Statistical Tables and Charts Second Series (1905), p. 5
11  Rowntree (1902), Table p. 253.
12  Oddy (1970), p. 314.
13  Reeves (1979) p. 97.
14  Roberts (1971), pp. 85–6.
15  Burnett (a) (1963)
16  Horder, Dodd & Moran (1954), p. 10.
17  Maunder (1969), p. 12.
18  Report from the Committee of the House of Commons on Laws relating to the Manufacture, Sale and Assize of Bread (1814–15), V, I
19  Jefferys (1954), p. 214.
20  Sheppard & Newton (1957), p. 170.
21  Fogarty (1948), p. 77.
22  Report of the Summer Committee on the Working Classes' Cost of Living (1918).
23  Barnett (1985).
24  Winter (1977), pp. 487–507
25  Fogarty, (1948), p. 77.
26  Orr, (1936), p. 14–15.
27  Crawford & Broadley (1938), pp. 165–6.
28  Crawford & Broadley (1938), p. 168
29  Rowntree (1941), pp. 188–191
30  Greene ed (1935), p. 69.
31  Sheppard and Newton (1957), Appendix A, p. 169.

32  Reekie (1978), pp. 34–5.
33  Jefferys (1954), p. 166.
34  Evely and Little (1960), p. 257.
35  Reekie, op.cit. pp. 36–7.
36  Wholemeal Bread is defined as containing 100% of the wheat: 'brown breads' contain 80–90% of the wheat and include 'patent' breads, eg Hovis, Vitbe, Allinsons
37  Domestic Food Consumption and Expenditure. Annual Report of the National Food Survey Committee for 1991 (1992), Table B6, p. 79
38  Warren (1958).
39  Domestic Food Consumption and Expenditure. Annual Report of the National Food Survey Committee for 1991 (1992), Table B14, p. 90.
40  Lang, Andrews, Bedale and Hannon (1984).

## Acknowledgement

This paper has drawn at several points on the work of Dr Sandra Hunt, who as a Research Fellow at Brunel University from 1978–83 undertook a major study of bread and the baking industry in the 20th century, sponsored by the Rank Prize Funds. I gratefully acknowledge her permission to use some of this unpublished material.

## Literature

Ashley, Sir William, *The Bread of Our Forefathers* (Oxford, 1928).

Barnett, Louise Margaret, *British Food Policy during the First World War* (London, 1985).

Board of Trade, Second Series of Memoranda, Statistical Tables and Charts . . . with Reference to British and Foreign Trade and Industrial Conditions. Cd. 2337 (London, 1905).

Booth, Charles. *Life and Labour of the People in London. First Series, Poverty* I (Reprint, New York, 1969).

British Association for the Advancement of Science. Report of the Committee . . . on The Present Appropriation of Wages (51st Meeting 1881).

Burnett, John (a) 'The Baking Industry in the Nineteenth Century'. *Business History*, Vol. V, No. 2, June, 1963 (Liverpool 1963) pp. 98–108.

Burnett, John (b) 'Trends in Bread Consumption', in Theodore Cardwell Barker, John Crawford McKenzie and John Yudkin (eds) *Our Changing Fare, Two Hundred Years of British Food Habits* (London, 1966), pp. 61–76.

Committee of the House of Commons. Report on Laws relating to the Manufacture, Sale and Assize of Bread. PP. 186 (1814–15).

Crawford, Sir William, and Herbert Broadley. *The People's Food* (London, 1938).

Domestic Food Consumption and Expenditure. Annual Reports of the National Food Survey Committee for 1950 (1952) and 1960 (1962):

Household Food Consumption and Expenditure Annual Reports of the National Food Survey Committee for 1985 (1987) and 1991 (1992) (London).

Evely, Richard and Ian Malcolm David Little, *Concentration in British Industry* (Cambridge 1960).

Fogarty, Michael Patrick (ed), *Further Studies in Industrial Organization* (London, 1948), citing Sir William Beveridge, *British Food Control. Economic and Social History of the World War* (London 1928).

Greene, Felix (ed) *Time to Spare. What Unemployment Means by Eleven Unemployed* (London, 1935).

Horder, Thomas Jeeves (Lord), Sir Charles Dodd and Thomas Moran. *Bread, The Chemistry and Nutrition of Flour and Bread, with an Introduction to their History and Technology* (London, 1954).

Jefferys, James Bavington, *Retail Trading in Britain, 1850–1950* (Cambridge, 1954).

Kirkland, John, *Three Centuries of Prices of Wheat, Flour and Bread* (London, 1917).

Lang, Tim, Hazel Andrews, Caroline Bedale and Ed Hannon. *Jam Tomorrow. Report of a Pilot Study of the Food Circumstances, Attitudes and Consumption of 1,000 People on Low Incomes in the North of England* (Manchester, 1984).

Maunder, Peter John, *The Bread Industry in the U.K. A Study in Market Structure, Conduct and Performance Analysis* (Nottingham, 1969).

Oddy, Derek John, 'Working Class Diets in late Nineteenth Century Britain'. *Economic History Review*, 2nd Series, 23, (1970) pp. 314–323.

Orr, John Boyd, *Food, Health and Income. A Survey of Adequacy of Diet in Relation to Income* (London, 1936).

Reekie, William Duncan, *Give Us This Day. An Economic Critique of Political Intervention* (London, 1978).

Reeves, Maud Pember, *Round About A Pound A Week* (London, 1913, 1979).

Roberts, Robert, *The Classic Slum. Salford Life in the First Quarter of the Century* (Manchester, 1971).

Rowntree, Benjamin Seebohm, *Poverty, A Study of Town Life* (4th edn, London, 1902).

Rowntree, Benjamin Seebohm, *Poverty and Progress. A Second Social Survey of York* (London, 1941).

Rowntree, Benjamin Seebohm and May Kendall, *How the Labourer Lives. A Study of the Rural Labour Problem* (London, 1913).

Sheppard, Ronald and Edward Newton, *The Story of Bread* (London, 1957).

Sumner Committee, Report on the Working Classes' Cost of Living Cd.8980 (London, 1918).

Warren, Geoffrey, *The Foods We Eat A Survey of Meals, their Content and Chronology* (London, 1958).

Winter, Jay Murray, 'The Impact of the First World War on Civilian Health in Britain', *Economic History Review*, Second Series, 30. (1977), pp 487–507.

# 7

# CONCENTRATION PROCESSES IN THE DRESDEN BAKING TRADE, 1949–1989

*Rudolf Weinhold*

In the former centrally planned economies of middle and eastern Europe, the food industry was mainly concentrated in a number of large-scale state owned enterprises. The purpose of this study is to give an analysis of the concentration processes in the baking trade of the former German Democratic Republic, taking the city of Dresden as an example. There are, however, some methodological problems. There is a deficiency on this subject, especially in the *Statistisches Jahrbuch der DDR* which was issued on a regular basis from 1955 until 1990[1]. Unfortunately, documents with information on steps and consequences of these concentration processes have been lost or are not yet available for research. It was therefore necessary to make use of key informants.[2] This approach has, however, some limitations.

The 35 volumes of the *Statistisches Jahrbuch* list the data that are interesting for the topic addressed, within different subject groups. This coordination changed in part during a third of a century, so that very time-consuming research and retrospective comparisons were needed to get hold of a rather concrete picture of the conditions in question. It is very difficult – almost impossible – to differ between the contributions of the industry and the craft[3] (including the so-called production cooperatives of the craft) of the production of bread and biscuits, as well as the making of pasta products during a particular span.

This can be explained by the procedure applied by the statistics.

In the yearbook of 1955 for example, only the gross production of all businesses is revealed altogether for the span of 1936 until 1954,[4] whereby the foodstuffs and luxury foods produced by them, like flour and processed foodstuffs of all kinds are joined for example by meat, sausages, different kinds of fats and oil, dairy products, fish and fish foods, sugar malt and beer.[5] Not before the year 1955 did a division of the production according to forms of businesses take place,[6] which at that time still revealed the output of the (mainly craftsman's pride) private businesses in terms of figures:2127 with altogether 59,800 employees. This group was opposed by 945 publicly owned businesses (i.e. between 1945/6 and 1955 production plants withdrawn from their owners) with 132, 100 and 294 Cooperative Societies of Handicraft (hereafter:PGH) with 32,500 employees. In view of the number of businesses the proportion turns out at 63% (private), 8,7% (PGH) and 28,3% (publicly owned businesses). A look at the number of employees changes the proportion slightly; publicly owned businesses (58,9%) dominate, lying above the private businesses (26,6%) and the co-operatives (14,5%). This represents the condition of the entire food industry. But it is necessary to gain more concrete insights for the following years on the basis of these statistical figures, as long as they refer to the industrial and craftmen's baking production. Thereby the entire former GDR inevitably forms the regional frame. For a better understanding of these processes it is necessary to have a look at the population development of this already historic territory. It shall be supplemented by excerpts from the craft's statistics of the same span. Both developments do not really have an immediate connection, but cannot be considered in isolation either, because they ultimately result from political-ideological conditions and from governmental measures these conditions direct. On the later territory of the GDR 16,745,000 million people lived in 1939.[7] After the end of the Second World War this number rose to 19,044,000 (1948).

This growth can primarily be attributed to the rush of refugees from the former German Eastern areas as well as Poland, Czechoslovakia, Hungary, Yugoslavia and Rumania. Since 1949 a continuous decrease of the population figures can be observed, which was caused mainly by the increasing stabilization of the economic and social conditions in the Federal Republic of Germany (FRG), founded in 1949, which from the very beginning could not be equated with the same attractiveness by the German Democratic Republic (GDR), which had been founded simultaneously on the territory of the Soviet-occupied Zone. The consequences of this incongruity was a constant exodus of people from the East to the West. Already in 1949 the figures fell under the 19-million-limit (18,739,000). In 1955 it fell short of the 18-million-limit (17,832,000). Surely, the consequences of the violently suppressed insurrection on 17 June 1953 played a decisive role. The population figure held the 17-million-level until 1972 (17,011,000). A decisive factor for this temporary slowdown of the exodus was the erection of the Berlin Wall on 13 August 1961 and the resulting draconic 'border protection measures', which made unknown number of people, who despite all this dared to flee, lose their freedom, their health or even their lives. In 1973 the population figure fell short of the 17-million-limit (16,351,000).[8] Since then the number of inhabitants fell continually to 16,661,000 until 1987. In 1988 a slight increase to 16,675,000 was noticed, but since 1989[9] the East-West migration increased again.[10] Until today one has to reckon with a new exodus of more than a million people.

These processes logically signal the decrease of the consumer figure for the products of the baking trade. Up to a particular degree they are also reflected by the decrease of the total number of craftman's businesses between 1950 and 1989. During this span the figure decreased from 303,821 to 82,672, (5,426 of which belonged to the occupational group of bakers, confectioners and producers of cakes that keep), i.e. by about 73%.[11]

A precise interpretation of this process requires an analysis of simultaneous processes in the craft of the FRG. It can be established in general, that contrary to the West the prime mover for the decrease of the craft in the GDR was not the competition of the large and medium-sized enterprises, but the political-ideologically motivated intention to choke the small production as a 'basic union of capitalism'. Reformative efforts did not alter this principle during the eighties, either, probably taking place under the impression of the political processes in Poland.

Despite such efforts the single example of the Dresden baking trade can confirm this trend: of about 520 businesses in the baking trade in 1945 only 120 survived until 1989.

The question about the development of the second, co-operatively organized producer group of the trade remains. As far as the particulars of the baking trade are concerned, the official statistics let us down almost completely. Only the total number of PGH for the production of luxury foods and other foodstuffs are listed. In the GDR in 1953 and 1954 only one and two associations, respectively, are registered. In 1960 131 were counted, in 1964 146.[12] The Dresden district registered 4 PGH in the latter year having a share of the total production of the branch of trade of 6.6%.[13]

The peak of the PGH development in the area of food production was probably reached during the sixties. The data for this category – now called 'other producing craft' (with the exception of food processing)[14] – signal at least since 1972 an obvious decrease in terms of figures (69 PGH) and a stagnation (between 73 and 77) until 1988.[15] In the GDR in that year still 7003 private businesses of the category 'other producing craft' were counted. It seems that at least within this area the socialist co-operative experiment was only little successful. The governmental compulsory measures of 1972 with the aim of liquidating all remaining private medium-sized enterprises might have had a bearing, because even for the existence of numerous PGHs they evoked negative consequences.

A relatively concrete survey about the topic 'baking industry', which was very anxious to be objective, can be found in the first and only *Statistisches Jahrbuch 1990* to be published after the political turning point in the GDR.[16] This survey – with the level of 1989 – refers to the number of businesses, workers and employees in the mills, foodstuff and baker's ware industry. In the whole country at that time 63 enterprises of this kind existed. The share of the entire large-scale enterprises of the food industry (579) was about 11%. They employed (apprentices excluded) 39,504 workers and employees, and the value of their production was estimated at DM3144 million. Compared to this the 5426 craftman's bakeries and confectioneries with their 27,061 employees produced – again the apprentices in the factories are excluded – products worth DM1104,2 million.

The ad valorem output of the industrial sector can be explained by the fact that the statistics add the products of the mill to it. On the other hand the fact that the production of bread and similarly small products (breadrolls, etc.) was concentrated in the hands of the baking industry, probably plays a role, too. They represent, as the statistics of 1988 show,[17] the output of the product range: in this year 803,110 tons of rye bread and small baker's ware. On the other hand 382,600 tons of fine and confectionery ware were produced as well as 512,600 tons of wheat bread and small baker's ware. This amounts to a proportion of 77,5% and 22,5% between bread and other ware.

Unfortunately for the time being we lack figures for a comparison of the craftman's businesses, which are needed to allow for well-substantiated conclusions. As far as quantity is concerned we can conclude that the trade's share of bread supply in the western industrial countries was very much higher (80%) at the end of the eighties than the present level in the GDR (50%). Presumably the figures have not changed since then.

The two large-scale enterprises in the Dresden district were privatized and closed down. The 'Konsum-Backwarenkombinat' had the firm name 'Sächsische Backwaren GmbH' from the turning point of 1989 and stopped work completely at the end of 1992, but the Dresden business part of the former publicly owned Backwarenkombinat, which was changed into the 'Dresdner Brot und Konditoreiwaren GmbH und Co' still covers about half of the bread production in the capital of the Free State of Saxony. The entire market of baker's ware is shared by the craft and the GmbH at the rate of 50 to 50.

In respect of quality – the author has to rely on own observations and practical experiences in the Dresden area – there were locally and temporarily considerable differences between the baker's bread and its industrially produced twin. Quite a few craftman's enterprises were hardly or not at all able to satisfy the demand of the population for their tasty and fresh product.

A certain differentiation between town and countryside developed in terms of bread supply – again we are referring to Dresden and its surrounding areas. Although the baker's trade of the town had to put up with considerable losses in terms of the number of businesses after 1945, it nevertheless contributed immensely to the supply of the population.[18] The situation in the surrounding areas after the end of the Second World War turned out more unfavourably. Many villages sooner or later had to dispense completely with formerly existing bakeries: the training of the junior staff necessary for maintenance was heavily limited by government regulations affecting the trade in a very negative way until into the eighties. Further similarly working disadvantages of this kind affected the subsidies of private small businesses in the towns and in the countryside. Contrary to the subsidised large-scale baking industry, which dominated increasingly over the government trade in the field of village supply, they were almost unable to pursue the necessary measures for a modernization of their production. Today this lack still has a negative effect on efforts to catch up gradually with the technology of West German craftmen's businesses.

Before 1990 the price of the baker's ware was also governmentally subsidized, primarily bread and biscuits. Thereby this area showed an incongruity between East and West which was often and gladly exploited by the official GDR authorities for propagandist reasons. While in the GDR prices were kept constant in this way (2 pounds of ryebread cost SDM 0,52)[19], prices for the same products rose in the FRG between 1985 and 1989 from DM3,04 to DM3,26. Consequently the per capita consumption of products made of bread-grain flour was much higher in the East than in the West.[20]

Negative consequences of these low bread prices in the GDR and the underestimation incident to it was its mass consumption as fodder. Especially owners of small animals exploited this cheap source. Their products, like meat and eggs, were bought by the government's registration offices at high prices, only to be distributed in the trade at much cheaper, and again subsidized prices. Thereby possible gaps in the supply of agricultural products were avoided. It can easily be seen that the large-scale enterprises of the baking industry finally benefited from this proces. In the former district of Dresden there were two such institutions: the publicly owned Backwarenkombinat and the Konsum-Backwarenkombinat. The former business with its centre in Dresden comprises branches in the towns of Pirna, Heidenau, Meissen, Riesa, Grossenhain, Bischofswerda and Görlitz.

They were gradually created in the fifties by means of the takeover or expropriation of private businesses with different levels of technical equipment and size[21] – from primitive 'cellar bakeries' to factories which at that time were in all ways modern (in Dresden for example the bread factory Wilhelm, the large bakery of the Bienert-Mill situated in the Plauenscher Grund, the businesses of Kuchen-Kramer and Kuchen-Jung). The consumer collective combines meanwhile developed from the association of businesses which belonged to consumer co-operatives for some time or that had been started after 1945 (like Bautzen and Riesa).

These large-scale enterprises dominated the baking trade increasingly. This did not remain without consequences for the range of the supply, but also for the quality of the products. These consequences have to be examined in particular. Only a few details will be sketched concerning this question, and attention shall be paid primarily to the state and differentiation of the choice of raw material and also to the processing techniques of the baking trade.

What should be stressed in the first place is the 'ton ideology' of the socialist industrial leaders (the work done in the food industry was accounted for according to weight), which caused an increasing reduction of the product range. In other words: the sorts of bread and biscuits were restricted decisively. Despite the first considerable imports of Hungarian and Canadian wheat, which were primarily for the benefit of Christmas bakery, types of flour made of home grain still dominated production. The main supplier for the Dresden baking trade was the Lommatzscher Pflege west of Meissen, which of old had been famous for its fertile soil. During the last years before the political turning point imports were completely given up and flour was processed exclusively of home grain, which was partly mixed with stabilizers or enriched in some other way. For rye bread the flour types 997 and 1150 were used, for wheat bread the types 630 and 812, for confectionery type 405.

The mills supplied the consumer with certificated products, and an exchange was prohibited on principle. The baking characteristics of the flour were checked in the factories with a sensor or 'ball test' or the washing-out of the gluten. Both collective combines had installed laboratories for this purpose.

The preparation of the dough was done in the smaller enterprises by using the leaven in so-called continuous processes. In the collective combines this was done by kneading machines which shaped dough cords. These production plants were imported from Hungary and Czechoslovakia. Corresponding installations for the processing and shaping of breadrolls were constructed in the GDR itself. The production plants brought into action were very large, but still could only produce one kind of pastry. Unlike Western equipment with the same function they were only capable of processing firm dough. The result was a thick product, aging within several hours and because of their viscosity jeered at popularly as 'rubber rolls'.

The leaven was used for the fermentation of the dough, and yeast was used for rolls and other white pastries. Furthermore special baking aids were used, like bio malt (powder or syrup) in the craft and industry. The bakeries would also add margarine and sugar to white pastry dough to improve its smoothness. In craft and industry the ready dough for breadrolls was prepared by portioning and kneading machines which shaped and portioned the products.

The types of ovens usually vary. In the bakeries one traditionally, and still, used a stone-built so-called peel oven, but ovens were also built according to a skeleton steel construction. They contained pipes which were filled up to a third with water and provided continuous transport of heat, the hot plates having a size of between 25 and 80 square metres.

All installations were heated with coal, gas or electric power.

The ovens used in the collective combines used infra-red rays to produce cookies. So-called oil fired ovens were put into operation at the Dresden Brot- und Konditoreiwaren GmbH after the political turning point. This company arranged its work in a three shift system. The technical equipment of the local bakeries, which compared to West German standards was frequently insufficient, proved to be problematic as far as the present production was concerned. Furthermore the owners were worried about the intentions of institution's superiors to transfer the West German interdiction of work before 4 o'clock in the morning to the territory of the former

GDR, because the bakeries in that area lacked techniques and processes that would allow such a late start of work. The management of the Federal Guild Association has protested against the acceptance of the relevant regulations and has asked for a time-limit of five years. This span is needed to give the businesses of the craft association of bakers and confectioners in the guild time to purchase the technical equipment necessary for such a change.

Before 1989 the government restrictions on the import of subtropical fruits and concentrates also had a diminishing effect on the quality of their products. During the fourth quarter of each year the Dresden bakery enterprises – industry as well as craft – suffered from this shortage, because they lacked candied lemon and orange peel, two ingredients which are absolutely necessary for the famous *Dresden Christstollen* (Christmas loaf) speciality.

Forced by the authorities bakeries hit upon the alternative to prepare green tomato and carrot pieces with sugar as a substitute for these imports. Instead of original ingredients aromatics played a decisive role in the production of biscuits. This kind of manipulation is reminiscent of processes familiar in Germany during the Second World War.

To supplement this complex of questions, it must be pointed out, that both industry and craft in the GDR suffered from a constant decrease in numbers of apprentices.

Compared to other branches of trade this profession remained relatively unattractive, not least because of the low income. Furthermore the apprentice hardly ever had the chance to equip a bakery which he could call his own. For the industry and its more or less mechanized production processes, this decrease in apprentice numbers had a negative effect. They had to rely extensively on training female workers. Here low income work in the food production sector was combined with shift work. For married women this was an additional occupational hindrance. A considerable number therefore gave up this job at an early stage. Thus during and after training the 'Dresdner Backwarenkombinat' suffered a loss of female workers of 80 to 85%.

Eventually an occupational differentiation between industry and craft turned out to be remarkable and until today proves to be grave. The question of training makes this quite clear. The certified master craftsman has to prove an expert knowledge on all sectors of the trade, the baker as well as the confectioner. On the other hand the master craftsman in the industry after 1945 was primarily expected to have skills in the field of technical equipment of production lines for mass production baking processes. Therefore the new literature about grain processing published in the GDR does not coincidentally deal exclusively with the production of bread.[22] Two Russian manuals about the technology [23]and biochemistry[24] of bread preparation were translated into German. A much wider-ranging manual about bakeries, [25]which was published in a first (1956) and a second (1958) edition in the GDR, was not reprinted in later years.[26] This is symptomatic of the whole development and relationship between the baker's trade and the baking industry.

Finally a look should be taken at the fate and perspectives of the Dresden baker's trade as well as the privatized successor organisations of the bread and confectionery collective combine in the course of the political turning point in 1989.[27]

In February 1990 the master craftsmen of the Dresden baker's trade united in a guild. Its predecessor, constituted in 1872, had in line with other organisations of trade yielded to an 'occupational group' of bakers and confectioners after 1945, which was only allowed to avail itself of limited functions of the former association. From the historical point of view the foundation in 1872 continued a much older tradition: a guild of bakers sanctioned by the council had existed in Dresden since the Middle Ages.

In the traditional sense today's association considers itself to be a representation of interests. Its head office and management is a constant point of contact for all organisational and legal problems as well as for questions about junior staff training. The guild represents the baker's trade in public.

About 120 master craftsmen with their enterprises were the founder members. Since 1989 this number has decreased slightly, because some bakeries had to cease work due to the high age of their owners or due to shortage of junior staff, but new businesses were also admitted to the guild. In particular these new entries are small enterprises in the form of a private limited company, which emerged from parts of the former bread and confectionery collective combine.

At the political turning point the Dresden baker's trade had a market share of about 50 percent. In consideration of the dictates and disadvantages to which it was previously exposed, and in comparison to quite a few other trades, this position was rather strong. The other half of the market share was in the hands of the bread and confectionery collective combine. Its successor organisations, which came into being as an economic consequence of the political turning point, could not maintain this high share. They fell back from 50 to 25 percent. The remaining craftsman's enterprises could not close this gap, because of a lack of their own abilities. The baking industry from West Germany stepped in.

As far as competition for market shares is concerned the baker's craft stands a good chance, because most consumers realize that bread and confectionery are first and foremost noted for their quality, freshness and large variety. Nevertheless, the prices represent a certain hindrance for a further development into this direction. After the political turning point they had to be raised considerably, because all subsidies were stopped. This burdened the consumer perceptibly, as the baker's ware as well as the rents and traffic tariffs were receiving the highest subsidies in the GDR. A total adjustment to the West German level, like foodstuffs, textiles, automobiles and services, has not been achieved yet.

It will remain the main aim of the baker's guild in Dresden to raise the number of shops in the city centre, maybe by establishing branches of already existing craftsman's enterprises. In two cases efforts have already been successful.

The understanding and the support of the town administration are needed, because Dresden has been famous not only for its *Christstollen* (now offered with the original ingredients), but also for the good quality of the entire baker's ware for a long time far across the town border. It is necessary to regain this reputation and to protect it imaginatively.

**Notes**

1  Berlin (1956–1990).
2  In this context I would like to give my warm thanks to Mr Hesse, managing director of the Saxonian baker's guild as well as the Dresden-Striesen, for their willingness to provide information.
3  The production cooperatives of the trade (Produktionsgenossenschaften des Handwerks – PGH) in the former GDR were to form an intermediate stage on the way to a so-called 'socialist reorganization of the small production of the craft'. Independent craftsmen and owners of industrial small businesses, who had enrolled in the trade register, as well as their employees, were members of these production groups. During the first step the craftsman made his machines and factories available for utilization and in exchange received a utilization fee from the cooperative, thereby remaining the owner of his production plant. During step two the cooperative would take the plant over and pay the owner off at least within 10 years. The indemnification of the work was always done according to quantity and quality. Above all every member shared in the profits. The profit was to be paid out to the members at the end of each year to the amount of at least 30 percent.
4  *Statistisches Jahrbuch,* 1 (1955), publ. 1956, pp. 154 ff.
5  *Statistisches Jahrbuch* 1 (1955), publ. 1956, p. 168.
6  *Statistisches Jahrbuch* 1 (1955), publ. 1956, p. 121.
7  *Statistisches Jahrbuch,* 18 (1972), p. 3 (for the span from 1933 until 1972).
8  *Statistisches Jahrbuch,* 34 (1989), p. 1 (for the span from 1973 until 1988).
9  *Statistisches Jahrbuch,* 35 (1990), p. 1.
10  The changing birth and mortality rates of the considered span could not be taken in account. The relatively small decrease in population between 1973 and 1989 can probably be explained by higher birth rate, resulting from the so-called economic and socio-political programme with great expenditure in the GDR during the Seventies and Eighties. It also shows that the encouragement of large families to compensate for the population decrease cause by the exodus and escapes, was not achieved despite strong financial support: the figure decreased between 1973 and 1981 by more than half million (517,000).
11  *Statistisches Jahrbuch* 35 (1990), pp. 208 ff.

12 *Statistisches Jahrbuch* 10 (1965), pp. 246 ff.
13 *Statistisches Jahrbuch* 10 (1965), pp. 248 ff.
14 *Statistisches Jahrbuch* 34 (1989), p. 175. Chemistry, building industry, mechanical engineering, electrical engineering and electronics, precision mechanics and optics, woodworking, printing trade, clothing manufacturing, leather, shoes, tobacco products, glass and ceramics, knitting factories, meat processing and service-rendering trade all belong to the groups (PGH) listed in the *Statistisches Jahrbuch*.
15 In the Dresden area in 1972 there was only one PGH of the category 'other producing craft'.
16 *Statistisches Jahrbuch* 35 (1990), pp. 158, 165.
17 *Statistisches Jahrbuch* 34 (1989), p. 232.
18 I must admit that during the reconstruction of the destroyed city centre in 1945 the responsible political authorities tried right from the start and systematically to prevent the establishment of private bakeries in this area.
19 *Statistisches Jahrbuch* 35 (1990), p. 309.
20 *Statistisches Jahrbuch* 35 (1990), pp. 480, 323.
21 The fate of the bakery Werner, situated at the south of Dresden and founded in 1893, is characteristic of this development. With a department for cakes that kept it going, it employed 70 workers until its temporary liquidation. After 1945 the business was 'publicly' owned, in 1947 it was finally assigned to the Backwarenkombinat.
22 Freund (1986), p. 269.
23 Auermann (1977).
24 Kosmina (1977).
25 Wernicke (1956, 1958).
26 Freund (1986, pp. 249–259.
27 The baker's guild Dresden introduces itself (1992).

**Bibliography**

Auermann, L.J., *Technologie der Brotherstellung* (Leipzig, 1977).
Berger, Emil, 'Quer durch die Stadt für Werners Waren', in, *Neue Zeit* (Dresden, 18.1.1993).
Freund, Walter, *Technologieentwicklung und Qualifikation des Bäckerhandwerks seit Ausgang des* 18. Jahrhunderts (Hildesheim/Zürich/New York, 1986).
Kosmina, N.P., *Biochemie der Brotbereitung* (Leipzig, 1977).
Wernicke, Walter, *Die Bäckerei* (Leipzig, 1956, 1958).
*Statistisches Jahrbuch der Deutschen Demokratischen Republik*, vols 1–345 (Berlin, 1956–1990).

# 8

# MILK AND MILK PRODUCTS IN SCOTLAND: THE ROLE OF THE MILK MARKETING BOARDS

## Alexander Fenton

This paper is concerned with the story of the Milk Marketing Boards in Scotland. To understand the forces that led to their development, it is necessary to look a little backwards in time; and the story also runs right up to the present (1993), because there is now before Parliament an Agriculture Bill which contains provisions for the ending of the Milk Marketing Schemes, not only in Scotland, but in England and Wales as well. The forces that have brought about this situation are, however, different from those that brought the Boards into being.

### Traditional techniques

Traditional techniques of processing milk reveal a double pattern of immediate drinking of fresh milk, and delayed consumption for drinks derived from fresh milk and secondarily from buttermilk and whey. All these practices were well known in the countryside. Distribution of these liquid products was relatively limited. Nevertheless, milk was exploited to its absolute limit at the level, mainly, of the individual family.

This situation remained firm in many parts of Scotland well into the twentieth century, but it had already begun to change near larger urban groupings, and communities of miners and other non-agricultural workers, by the end of the eighteenth century. The area first affected by the pressures of industrialisation was the South West of Scotland. Circumstances were favourable because the land suited grazing more than arable, and developing industry, at first water-powered and then based on coal and steam, lay close by.

It was in this area that moves towards a dairying industry first appeared in Scotland. Where the rest of the country was making cheese of sheep's milk, Ayrshire was already noted for cow's milk cheese by the 1660s.[1] By the late 1700s dairying was the dominant activity, and the making of Dunlop cheese, based on cows' milk, was spreading. There was a growing demand for butter and cheese in the markets of Glasgow and Paisley, and some of the supplies even reached the remoter Edinburgh market.

## The early 19th century pattern

If the urban industrial districts are thought of as fields of force, then these can be related to a threefold pattern that evolved in the first half of the nineteenth century:

1   Liquid milk became a major item of trade near such industrial centres. This coincided with a rapid spread of urban dairies within the built up areas, so reinforcing the cohesion of the liquid milk ring, which extended for two or three miles around the towns, within the range of access of a light horse-drawn vehicle.[2] In view of the relatively perishable nature of liquid milk, buttermilk was an equally common item of such trade. It became a widespread urban phenomenon. Every urban household had its **soor-dook**[3] cans to collect the daily ration from the buttermilk barrels on the farmer's cart. It was used as a drink considered to have therapeutic qualities, and was also much used in baking. An analysis of the locations of the numerous photographs of such milk carts in the Scottish Ethnological Archive in the National Museums of Scotland shows that they clustered around the main towns, and that the carrying of liquid milk in upright metal churns and buttermilk in horizontally placed barrels continued through the First World War and sporadically into the 1950s.

2   The outer and very much deeper ring concentrated more on the conversion of liquid milk into cream cheese or skimmed milk cheese.

3   In remoter districts still, butter and milk production was more limited and much of the milk was fed to calves. These were brought on to a certain stage, and were then sold to form parts of dairy herds elsewhere.[4]

## The late nineteenth century

From the mid-nineteenth century, zonal differences began to be eroded with the spread of railways. Transport improvements led to increased profitability, and this in turn to breed improvements. This was when the Ayrshire cow became Scotland's primary dairy animal. The Highland and Agricultural Society of Scotland also encouraged instruction in cheese-making and in butter-making. An early commercial creamery was set up a few miles south-east of Stranraer, in the 1880s; it could handle the milk of 2000 cows, and the by-product, whey, was fed to an associated stock of up to 500 pigs. A Dairy School was established at Kilmarnock in 1899.

These are pointers to the localised development of what was to become a leading Scottish industry, but for some considerable time, organisation on any scale was severely inhibited by the small size of the individual units, and the necessity for hand milking that continued far into the twentieth century.

In the 1870s, two thirds of the holdings in the South West were under 100 acres, because the pressures of hand milking could scarcely cope with anything else. On average, a milker could handle 10 cows in an hour and a half, but had to do so for 365 days a year and for 7 days a week. It is no surprise, therefore, that the South-West had a lot to do with the development of milking machinery from the late 1800s.[5]

## The Milk Marketing Boards: background

It was against the pattern of effort and enterprise in the South-West, but not only there, that the Milk Marketing Boards were set up in the 1930s. Formerly there had been sharp zoning around urban centres, in demonstration of J.H. von Thünen's concentric bands' concept which 'stresses the differential impact of concentrated urban demand and its propensity to generate zones of specialised land-usage in the hinterlands of cities',[6] but now with the setting up of the Boards came a more artificial set of man-made zones related to collection and distribution centres, especially after bulk milk collection was adopted.

By this period there was an increasing need for regulation of the milk industry. In the mid-nineteenth century, producer and consumer were closely related and physically adjacent; often producer and consumer were one and the same family. But as industrialisation proceeded, and with it an ever increasing degree of urbanisation, there grew a need for an ever widening circle of producers. Within the towns there appeared large numbers of retail and wholesale dairymen, who had little interest in the producer.

During the stressful conditions of the First World War, demand for milk was high. The wholesale dairies and powerful companies came to almost monopolise and control distribution. Producers found themselves forced to bargain with them as individuals. In general milk production was extremely unsatisfactory and uncoordinated. Such was the level of dissatisfaction, that central action had to be taken. Already in 1917, the Astor Committee was considering 'the general conditions of dairying and milk distributing industries, apart from the war, with a view to their being placed on a more satisfactory basis for the future'. As a result, the Ministry of Food took direct control of about 800 wholesale dairy companies, and implemented economies and improvements in handling and transport. A proposal for State control of milk wholesaling was put forward, but not adopted, Ministry of Food control came to an end in 1920.

The problems, on which an official light had thus been flashed, remained. They affected the relationships between the companies and the producers, for the former could control the retail price. The gap in the price paid to the producer and the price charged to the customer widened. The National Farmers' Unions tried to act as middlemen in getting agreements with the distributors' association; in 1922, Joint Milk Councils were set up, one in England and one in Scotland, with the aim of negotiating prices.

They helped to stabilise a fairly volatile situation, but could not control it. The main problem was the milk that was surplus to the needs of the liquid market, of limited sale value because of its relatively short keeping qualities. When manufactured into butter and cheese, it had to compete with foreign imports and fetched low prices. Worse, an agricultural recession ensued, and more farmers turned to dairying because the demand for liquid milk had not slackened and prices were maintained. The outcome was a greater surplus to be sold, sometimes at only nominal prices. There was also a rapid fall in the average world price of cheese in 1920–30. Producers began to undercut the price of liquid milk to avoid the excessively low prices for their surplus milk. The effectiveness of the Joint Councils was weakened, and they reached a state of almost complete collapse at this period.

Further efforts to control marketing were made. Disappointment with the Joint Milk Council in the West of Scotland led to 1100 producers setting up an association for marketing milk in Glasgow in 1927. This was the Scottish Milk Agency, the first large scale milk marketing organisation in Britain on a voluntary cooperative basis. Though it operated successfully, internal dissension weakened it and many members were too prone to make private arrangements in the hope of a better return. It failed after three or four years; but the Aberdeen branch, set up in 1927–28 with 300 members, remained in existence and in fact became autonomous.

## Milk Marketing Boards: setting up

Problems remained acute, and in 1931 came the Agricultural Marketing Act, in effect an attempt to prevent the collapse of the dairying industry. Not only was it concerned to regulate milk marketing, but it also sought to promulgate the concept of the health of the nation. A Commission appointed under Sir Edward Grigg made its Report in 1933, on the basis of which the Milk Marketing Boards were set up, as producers' organisations. The powers of the Boards included control of milk marketing, the arranging of prices, the prevention of selling without Board permission and, an excellent concept in terms of enhanced public awareness of food and diet, the promotion of agricultural cooperation and with it education and research.

Because, under the Board, producers got a guaranteed price, higher than before, milk production became one of the most profitable types of farming, leading again to an increased surplus over the retail demand, whence an increased production also of butter and cheese. This was an embarrassment to the Board because of the low market price of cheese. To try to level matters, they lowered the average 'pool' price to producers and raised the levy paid by producer-retailers. This was resented, since they had had a ready market for their milk before Boards were set up. A case was heard before the Court of Session in Edinburgh against the levy, and was decided in favour of Mr Ferrier on behalf of his fellow-producers. The view was held that 'we must have a Board but they must in future study the interest of all concerned in the industry' and not the producers alone.[7] The scheme was, therefore amended, and the levy fixed at a much lower rate. The Board had learned a lesson in public relations.

An outcome of the difference between the prices for liquid and manu-factured milk was that illicit private enterprise could develop. The Board set the price for liquid milk at 1/- a gallon in 1934, and milk for manufacturing at 5d a gallon. Some entrepreneurs bought at the surplus milk price and sold at the liquid milk price. Others bought the lower price milk, put it through a separator, then sold it to a small dairy as skimmed milk plus cream, which was put into a tank, stirred, and sold as whole milk. The wholesaling of milk needed a licence, and sales should be declared. Nevertheless private sales by drivers of milk vans to the inhabitants of blocks of Glasgow flats were not rare. In particular, milk supplies to ice cream merchants gave a lot of trouble. Many sales were not declared to the Board, and pilfering for private sale was rife.[8]

In England, where the same problem of surpluses existed, the Treasury made a grant to enable payment by the Board of a standard price, authorised by the Milk Acts of 1934 and 1936. A sum of £1,750,000 was also allocated by the Government for use in improving milk quality, in encouraging individual consumption of milk through publicity, and through the development of the milk-in-schools scheme. The effort was successful, and was later coupled with the Welfare Foods Scheme, through which pregnant and nursing mothers, etc, got milk at a cheap rate. The success of the scheme was such that during the 1939–1945 War it led to a shortage of liquid milk.

## The three Scottish Milk Marketing Boards

Three Boards were established in Scotland, the Scottish Milk Marketing Board (SMMB) at the end of 1933, the Aberdeen & District Milk Marketing Board (A & D MMB) in August 1934, and the North of Scotland Milk Marketing Board (NoS MMB) in October 1934. The reason for three Boards (as against one for the whole of England and Wales) relates partly to history and partly to terrain. During the formation of the Boards, the North-East of Scotland producers were doubtful about cooperating with producers in the South of Scotland, because of the bad experience they had already had with the Boards' precursor, The Scottish Milk Agency. They therefore formed their own Board, as did the North of Scotland producers who were getting a higher price for milk than the producers in the South, and did not have a surplus milk problem. An all-Scottish scheme would have led to lower prices for them.

The levels of operation in each of the Board areas mark regional differences. In the SMMB area, production rose from 109 million gallons in 1934 to 162.4 million in 1951 and payments to producers rose from

£3.8 million to £26.2 million over the same period. By 1951, there were 7966 registered producers in the Board's area. Of these, 7365 had Tuberculin Tested herds. Overall, there was a 60% increase in sales of liquid milk between 1939 and 1951, and of the total sold in the latter year, 5.25 million gallons were of 'Certified' milk. The average prices paid to producers were (excluding bonuses), 10.37d per gallon in 1939 and 32.50d in 1951. Between 1939 and 1947, there was a steady decline in the amount of milk manufactured, matching the increased consumption of liquid milk as the provision of cheap school and welfare milk spread. 43.8 million gallons were manufactured in the Boards' Creameries in 1939 (36.6% of the total produced), declining to 17.7 million gallons (14%) in 1947. There was then a surge in 1950–51, when 33 million gallons (33%) were manufactured into 2100 tons of cheese and 1200 tons of butter.

At the same time, the increasingly strong effect of the SMMB was seen on the decreasing levels of farm cheese production. The cheese presses of metal and of stone that had proliferated on the farms, spreading to other parts of Scotland from the South West from the end of the eighteenth century, began now to fall into disuse.[9] Individual farmers turned 6.5 million gallons into cheese in 1939, but only 1.4 million in 1950. By this date there were only 35 producers (registered), making their own cheese in the Board's area. None remained in 1974.

The NoS MMB started with the counties of Nairn, Inverness, Ross & Cromarty, Sutherland and Caithness in October 1934. Moray joined in July 1944, and Orkney only in October 1946, after the Second World War. By 1951, it had 493 producers and 7,588,900 gallons of milk were sold off the farms, 72% of this being from tested herds. It differed form the other Boards in carrying a large retail trade in milk, in addition to manufacturing cheese and butter. Its main depot in Inverness was used to pasteurise milk for the supply of areas such as the Fort William area, the West Coast and the Western Isles that were not self-sufficient in milk. A Creamery was added at Wick in Caithness in 1947 to pasteurise milk for local retail sale and to make butter from the surplus. By 1951 it was handling over 1 million gallons of milk and producing 126 tons of butter; most of this was Caithness milk. In this year also a new milk depot was set up in Nairn, getting its supplies from Moray and Nairn and acting as a retail distribution centre.

In Orkney, which in recent decades has become renowned for its cheese, the Board set up the first cheese factory in 1946. It handled 431,500 gallons in that year, and 1,168,000 by 1951, as Orkney farmers responded. 508 tons of cheese were made in 1951.

**Progress and improvements; organisation, hygiene, consumption**

At each of the creameries set up by the Boards, laboratories were established to test the milk and field officers were appointed to advise and assist producers. Such developments were part of an integrated chain of organisation that ran from the central decrees of the Government down to the consumer, and included forms of laboratory testing and general health care that brought with them new nutritional horizons.

Even in the 1920s, milk distribution and dairy manufacture was still small scale and only a step away from traditional farming practices. Hygiene was uncertain. Sales were mainly of raw milk, of poor keeping quality. But from that period, progress that can rightly be called revolutionary came into play. Chemical preservatives were prohibited in favour of hygienic handling c.1928, and dairy bacteriology became a science. Pasteurisation came in as the main new factor. Perhaps not surprisingly, cleanliness at the farm was at first hardest to achieve, and the spread of milking machinery itself created problems, because of the difficulty of washing and keeping clean all the parts. A strong propaganda and educational effort was required.[10]

In Britain as a whole, there was a 50% increase in the consumption of milk during 1939–52, due to cheap supplies for schools and for social welfare, a general increase in purchasing power, and perhaps also to the propaganda of the Boards that layed stress on the importance of 'safe' milk. Another factor was the excellent organisation of transport and retailing.

Britain was, in fact, the only country to have a daily delivery of bottles to the home, with all its accompanying technology in filling and sealing bottles and later washing and sterilising the returned empties.[11] In the early days, for example, 21 hauliers were licensed by the SMMB to haul milk, these employing about 47 lorry drivers in winter and 51 in summer when supplies were more plentiful. The heavy milk cans had to be manhandled at first. Each farmer had his name and address stamped or printed on the shoulder of each can. As each can was emptied at the creamery's dump tank the man in charge removed the farmer's label, kept it, and handed it in to the office at the end of the day. He broke the seal, made a preliminary test by smelling the milk to check for any unusual flavours, then passed it to be weighed and emptied. Office organisation was an essential element in the whole.[12] The overall labour involved began to be eased with the introduction of the Bulk Tank Pilot Milk Collection Scheme by the SMMB in 1952–53, as far, at least, as South West Scotland was concerned; economical collection areas were worked out through liaison between the Board, producers, distributors, hauliers and Creamery managers.[13]

Central government and local authority provisions marked the new order of things. There was a profusion of acts and orders relating to testing for bovine tuberculosis, pasteurisation, systematic milk testing, etc. In Scotland the administration of Acts and Orders on the production, handling, processing and distribution of milk was a function of the local authorities. Via the Department of Health for Scotland, the Secretary of State for Scotland had an immediate interest in the administration. This was done through a staff of milk inspectors who advised the local authority officials on milk and dairies administration. Local authorities in turn had their sanitary staff, and a staff of milk officers qualified in dairying, who visited farms and dairy premises and gave guidance on the hygiene of milk production and distribution. This relative immediacy of contact through the bureaucratic chain differed from England, where the administration of the regulations on the production of milk were implemented by the Ministry of Agriculture, and those on distribution by the local authorities.

The Boards were to some extent instruments that helped to facilitate the operation of such acts and orders, but the administrative beginnings preceded the Boards by over 20 years. The Milk and Dairies (Scotland) Act of 1914 (implemented 1925) established the annual (at least) inspection of all dairies, the registration of all dairymen, the making and enforcing of dairy by-laws by local authorities, and gave the Secretary of State powers to make general or special orders for the protection of milk against infection or contamination, for the prohibition of the adding of colouring matter, for the conveyance, sealing and labelling of cans, etc. The interim Milk and Dairies (Amendment) Act of 1922 made the same points, including also the obligation on local authorities to maintain a separate register of milk retailers. In 1934 came the Milk and Dairies (Scotland) Order with a number of additional requirements concerned with hygiene, and in 1951 the Milk (Special) (Designations) (Scotland) Order consolidated and replaced similar Orders of 1936–49. It provided for the granting of licences by local authorities to dairymen using special designations of milk: Standard, Certified, Tuberculin Tested, Pasteurised and Sterilised, each defined in relation to testing and bacterial content. It was the aim of the Government that only milk of a special – and therefore controlled – designation should be sold to the public. The Milk (Special Designations) Act 1949, made arrangements for four areas to be covered initially by the specification – significantly, these were Scotland's major towns, Glasgow, Edinburgh, Dundee and Aberdeen. These and the Tuberculosis (Attested Herds) Scheme 1950, which allowed for the scheduling of areas where tuberculosis had been eradicated, laid the administrative basis that ensured a clean, safe milk supply to the public for the future.

### The nation's health

All of this meant a great deal in terms of public nutrition. By 1930, the value of milk for the health of the nation had been fully realised. The investigations of the Milk Supply Committee showed that in the lowest income groups, milk consumption was under 1½ pints (0.9 l) per head per week, but in better-off families up to 5 pints (2.84 l). The work of Sir John Orr indicated that the lower the income, the greater the reliance on foods rich in carbohydrates, but poor in protein of high biological value, in fat and in natural salts and vitamins. A large part of the population was seen to be living on a diet dangerously low in these, and milk was recommended as a main antidote. This view was reinforced by experimental work in an English Public School and in Scottish schools. The Boards were able to cooperate with nutritional experts and in this way moved towards a solution to the surplus milk problem. In 1935, 402,689 children took milk at school, at half the retail price (313,645 gallons a month). In 1951, the number was 651,180, c.87% of those on the roll of grant-aided schools (600,000 gallons a month). Good results led to an extension of the scheme to children under five and to nursing and expectant mothers, at 1 pint (0.57 l) a day for 1½d or free for those on low incomes. Alternatively, an equivalent amount of dried milk could be supplied.[14]

By the 1950s, the Boards had settled into the form that continued, though always subject to development along the line of business and commerce, within the framework of their cooperative composition. Of the Scottish Boards, the SMMB was far and away the most important, serving the major population concentrations. The remainder of this paper, therefore, concentrates on the SMMB.

**Rationalisation and innovation**

Part of the process of rationalisation that went on lay in the acquisition of creameries, which allowed the Board to manufacture the milk of its own producers. It took over 19 creameries in Glasgow, Ayrshire, Dumfriesshire, Lanarkshire, Kirkcudbrightshire and Wigtownshire. These were producing cheese, fresh cream, butter, skim milk, whey, condensed milk and cream and casein. Several had been sold off by the early 1940s as part of an intensive rationalisation process. New creameries were built at Hogganfield (Glasgow) and at Mauchline (Ayrshire). Having decided against the liquid milk market, the Board at first continued with the products of the creameries they had been taking over, but gradually widened the range as technological innovations were introduced. These included much larger cheese vats, the replacement of the traditional cylinder shaped cheese by blocks, improved starter cultures for cheese making that gave a closer texture and was good for cut portions for the retail trade, continuous butter-making machinery, further mechanisation of cheese-making, the installation of a plant for ultra-heat-treated (UHT) 'Long Life' milk, and the replacement of open vats by automatically controlled cylindrical units.

Innovations continued, but these examples show the continuing pattern. By 1979, there were 9 creameries instead of 19, manufacturing a range of products in line with the needs of modern times, for individual consumers, for animal feeding and for commercial purposes. In sum, these were Cheddar and Dunlop cheese in the traditional cylindrical form (which customers like and which still enjoys popularity), in blocks and also prepacked for shop sales; salt and unsalted butter, in bulk or packeted; UHT products such as milk, pouring cream and whipping cream, and, to satisfy the tastes of the younger generation, flavoured milk drinks; spray skim powder; edible casein; sodium caseinate; calcium caseinate and calcium precipitate; whey spray powder; demineralised whey powder; and whey/skim powder mixtures.

## Marketing and consumption

Control of the Board by the Ministry of Food ended in 1954, after 15 years. The marketing of products – powder, cheese and butter – then fell to the manufacturers themselves. The Board collaborated with private manufacturers in setting up the Company of Scottish Cheese Makers to buy all the cheese from the manufacturers and market it through approved factors. The cheese market was already overloaded, and prices slipped, though they later firmed up. One result was that the Cheese Bureau was set up to do generic cheese advertising, marking not only an advance in the advertising of food products, but also widened forms of international cooperation, for the Bureau included Scotland, England, New Zealand, Australia, and later Ireland, as well as Canada, which did not, however, become a full member. For the butter market the Board worked with New Zealand and Australia and cooperated with Ireland, Denmark, Finland, Norway and Holland in the Butter Information Council (eg advertising butter as against margarine; in the late 1950s, advertising in the UK was up to £700,000). Cooperation between the Board and the trade also touched on liquid milk; the Scottish Milk Publicity Co worked with the National Milk Publicity Co in London, even using the same advertising agents (Mather & Crowther Ltd, later Ogilvy, Brown & Mather Ltd).

Advertising and promotion went hand in hand. An active Sales Development Staff led to further aspects such as the setting up of the Scottish Milk Centre in Glasgow in 1958, with a self-service restaurant, coffee lounge and dairy shop, the organisation of dairy cookery demonstrations, the provision of a Roving Milk Bar at major agricultural shows (the SMMB now has a large, permanent stand in the Royal Highland Showground), and in the 1960s sponsorship of a sporting event, the Scottish Milk Race, began[15]. All of these devices were calculated to raise the level of consciousness of milk and milk products amongst the populace, and to increase consumption. The following table gives the per capita milk consumption of liquid milk in Scotland from the early days of the formation of the Boards, though it should be understood that these are minimum figures; milk was also absorbed in a range of other ways, as cheese, in milk chocolate, etc, though these have not been calculated.

The picture shown here is one of fairly level consumption, highest between 1974–84, and subsequently tending to fall, but nevertheless maintaining a higher level in Scotland than in the UK as a whole.

*Table 1:* Per Capita Milk consumption in Scotland

| Year to March | Litres per Week | UK Consumption |
|---|---|---|
| 1938–39 | 1.64 | |
| 1944–45 | 2.35 | |
| 1954–55 | 2.56 | |
| 1958–59 | 2.46 | |
| 1959–60 | 2.48 | |
| 1960–61 | 2.48 | |
| 1961–62 | 2.49 | |
| 1962–63 | 2.49 | |
| 1963–64 | 2.48 | |
| 1964–65 | 2.49 | |
| 1965–66 | 2.47 | |
| 1966–67 | 2.45 | |
| 1967–68 | 2.44 | |
| 1968–69 | 2.41 | |
| 1969–70 | 2.41 | 2.67 |
| 1970–71 | 2.41 | |
| 1971–72 | 2.35 | |
| 1972–73 | 2.39 | |
| 1973–74 | 2.44 | |
| 1974–75 | 2.60 | 2.69 |
| 1975–76 | 2.68 | |
| 1976–77 | 2.61 | |
| 1977–78 | 2.50 | |
| 1978–79 | 2.53 | |
| 1979–80 | 2.50 | 2.52 |
| 1981–82 | 2.48 | 2.44 |
| 1982–83 | 2.47 | 2.40 |
| 1983–84 | 2.45 | 2.43 |
| 1984–85 | 2.41 | 2.38 |
| 1985–86 | 2.41 | 2.35 |
| 1986–87 | 2.36 | 2.30 |
| 1987–88 | 2.34 | 2.27 |
| 1988–89 | 2.32 | 2.26 |
| 1989–90 | 2.33 | 2.27 |
| 1990–91 | 2.35 | 2.25 |
| 1991–92 | 2.37 | 2.24 |

From *UK Dairy Facts and Figures*, 1992, 184

A new phase came with membership of the EEC on 1 January 1978. The period of commodity guarantees came to an end, and UK farmers had to get their whole milk income from the market by way of the Boards. The five UK Boards (England & Wales, Northern Ireland, the three Scottish ones) were retained, and a poll undertaken amongst the producers showed that this was the common wish. The production of milk from Scottish farms, however, is now controlled by EC quota rules at 1200 million litres a year. This is organised through the three Boards, and provides the basis for a processing and marketing industry that comprises 155 establishments, with an annual turnover of over £500 million and employing 5000 people directly, and a further 4000 in related activities.

As a result of rationalisation, the number of establishments has been declining since 1980. Over a hundred have vanished, and the process is likely to continue, particularly since the quota system does not permit expansion in production. At the same time, there has been much concentration; the bulk of the milk is handled by only a few establishments, in fact 50% by five of the biggest plants.

Slightly over half the Scottish product goes as liquid milk, now largely packaged in cartons, though the milk bottle is not quite extinct. Much of the remainder, over a quarter of Scottish milk production, goes into the making of hard cheese in 10 factories. Mozzarella, produced near Edinburgh, is the second most important cheese variety. The rest goes into evaporated milk and chocolate crumb, which represents an interim stage in the making of milk chocolate. In general terms, Scotland is self-sufficient in milk products, which represent 15% of the total food expenditure of Scottish households. The milk industry is a major element in the food and drinks industry and in the economy as a whole, providing a higher level of employment and a greater value of output than any other sector.

## The end of the Boards

However, new influences are coming to bear on the Boards. As a result of market pressures, the opening of EC milk markets to cross-border trade, and pressure from the EC and from the UK Government itself, it has become clear that the Boards must move away from their present regime and lose their statutory monopoly buying powers. These powers have made others in the industry, represented by the powerful Scottish Dairy Trade Federation (SDTF), discontented. Under earlier conditions, they were appropriate and of much value, and possibly essential under wartime and post-war conditions. In summary, they mean that in the Board areas, all producers are obliged to sell all milk produced by them to, or through the agency of, the Boards. The Boards are legally required to accept all milk of the requisite legal quality from registered producers, both organising its collection and its delivery to buyers who may be manufacturing products made with milk or selling pasteurised milk as such. The price at which milk is sold is determined by a statutory joint committee representing Board and buyers (through the SDTF). The SMMB itself carries on its own manufacturing operation, and in compliance with the statutory scheme has established a commercial operation ('Scottish Farm' and 'Scottish Pride') which buys milk from the SMMB in the same way as an independent buyer. This situation is viewed by the SDTF as monopolistic, and there is, therefore, considerable opposition to the SMMB's staying in business, after the Agriculture Bill comes into force in 1994, as 'son of milk board'.[16]

What the SMMB proposes is that a voluntary cooperative should be established, 'Scottish Milk Marketing Ltd', to which all the present activities and assets of the board should be transferred without interruption, and which would also assume all liabilities. Legislation would be necessary to put these proposals into effect. The cooperative would be owned and controlled by milk producers; membership would be voluntary, and producers would be free to contract to sell their milk on the open market in the absence of a statutory scheme. The objectives the cooperative would seek to achieve are as follows:

1   the retention of voluntary producer involvement by establishing a body controlled by producers to allow the development of the Scottish milk industry over the longer term.
2   to retain sufficient size to be able to negotiate reasonable terms for all producers.
3   to provide the scale of organisation required and facilities necessary to collect and supply the increasingly large volumes dictated by the larger dairy companies.
4   to retain and maintain the existing commercial activities undertaken by the Board so as to ensure their ability to compete effectively in a market place dominated increasingly by significant companies of international reputation, such as Dairy Crest and Northern Foods.
5   to provide competitive access to milk supplies for all buyers and to operate an open pricing system.[17]

These proposals are basically in line with the requirements of the appropriate sections of the Agriculture Bill, currently being considered, by which the milk marketing schemes in the UK would be revoked in 1994, so ending one long story in the provision of an essential food item to the consumers of Britain, and opening another that will be increasingly affected by the requirements of European and even wider international trade. However the story is written, it will be carefully looked at by the consumers themselves, whose voice, through Consumers' Associations, is no longer without influence.

**Notes**
1   Fenton 1963, p. 69.
2   Robertson 1994, p. 641.
3   *Scottish National Dictionary* sv *Dook*, n, 2, ie sour milk, buttermilk, first recorded in the Lothians, 1825.
4   Coppock 1976, p. 125.
5   *The Scottish Farmer*, 6 July 1946, pp. 834–35; Peacock 1958, pp. 18–19; *Farming News*, 7 Jan. 1961.
6   Campbell et al, 1992, pp. 1–22.
7   Paul, Typescript (SEA 1975/43).
8   Paul, Typescript (SEA 1977/3).
9   Fenton 1976, pp. 150–156.
10  Crossley 1952, pp. 324–25, 328.

11  Ibid, 326.
12  Paul, Typescript (SEA 1976/1).
13  Paul, Typescript (SEA 1976/2).
14  Chalmers, n.d. (a source of much of the detail in this paper).
15  Urquhart 1979.
16  Maxwell 1992.
17  *Scottish Milk Marketing Board Reorganisation. Summary of the Proposals of the Board.* n.d. (typescript).


**Literature**

Campbell, B.M.S. J.A. Galloway and M. Murphy, 'Rural Land-use in the Metropolitan Hinterland, 1270–1339: the Evidence of the Inquisitiones Post Mortem', *Agricultural History Review* 40/i (1992), pp. 1–22.

Chalmers, C.H. *A Review of the Milk supply of Scotland*, Department of Health for Scotland 1952 (typescript).

Coppock, J.T. *An Agricultural Atlas of Scotland*, Edinburgh 1976.

Crossley, E.L. 'Developments in Milk Distribution in Britain', *British Agricultural Bulletin* 4/18 (March 1952), pp. 324–329,

Federation of United Kingdom Milk Marketing Boards, *United Kingdom Dairy Facts & Figures* (annual).

Fenton, A. 'Skene of Hallyard's Manuscript of Husbandrie', *Agricultural History Review*, XI/ii (1963), pp. 65–81.

Fenton, A. *Scottish Country Life*, Edinburgh 1976.

Maxwell, F. 'Dairy trade comes to terms with ruling by monopolies board', *Scotsman*, 10 December 1992.

Paul, W. Life Story, in Scottish Ethnological Archive 1975/43 (typescript).

Paul, W. Handling Milk from Farm to Creameries in the 1930–1950 Era, in Scottish Ethnological Archive, 1976/1.

Paul, W. Bulk Tank Pilot Collection Scheme, in Scottish Ethnological Archive 1976/2.

Paul, W. 'Dodger' in 1934, in Scottish Ethnological Archive, 1977/3 (typescript).

Peacock, J.W. 'Milking Machine's 70th Anniversary', *The Farming News*, 22 March 1958, pp. 18–19.

Robertson, U. 'The Supply and Sale of Milk in 19th Century Edinburgh', in P. Lysaght, ed., *Milk and Milk Products from Medieval to Modern Times*, Edinburgh 1994, pp. 63–70.

Urquhart, R. *History of the Scottish Milk Marketing Board*, Paisley 1979.

# 9

# MILK: NUTRITIONAL SCIENCE AND AGRICULTURAL DEVELOPMENT IN NORWAY, 1890–1990

## *Unni Kjærnes*

This chapter will deal with the relationship between nutritional science, food industry and consumption trends. Levenstein has shown how changes in American food habits around the turn of the century should be seen as the outcome of a number of forces, where socio-cultural as well as material and economic factors influence the development in very dynamic and complex ways.[1] Nutritional science has played an important part, but its role has been interlinked with that of the food industry.[2] While this alliance proved very useful for certain industries, the outcome for the promotion of nutrition was more mixed. This contribution takes a similar approach, but the time perspective here is much longer – a full century – and the discussion is limited to one specific food item: milk. Central questions are: To what degree can consumption trends be explained by changes on the demand side (in household economy, demography etc.)? How do production trends relate to consumption? To what degree have dairy producers attempted to reinforce or redirect existing consumption trends and have they succeeded? Have spokespersons for nutritional science managed to influence consumption contrary to producer interests, or have they succeeded only when their advice has supported established interests?

The approach is historical and rather open. Data are limited mainly to Norway, based on general statistics, special studies performed by others and research at SIFO.[3]

I begin by presenting consumption trends with respect to milk and the various milk varieties. Here I will also include butter, the economically most important 'by-product' of dairy production. To understand conflicts over butter, we need data on its substitute, margarine. The second part will deal with the market and economic interests, mainly the dairy industry, focusing on hallmarks in the development of production and market. The third part will present the issue of milk and health. Here I highlight central shifts or phases in the development of this issue, as well as its relationship to production and production interests. Finally, I discuss consumption trends in the light of these two interests, those of science and those of production.

## Consumption

Milk and dairy products are regarded as central components of the traditional Norwegian diet. And indeed they probably are, at least in some
population segments and in certain parts of the country.[4] A frequently
cited example is the remote rural area of Setesdal, which was modernised
only recently.[5] As recently as in the inter-war period, subsistence farming was
dominant in this area. In 1937 the local diet included 1246 grams of skimmed
milk and 355 grams of whole milk a day for adults. Consumption of other
dairy products was, however, very low. The case of Setesdal is the extreme,
and it clearly shows a quite traditional community. I say quite, because the
consumption gap between skimmed and whole-fat dairy products indicates
that sale of butter must have been an important source of income here, and
this was common among farmers at that time. The example indicates that
with food traditions as a 'frame of reference', milk holds a strong position in
the Norwegian diet. I will later show that milk consumption is still high
compared to other countries.

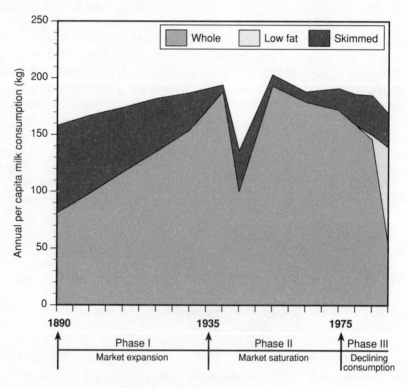

*Figure 1.* Milk consumption trends in Norway, 1880–1991.
*Sources:* Ministry of Agriculture (1975)
National Nutrition Council

Figure 1 shows consumption trends in Norway over the past century.[6] We can identify three distinct phases. With industrialisation and urbanisation starting rather late in Norway, it is reasonable to start our description around 1890. The demand for marketed food was at that time restricted mainly to urban, industrialised areas, where increasing numbers of poor workers required cheap, energy-rich foods. For them it was rather expensive to buy milk and dairy products, especially products rich in fat. The first phase of *market expansion*, then, starts with a relatively low consumption of dairy products, only skimmed milk being consumed in substantial quantities. Figure 1 shows how consumption of whole milk more than doubled from 1890 to the 1930s, while skimmed milk nearly vanished from the menu. The total increase was also considerable.

The next phase, *market saturation*, lasted from the late 1930s until around 1970. During World War II there was a substantial drop in consumption of milk. Supply was reduced, mainly due to lack of fodder. After the war, pre-war consumption patterns were soon restored. If consumption during the actual war years is disregarded, this period represents only minor changes in milk consumption. Even the pattern concerning milk varieties changed very little in this phase. However, a peak in milk consumption can be detected in the early 1950s. At that time milk provided a substantial amount of the caloric content in the diet and also of the fat intake.

The third phase, from the 1970s to date, shows quite different consumption patterns. Overall milk *consumption* has been *declining* slowly but steadily. More important is the dramatic shift from whole milk to skimmed, and then to low-fat milk. Here it should be noted that low-fat milk (1.5% of fat) was not introduced on the Norwegian market until 1984. This recent shift is regarded as the main explanation for the reduced percentage of fat in the contemporary Norwegian diet (from 40 to 35 per cent of energy intake).[7]

*Table 1.* Consumption of margarine and butter in urban working class households in Norway (grams per person per day)

| | 1906–07 | 1918–19 | 1927–28 | 1935–37 | War rations |
|---|---|---|---|---|---|
| Margarine | 40.8 | 48.1 | 67.5 | 60.4 | |
| | | | | | 45.0 |
| Butter | 11.0 | 8.5 | 7.0 | 21.1 | |

*Source:* Wold (1941)

The food market has changed in other ways as well. Consumption of butter and margarine have increased steadily, with margarine as the clear winner. A special situation occurred in the 1930s, when butter was increasingly mixed into all margarine on a mandatory basis. The result was a substantial increase in overall butter consumption. While this mandatory adding of butter to margarine was discontinued after World War II, the shift from margarine to butter continued until the early 1970s (Table 2).

*Table 2*   Total annual consumption of butter and margarine 1930–1990 in Norway
(mill.kg)

|           | 1938 | 1949–50 | 1970 | 1990 |
|-----------|------|---------|------|------|
| Margarine | 55   | 82      | 73   | 56   |
| Butter    | 24   | 13      | 21   | 14   |

*Sources:*   Ministry of Agriculture (1975) National Nutrition Council (1992)

Parallel to the recent shift in milk consumption, margarine consumption – and to some degree butter consumption – have also gradually declined.

How can these shifts be explained by changes on the demand side? Economists have explained consumption changes before World War II by reference to improved economic conditions in the Norwegian population.[8] This is supported by studies of social inequalities in food consumption in this period. Prior to World War I, consumption of dairy products was generally low in working class households, and involved mainly skimmed milk. In addition these households had a high consumption of margarine. White-collar workers, by contrast, consumed more whole milk and more butter. In the rural population consumption of dairy products was generally higher than in other social groups, but even here consumption of fat dairy products varied according to household finances. These social differences were to become an important issue on the political agenda in the 1930s.[9]

During the 1950s and 1960s, income and welfare increased for most or all population groups in Norway. That the second phase (disregarding World War II) was marked by only minor changes in milk consumption may support the view that income was no longer the main limiting factor for this consumption. On the other hand, the shift from margarine to butter has been explained in terms of improved household income. The declining consumption of milk in the third phase may actually also be explained by income changes.[10] Since the 1970s, milk has increasingly been replaced by drinks with higher income elasticities, such as orange juice and coca cola. Social inequality in the consumption of different milk varieties, however, is related to education rather than to income. Lower social strata have a higher consumption of whole milk. Furthermore, it is recognised that changes in dietary habits in line with new nutritional recommendations are more common in social groups characterised by high education, high income, etc.[11]

Contemporary milk consumption patterns in Norway show similar features to those of other Northern European countries.[12]

Figure 2 indicates a substantial shift from whole milk to low-fat and skimmed milk in most of the countries included. Changes from 1989 to 1990 indicate that this change is still in progress, along with a decline in the consumption of liquid milk. Total consumption of milk fat in Norway in 1990 is at a medium level, compared to these other countries.

Are the changing patterns in the consumption of milk and dairy products merely a reflection of improved welfare in the Norwegian population? Until

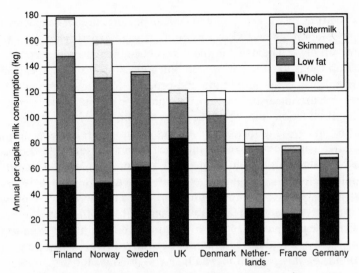

*Figure 2:* Milk consumption in 1990 in some European countries.
*Source:* International Dairy Federation (1992)

World War II a higher income implied a higher level of consumption, especially of the more expensive and more appreciated whole-fat milk and dairy products.[13] According to a micro-economic way of reasoning, the demand for basic foods was satisfied for most groups by the late 1930s, and a higher income was no longer accompanied by a corresponding increase in consumption of milk. In the third phase, the shifts can hardly be explained by changing incomes.[14] So, while changes in the inter-war period may require *some* additional explanation, quite different factors would seem to have caused the post-war development. Below I will discuss the role of milk supply, its adjustments to and/or influence on demand.

**The milk market in Norway**

This history starts with the profound changes in food production which took place in the final decades of the 19th century. Agriculture shifted to market-orientated farming, based on a mechanised, specialised and more intensive form of production.[15] Milk emerged as the dominant product, one reason being that grain could be imported cheaply from abroad. At least for some time the expanding market and slowly improving income levels ensured the sale of the increasing agricultural output.[16] Distribution and marketing gradually became better organised, through dairies owned co-operatively by the producers. Sale of fresh milk was most profitable, compared to other dairy products. But there was an increasing production of butter, mainly because the market for fresh milk was limited. Butter was far easier to handle for storage and transport, and for a while surplus butter could also be exported.

After the turn of the century, however, exporting butter became an unsatisfactory solution, as several other countries were experiencing similar problems of surplus.[17] The dairy farmers also encountered serious competition when cheap foods like margarine were introduced to Norwegian consumers. Margarine became an important end-product for the emerging whaling industry and herring fisheries, and the conflict over fat started. When the increasing production (Fig. 3) of the 1920s was no longer accompanied by a parallel rise in consumption, the result was extensive problems of surplus in supply and falling prices.[18] Around 1930 the farmers and farmer-owned dairies managed to gain control over the market, by organising and by measures of public policy,[19] and prices again started to rise. From 1930 and up to the present, the dairy industry has concentrated on controlling a market situation of surplus supply in order to ensure a reasonable income for the producers.[20]

One example is an act of 1931, which stipulated that the surplus was to be handled by the mandatory addition of butter to all margarine.[21] The background for this regulation was farmers' pressure for protection – but, perhaps surprisingly, also most of the margarine industry supported this. The reason was threat of competition from imported margarine, with Unilever as the main actor. In practice, the mandatory mixing of butter into margarine functioned as a technical barrier to trade. The percentage of butter in the margarine was gradually raised towards the end of the 1930s, starting at 0.5% and reaching a maximum of more than 20%. The overall result of these various measures was that not only did the surplus of milk and butter disappear, but also a steep rise in dairy production was triggered off.

After a temporary reduction during World War II, dairy production continued to increase, peaking in the 1950s. In the post-war period, dairy production and marketing has been strictly regulated through negotiations between farmers' organisations and the Norwegian state.[22] Agreements are made concerning the total level of dairy production for the following year, milk prices from the farm, consumer prices, and subsidies. Milk prices to the consumers are kept at a relatively low level by means of heavy subsidies from the state. From the farmers' side, the point is to guarantee dairy farmers' incomes while at the same time ensuring the sale of the total production.

Innovations in breeding methods etc. have resulted in more efficient production, and output has been growing steadily (Fig. 3). This has led to a tremendous pressure on the market – and on the negotiated production goals. The declining demand has aggravated the situation. As noted, demand has also shifted to low-fat varieties. Since surplus milk is stored in the form of butter, the shift to low-fat milk was for a long time conceived as very threatening to the producers. When low-fat milk was introduced in 1984, it soon replaced a substantial portion of whole milk consumption.[23] This development has not yet levelled off. Producers have tried to compensate by active marketing of butter and other full- or high-fat dairy products, but the results have been mixed. In total, fat intake has been reduced in Norway.

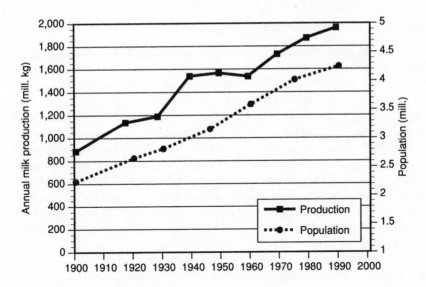

*Figure 3:* Total production of milk, and population growth in Norway, 1900–1990.
*Sources:* National Bureau of Statistics (1978)
National Nutrition Council (1992)

Even the introduction of low-fat milk may be regarded as a strategically rational action from a producer perspective, given the market situation at that time with declining consumption of milk. First, it would give the dairy industry a more positive image. But there are more practical considerations as well: 107 litres of whole milk is needed to produce 100 litres of low-fat milk. Thus, shifting to milk with less fat requires higher overall dairy production.[24] It was also assumed that low-fat milk could restrain the increasing demand for skimmed milk. With overall consumption levels falling, it may have been in the interest of the producers to support the sale of low-fat milk.

Over the past decade the dairy industry has invested massively in advertising milk, trying to keep a high profile against coffee, soft drinks and others. Other big campaigns have tried to capture market shares from the margarine industry, by promoting the dairy industry's own 'margarine' consisting of 80% butter. This 'margarine' is mainly marketed in a low-fat version which provides a 'healthy' image to the product.

To sum up, then, the overall impression is that the dairy industry benefited greatly from changes in consumption until the early 1970s. But as a market surplus was experienced already in the 1920s, the increase in consumption cannot be explained by changes on the demand side alone. Rather, the Norwegian dairy industry seems to have been very successful in influencing demand, so as to ensure the sale of a growing output. However, the decline in the 1970s cannot be explained in this way. In the following, I will discuss the changing role of science in the history of milk.

### The role of nutritional science[25]

Nutrition is important not only for the well-being of consumers, but for industry as well. For most application purposes, knowledge about the relationship between food and health has to be translated into dietary recommendations.[26] Such recommendations will state that some foods are more healthy than others – in other words a priority list with immediate consequences for the market.[27] In this way, translating scientific findings into recommendations and policy goals will therefore logically become an arena where conflicts between interests unfold, conflicts between different economic interests as well as between the supply side and the consumers. Nutritionists' views on milk have shifted several times – milk has been deemed both 'healthy' and a 'health hazard' over the years – making this a useful case for discussing the role and influence of nutritional science in a market context.

Urbanisation is generally accompanied by a need for better food distribution systems – to ensure regular supplies and acceptable quality of perishable foods, and also to avoid speculation and high food prices.[28] Just before the turn of the century it had become acknowledged that contaminated milk represented a considerable health problem in Norway.[29] The idea of centralised distribution through producer-owned co-operatives gained increasing support. Physicians as well as veterinarians and health authorities held that such centralisation would make possible hygienic improvements in premises and in transport, as well as simplifying control. Around 1910, several co-operatively owned dairies were established, and control was improved considerably. Clearly, this had beneficial effects on milk quality, but it also had other consequences for the consumers – in terms of higher prices.

A new phase started in the 1920s, when perceptions of milk changed – what had been a health hazard was now seen as essential nourishment. In the early days of nutritional science, milk seems to have played a rather minor role. It was not until the discovery of vitamins, mainly after World War I, that milk developed into a kind of nutritional 'miracle food' in Norway. Whole milk came to be *the* source of vitamins par excellence in Norwegian nutrition. By 1930 most experts had come out in great favour of whole milk and butter. It was a question of 'the more – the better'. The official Norwegian norm became 1 litre of whole milk per person per day.[30]

Milk could be marketed as clean *and* nutritious. But there was more to it than merely a scientific reorientation. To drink milk showed a positive, national spirit. This redefinition of the role of milk in the light of new scientific findings took place in the mid-war period, when the general attitude in society was favourable to science and scientifically based progress. Co-operation between agricultural policy and nutrition policy was based upon these new ideas, where different interests were to join hands in common efforts towards a more rational use of production resources, at the same time improving the general welfare of the population. Through public policy, dairy surplus was to be used to satisfy the need for milk *beyond* the existing market demand.[31] Indeed, calculations of total 'needs' according to the new norms even showed that production should be increased. Improved welfare could be obtained while at the same time supporting a crisis-ridden industry.

The promotion of milk was successful. Milk consumption increased steadily, reaching new heights in the 1950s. On the other hand, cardiovascular mortality rates increased dramatically as well – for Norwegian men, a 40% rise in the course of 10 years from the early 1950s to the 1960s.[32] The issue of coronary disease and its possible relationship to certain types of diets was becoming a topic of medical discourse. Gradually the dietary fat-cardiovascular disease hypothesis gained acceptance.[33] In line with this came new recommendations which changed perceptions of good nutrition completely, in that total fat intake was now to be reduced considerably. A lower intake of saturated fats was seen as most important, with fat from milk and other dairy products as one of the main sources (along with margarine). This meant that the consumption of all high-fat dairy products should be limited, whole milk as well as butter. Once more milk had become a hazard.

Questioning as it did the existing alliances and the milk policy rooted in these alliances, this change in the nutritional understanding of milk was not easily accepted.[34] It took more than 10 years of debate and quests for a reformulated policy, before the issue was put on the political agenda and new policy goals were formulated in a White Paper.[35] The setting for this formulation process, however, was not what had been intended by the advocates of a new policy. Once again, a main issue was dairy production and the threatening surplus of fat. The goal of lower fat intake was maintained, but it was moderated from 30 to 35% of calories. Intricate calculations were employed to show that this could be obtained by reducing the consumption of *imported* fats. Not only was the existing level of dairy production to be ensured, but also other national sources of fat for margarine production, such as herring oil, were protected.[36]

Experts have changed their minds only marginally after the reformulation of nutritional recommendations in the 1960s and 70s. First of all, more documentation has been collected on the importance of a diet with a low intake of fat and a high proportion of polyunsaturated fats. The public debate on the nutritional qualities of milk has, however, continued – with representatives from the dairy industry as active participants.

The first phase discussed in relation to milk consumption commenced in a period when milk was generally regarded as a nutritious food, albeit a luxury. But with the discovery of vitamins, the conception of milk changed: it became essential for all – and especially for children – to drink large amounts of whole milk daily. In that way nutrition experts actively supported milk marketing and milk promotion. Then, in the 1960s, the role of nutrition changed again, as the result of experts presenting arguments against milk fat. Since then, demand has slowly declined. This is due both to demographic changes and to lower milk consumption. However, it is difficult to disregard new nutritional recommendations when trying to explain the shift in demand from whole milk to low-fat and skimmed milk. Attitudes related to the ideal of a slim and fit body have probably also promoted this trend.

## The relationship between nutritional science and the dairy industry

After an initial period of conflict, there was for a long time harmony between the interests of the dairy industry and nutritional concerns in Norway. The dairy industry found nutrition and health experts to be useful allies. They could refer to obligations concerning general health and welfare – common goods in the society. Arguments as to the essential role of milk in nutrition, and studies of insufficient nutrition among certain population groups were utilised in this way – to legitimise regulations which (among other things) increased the industry's control of the market. Secondly, nutrition proved useful in milk marketing campaigns. However, it is difficult to determine the importance of nutritional science as such, as its recommendations supported the existing development of both demand and supply. In the third phase, however, consumption trends have not developed in accordance with agricultural interests.

The milk market is embedded in public policies. Analysis of these policies has shown that producer control has increased, and that nutritional arguments invariably had to yield when other strong interests were challenged. Focusing market processes, on the other hand, the outcome seems more successful from a nutritional point of view. The composition of the milk intake can be explained by nutritional science arguments. The decline is also in accordance with nutritional advice. The major explanation for this total decline, however, should be related to the increased welfare and the new situation of competition with income elastic substitutes to milk. Through political pressure and active marketing the dairy industry has only partly succeeded in postponing and subduing this development of demand. The market pressure produced by the surplus of milk production continues, as has been revealed on several occasions. A recent example is a statement made by the launchers of a large – partly publicly supported – marketing campaign to buy 'good Norwegian food':

*'Norwegians prefer low-fat milk. In 1988 each person consumed 52 litres of whole milk annually, in 1993 the figure had been reduced to 35 litres. The 'Good Norwegian' sign is to contribute to correcting our consumption habits. The 'light' – low-fat – revolution has created a fat surplus which the Norwegian dairy industry is striving to get rid of.'*[38]

The citation shows that the goals of the dairy industry have not changed, and that conflict between consumers and this industry persists.

In summation, then, this chapter has discussed some explanations for the dramatic changes in milk consumption over the last century in Norway. Others might be added. The structural factors that influence people's way of life are important here, as are economic interests. But seen in a long-term perspective – and disregarding a public policy captured by producer interests – consumers have acted in accordance with changes in the scientific understanding of the nutritional role of milk. This independent and active role of consumers should not be disregarded.

**Notes**

1  Levenstein (1988), p. 173.
2  Ibid, p. 160
3  The following reports refer to a SIFO study of Norwegian nutrition policy: Fjær (1990a, 1990b), Hansen (1990), Kjærnes (1990), Lien (1990), Jensen (1994), Kjærnes (1993). Material has been collected through archive studies, official documents, and interviews with key persons.
4  Gron (1942), Wold (1941).
5  Wold (1941).
6  The figure should be regarded as a broad outline. Data sources are not fully compatible, and data for the first 50 years are incomplete.
7  National Nutrition Council (1992).
8  See for example Frisch and Haavelmo (1938), Wold (1941), Vale (1984).
9  Kjærnes (1990).
10  Demographic changes have also been discussed (Vale, 1984).
11  Changes in the relative levels of prices have also favoured this development.
12  Lien (1990).
13  International Dairy Foundation (1992). Participating countries are mainly industrialised, developed countries, of which some are selected for comparison in this paper.
14  Frisch and Haavelmo (1938), Vale (1984).
15  Vale (1984).
16  Nordby (1990).
17  Munthe (1986).
18  Viinisalo (1993), Fjær (1990b).
19  Erland (1981).
20  Tennbakk (1988).
21  Munthe (1986).
22  Hovland (1979).
23  Munthe (1986).
24  Skimmed milk had existed as a variety of choice all the time. Low-fat milk was introduced in Sweden in 1969, and in Denmark in 1973 (Fjær 1990a). The fat content in whole-fat milk is 3.8, low-fat milk 1.5, and in skimmed milk 0.05.

25  Tennbakk (1988).
26  This has been more thoroughly discussed in Kjærnes (1993), pp. 91–106.
27  Botten and Kjærnes (1987).
28  Levenstein (1988).
29  Hirdman (1983).
30  Flateby (1979).
31  Rustung (1940).
32  Frisch (1941).
33  Central Bureau of Statistics (1987).
34  Lien (1990a).
35  Lien (1990a).
36  Ministry of Agriculture (1975).
37  Hansen (1990).
38  Interview with the Director General of the 'Good Norwegian' campaign, in *Dagens Næringsliv* 12 April 1994.

**Literature**

Botten, Grete, Kjærnes, Unni, 'Behov for mat og ønske om matvarer'. [Need for food and wish for food items], *Scand J Nutr* 4 (1987) pp. 116–120.

Central Bureau of Statistics. *Historical Statistics* (Oslo, 1978).

Central Bureau of Statistics. *Annual Report* (Oslo, 1987).

Erland, S. 'Norske Melkeprodusenters Landsforbund'. [The Norwegian Dairy Producers' Association] In: Hans Borgen, Erland, S., Ringen, Anders (eds.) *Norske melkeprodusenter gjennom 100 år.* [Norwegian dairy producers through 100 years]. Norwegian Dairy Producers' Association (Oslo, 1981), pp. 41–196.

Fjær, Svanaug, *Fettkabalen som ikke gikk opp. Lettmelkens historie.* [The fat puzzle that didn't work out. The history of low-fat milk]. Working Paper no.2, National Institute for Consumer Research (Oslo 1990a).

Fjær, Svanaug, *Makt, marked og margarin. Fettreguleringens politikk.* [Power, market and margarine. The politics of fat regulation.] Working Paper no.6, National Institute for Consumer Research (Oslo, 1990b).

Flateby, Anne M., *Opptakten til en norsk næringsmiddellovgivning. Ca 1880–1910.* [The emergence of a Norwegian Food Law. c.1880–1910]. Thesis. Department of History, University of Oslo (Oslo, 1979).

Frisch, Ragnar, 'Sosialøkonomiske problemer ved kostholdet'. [Social-economic problems in connection with the diet]. Introductory chapter in Wold, K.G. (1941), pp. 1–23.

Frisch, Ragnar, Haavelmo, Trygve, 'Etterspørselen etter melk i Norge'. [Milk demand in Norway.] *Statsøkonomisk Tidsskrift* 1938, no.1.

Grøn, Frederik, *Om kostholdet i Norge fra omkring 1500-tallet og op til vår tid.* [Dietary habits in Norway from the 16th century and up to the present time.] Jacob Dybwad (Oslo, 1942).

Hansen, Ranveig I., *Den hensiktsmessige ernæringspolitikken. Prosessen fram til stortingsmeldingen om norsk ernærings- og matforsyningspolitikk.* [Appropriate nutrition policy. The process leading to the Norwegian food and nutrition policy]. Working Paper no.8, National Institute for Consumer Research (Oslo, 1990).

Hirdman, Yvonne, *Matfrågan. Mat som mål och medel Stockholm 1870–1920.* [The Food Issue. Food as objective and means, Stockholm 1870–1920.] Raben & Sjögren (Stockholm, 1983).

Hovland, Einar, 'Smør og margarin blir ett fett'. [Butter and fat – one and the same thing]. *Historisk Tidsskrift 58* (1979), pp. 305–325.

International Dairy Foundation. Consumption statistics for milk and milk products. *Bulletin of the International Dairy Foundation* (1992) no.270: 1–22.

Jensen, Thor Ø. The political history of Norwegian nutrition policy, in John Burnett, Derek J. Oddy (eds.), *The origin and development of food policy in Europe*, Leicester University Press (London, 1994), pp. 90–111.

Kjærnes, Unni, *Velferdskrav og landbrukspolitikk. Om framveksten av norsk ernæringspolitikk.* [Welfare demands and agricultural policy. On the emergence of Norwegian nutrition policy]. Working Paper no.7, National Institute for Consumer Research (Oslo, 1990).

Kjærnes, Unni, 'A sacred cow. The case of milk in Norwegian nutrition policy'. In: Unni Kjærnes, Lotte Holm, Marianne Ekström, Elisabeth L. Fürst, Ritva Prättälä. *Regulating markets, regulating people. On food and nutrition policy.* Novus Forlag (Oslo, 1993), pp. 91–106.

Levenstein, Harvey, *Revolution at the table. The transformation of the American diet.* Oxford University Press (New York, Oxford 1988).

Lien, Marianne, *The Norwegian nutrition and food supply policy. Accomplishments and limitations of a structural approach.* Working Paper no. 4, National Institute for Consumer Research (Oslo, 1990).

Ministry of Agriculture. *Om norsk matforsynings- og ernæringspolitikk.* [On Norwegian food and nutrition policy.] Report to the Storting, No.32 1975–76 (Oslo, 1975).

Munthe, Preben, *Norsk jordbruk, politikk og utvikling.* [Norwegian agriculture, policy and development.] Norwegian University Press (Oslo, 1986).

National Nutrition Council. *Annual report 1991* (Oslo, 1992).

Nordby, Trond, *Det moderne gjennombruddet i bondesamfunnet.* [The modern breakthrough in rural society]. Norwegian University Press (Oslo, 1990).

Rustung, Erling, *Kostholdsstudier.* [Dietary studies]. Johan Grundt Tanum (Oslo, 1940).

Tennbakk, Bodil, *En analyse av produksjonsmålet for melk.* [An analysis of production goals for milk]. Thesis. Department of Economics, University of Bergen (Bergen, 1988).

Vale, Per H., *Melkeetterspørselen i Norge i perioden 1975–1982.* [The demand for milk in Norway in 1975–1982.] Agricultural University of Norway,

Department of Agricultural Economics. Report No.49 (Ås, 1984).

Viinisalo, Mirja, 'Butter-margarine issues in Finland before the Second World War', in Kjærnes, Unni et al (eds.) *The Politics of Nutrition.* Novus Forlag. (Oslo, 1993), pp. 107–122.

Wold, Knut G., *Kosthold og levestandard. En økonomisk undersøkelse.* [Diet and standard of living. An economic inquiry]. Fabritius & Sønners Forlag (Oslo, 1941).

# 10

# THE DEVELOPMENT OF CHEESE CONSUMPTION IN FRANCE IN THE PAST 150 YEARS

## Jacques Pinard

Cheese has always formed an important element of the food of the French lower classes, but it has become for some decades a significant part of the meal throughout all levels of society, as a consequence of which its consumption has strongly increased from the beginning of this century. The consumption of cheese in Paris at the eve of the First World War was estimated at 3 kilograms per head annually – an amount comparable with or a little above that at the end of the 18th century – and doubled between the inter-war years, reaching an average of 8.8 kilograms for the entire French population by 1959. In this way France had to import some kinds of cheese, while at the same time exporting certain qualities of cheese, due to the wide range of types that are produced all over the country. Nowadays consumption is about 18 kilograms (Fig.1).

The following question will be addressed: in which way has cheese, a food product that has always been an essential element in the daily food pattern of the French, undergone a transformation in its technical, economic and social aspects, as part of the general development of the foodmarket over the past 150 years?

### Before 1850: traditional and mainly popular cheese consumption

Until the middle of the last century the food of the rural population remained limited in the choice of consumption available, even considering the availability of a certain range of local products. Vegetables, either raw or cooked as in the case of starch products, were often the basis of the diet, for example in the form of soups, or as a garnish with some meat.[1]

Meat as part of the meal consisted mostly of poultry or pork, according to social class, season, feast meal or rural/urban differences; the so-called red-meats (beef, veal, mutton) were more rarely on the table.[2]

The required protein-level for a balanced diet was – though not on a conscious level – obtained from eggs, freshwater fish from lakes, ponds and rivers, as well as from the sea and occasionally from game. The pleasant complement of today's sweet dishes seldom occurred on the everyday menu of ordinary people.

Yet, there was one dish that appeared almost daily on the table of even the poorest people, rural or urban, namely cheese in its most varied forms, according to the regions and seasons. The reason for this omnipresence is simple enough: in rural areas where milk was produced on every farm, from cows, ewes and goats, cheese in the form of cream cheese ('fromage blanc') was easily produced. It was sufficient to have the milk curdled and drained and salt added before drying in a preferably cool place, like a cellar, when not eaten immediately.

Soon some other operations evolved and completed this simple preparation through fermentation by adding 'noble' moulds, as yet unknown, or by pressing the cheese and, even better, by heating in an oven, for example in the household kitchen, to change the components.

As early as in the Middle Ages, there was a large choice of cheeses in France, nowadays labeled as fermented, pressed or 'cooked' cheeses, some of which were sold already in urban markets. In towns of every region, housewives could find, apart from cream cheese made by themselves from bought milk, an assortment of cheese products from neighbouring regions, sold by peasants alongside their other farm products.

Some cheeses were already famous at the end of the *Ancien Régime*, such as *Brie*[3], *Munster*[4], and *Roquefort*; cheeses that were sent off to markets of faraway cities, where they were appreciated by wealthy people from the upper class.

At this time the size and amount of cheese consumed in the countryside was small. The herds were mostly restricted to one or two animals and usually employed for draught, which meant a low milk production. The average peasant family would have a similar number of sheep and goats.

The making of goat's cheese was widespread in earlier times, because the frugal animal was satisfied with the grass of roadsides and gave enough milk to produce a cheese every two or three days. However, traces of marketing are not found before the end of the last century.[5]

The more important herds belonged to secular and religious manor estates, or village communities, where animals were herded on meadows called 'alpages' at the higher altitudes in the mountains, like the Alps.[6] Milk from those herds produced larger cheeses generally stored for a longer time to mature, in places with a more or less constant temperature (cellars belonging to an abbey or a castle), after which they were transported over longer distances. This was the case for *Gruyères*, *Fourmes* and other mountain cheeses, which were produced far from the big centres of consumption and were transported in large numbers by carriers from remote regions. Monasteries dedicated themselves to the production of cheese in the 'Bassin Parisien' and in the western part of France, as in the case of the Trappists in the province of Maine, from which came the famous *Port-Salut*. In those

## LES GRANDS FROMAGES TRADITIONNELS FRANÇAIS

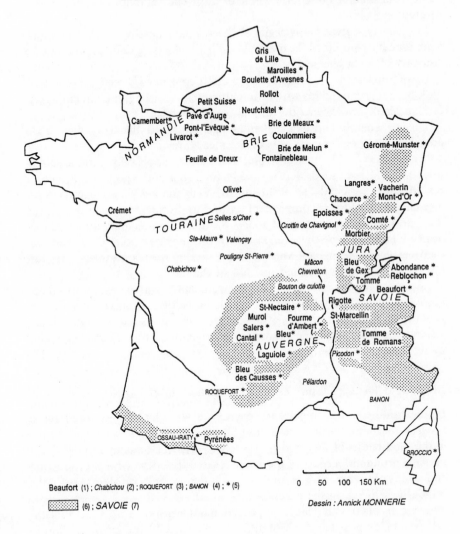

Fig.1 – Main French cheeses and regions making them. (By courtesy of J.R.PITTE 1987). 1– cow's cheese; 2 – goat's cheese; 3 – ewe's cheese; 4 – goat or ewe's cheese; 5 – Cheese A.O.C. (Appellation d'Origine Contrôlée); 6 – Main cheese producing region.

regions peasants in the first half of the nineteenth century were beginning to sell their cheese products and soon applied much of their dairying efforts to this product, sometimes adding those from neighbouring farms to produce the famous local cheeses, while keeping for themselves low-grade cheese made from skimmed or churned milk or those cheeses that turned out wrong or grew too old.

In this way a great many regional cheeses have developed; cheeses which since then have obtained the mark of nobility and have gained entrance to the category of great cheeses.

In addition some by-products were often consumed directly, like butter-milk in the form of soups with different names according to the regions, e.g. *la barattée* or *la caboussa* on the hills of the Perche.[7]

This consumption provided casein and improved the daily diet, when added to the other constituents of the meal (bread, butter).

It is true, as C. Thouvenot wrote, that: 'This humble daily pittance could not be considered as a dessert for the larger strata of the population, since it remained the principal dish of the supper'. Only among the privileged classes was cheese considered complementary and appreciated as such during the meal and sometimes eaten, as today by the Anglo-Saxons, after a sweet dessert. This explains the French expression 'entre la poire et le fromage' (between pear and cheese), which denotes a business to be handled during an important moment of the meal, if not of the day.

At the beginning all these cheeses were made on the farm, produced according to traditional methods, even when the first initiatives of industrial production came from large cattle breeders, who gathered the milk for the larger-scale production of cheese with a more uniform quality, made possible by technical improvements.

### 1890–1950: The appearance of industrial cheeses on the market

In the middle of the nineteenth century new technology allowed for a progressive change in the conditions of that way of life and more specifically in the food habits of the French. There was greater access to a much larger range of products, because of the lower prices due to new ways of production and means of transportation on the one hand, and the general increase in the standard of living on the other.[8]

As means of communication improved, mass transport across the country-side was made possible. First of all, the emergence of the railways allowed agricultural products to reach out to more and more remote markets. In that way competition increased and producers were compelled to improve their technology in making an acceptable product. This was particularly true for cheese, the making of which was in the hands of manufacturers; big merchants often progressively eliminated cottage cheeses through utilization of new equipment and processes.

At the end of the 19th century, the introduction of a continuously working centrifugal cream separator replaced the ancient method used at the farm of separating cream by decanting. This allowed the collecting of milk in cans instead of, as previously, only cream. However, the skimming of milk was more rigorously undertaken in the dairies, so this also changed the composition of the cheeses and affected the quality and the taste. On the other hand, research was carried out by biologists, who were linked to these new industrial dairies and who applied principles of lactic fermentation, discovered by Pasteur. This led to the use of purest fermenting agents, resulting in the production of a more homogeneous cheese with a more consistent quality, taking the character of famous cheeses from other regions. *Brie* and *Camembert* are produced in all the big dairy regions: Lorraine, Touraine and Poitou. Some decades later, during the inter-war years, it proved to be necessary to promulgate a law (1935) defining guaranteed places of origin (appellations), rules and conditions governing the production of every type of cheese under a particular label, and which compelled – in some cases with the help of the Court – imitators to respect the rules. It took some time for the manufacturers to submit themselves to the law, but the guaranteed cheeses met with success and numerous regions applied for labels on their cheese: in these days the number was about thirty.

The use of lorries instead of former horse-drawn carts to collect the milk from the farms, allowed dairies to extend their areas. As a result, there was tough competition between collectors, caused by the increasing demand for milk by the consumers as well as by the producers of dairy products and the demand for milk by cheese producers.

The necessity to go and collect the raw material from larger and larger areas, was eventually relieved by agreements about the precise delineation of the boundaries of the monopolized areas, within which every dairy was to collect milk. Not only did this have a cost-reducing effect, but also in-fighting ended. Also, the wider expansion of the dynamic enterprises was halted, though in some instances they set up other dairies, not too far from the first plant, in productive but not yet explored areas. These newly-founded dairies were more or less autonomous[9], producing often the same cheese by the same processes, but under a different label, giving the consumer the impression that they were being offered a wider range of products. It is only in the last few decades, for reasons of economy of scale and thanks to new methods put into operation, that we see a regrouping of the diversity into one single firm, or the creation of a new company through the merging of small enterprises. However, the more famous products keep their own trademark.

In the second half of the nineteenth century growing urbanization and industrialization led to a high concentration of population in a limited space. These urbanized populations themselves produce only a small part of foodstuffs they consume (vegetables raised in small kitchen gardens, some bottled preserves) so they have to resort to industrial processed foods. To market their products, factories have to observe very strict health rules, and moreover, adapt themselves to the taste of large numbers of consumers. The aim was to retain the consumer, who originally came from the countryside from regions like Normandy, Auvergne and Savoie. This resulted in a generalization of consumption of the most famous cheeses, often those with a less strong flavour. Cheese continues to play an important part in everyday meals and as a snack that workers bring along to eat at the work site in mills, yards or pits in the same way that craftsmen and peasants did during agricultural labour.

Likewise, in meals eaten at home and prepared by the housewife, cheese has always been of some importance, despite the increasing consumption of meat, vegetables and fruits, because it was cheaper and allowed the eating of bread, in other words 'il faisait du profit', as was said formerly (probably the meaning of which was to have a nourishing and substantial meal) (cit.C. Thouvenot).[10] However, in towns where the population was socially more differentiated, the consumption of cheese became more varied: next to the hard cheeses which were still in the middle of the nineteenth century the only ones to qualify for transport over long distances – the means of transport were relatively slow – there was a rise in consumption of fresh cheeses.[11]

Up to the second half of the last century, fresh cheeses were consumed during Lent by religious families to replace meat. They were produced in regions that became more accessible through the construction of railways, as for example the Pays de Bray northwest of Paris, where dairies began from the 1870s to make new products, like *Petit Suisse*, *Demi Sel*, and later *Double Crème*. These products were inventions of Charles Gervais[12], founder of the still famous company and owned by the firm B.S.N. Danone. Well-prepared and refined cheeses produced by more and more mechanized dairies were now asked for by middle classes for whom they replaced the sweets and also increasingly by wealthy classes who added them to their menu. The production in these modern dairies was made easier by the use of the steam engine, which enabled the mechanization of cream separation, churning and pasteurization by treating the whole of the milk. The plants were proud of this equipment and they showed it in their advertising.

One could say that the consumption of cheese became popular and this showed in the demand by new types of customers – wealthy as well as less wealthy –, made possible by improvement of transport and techniques of packaging in boxes made from wood (a technique claimed by Lepetit in 1870 and later by Ridel in 1890) as well as preserving by cooling techniques, so that seasonal conditions could be accommodated.[13] The cheese of *Roquefort* took advantage of these developments. One could speak of a democratization of consumption, mainly because the price decreased, at least in relative value. New cheeses from abroad appeared at that time, at least on the urban market: *Parmesan* which accompanied the Italian immigration to several industrial regions also spread to the South of France.

At the same time some of the French cheeses were copied by dairies abroad, like the blue cheese of Auvergne by the Dutch, and *Roquefort* by the Danes under the name of *Danablu*. The import of these cheeses to the United States replaced the French export during the First World War. But it is only after the Second World War that conditions under which consumption took place changed significantly.

## After 1950: a dual consumption of current cheeses and refined cheeses

In France the consumption of cheese and food consumption in general since the last 50 years has fundamentally changed under the influence of a new way of life. After the restrictions of the war and the post-war period, when cheeses made from skimmed milk were the only ones available, the French were once again able to eat to their heart's content. So again families had a full meal, that is to say with cheese and sweets at the end of each meal.

This remained until medical and aesthetic considerations curbed the consumption of foods that were claimed to be responsible for their lipid content or for supplying too many calories, both being the origin of so-called diseases of the century (cardiovascular diseases, overweight, diabetes). Cheeses are the first among the high fat-containing foods aimed at. But even if many a big eater was willing to reduce the quantity, he was not inclined to give up the quality.

Like wines, new cheeses appeared on the market during the 1970s and 1980s and can be classified in two groups. The first comprises industrial cheeses made from pasteurized milk in the form of a more or less soft consistency, mainly tasteless[14] and comparable to some foreign imitations that are trying with little success to gain access to the French market. These cheeses produced by the large-scale food industry are endowed with a label bringing to mind some prestigious site, where for example an abbey is situated, but which does not refer to any geographical region. Neither being able nor wishing to do so is a strong handicap in getting the product accepted by the French consumer, as is also the case with wine. The second group corresponds to cheeses 'de pays' or local cheeses. Some of them are already famous and are also produced again by industrial dairies according to ancient processes, that is to say essentially 'au lait cru' (with raw milk). The pasteurizing process eliminates the flavours that make the reputation of good cheese. Cottage cheese is in this category: the different operations are in principle carried out by hand, for example the moulding of curdled milk with a ladle instead of automatically by machine. To be sure, these cheeses are more expensive, but as the gustative quality is better by far, they will find their way to the connoisseur.

Since the 1960s the marketing of all consumer goods changed rapidly with the expansion of supermarkets, selling cheese nowadays for 80 percent against only 20 percent through cheesemongers.

Manufacturers are very soon subjected to financial conditions (prices and terms of payment) imposed on them by the wholesale trade, which employs new means of delivery and slashes prices by raising competition to a maximum for current foodstuffs, like cheese.

Manufacturers aim at the mediocre to satisfy a wider range of customers, launching grand-scale advertising in the media, occasionally inspired by foreign fashions. Those consumers, whose palate is becoming less and less educated, partly because the majority of them have no reference point to distinguish between good and bad products, are easily deceived and often accept any product as long as it is cheap. However, the total amount of money those consumers spend on shopping in supermarkets is fairly high, which is a sign that they are in a comfortable position to afford a luxurious diet. The high-grade cheeses, and particularly cottage cheeses, are hence sold by specialist merchants, like cheesemongers, delicatessen shops, local shops in the countryside and suburbs, or at daily or weekly markets, directly supplied by reputable producers, who themselves deliver or offer their cheeses. It is also possible to taste them in some gastronomic restaurants; especially those that are able to compose a varied and carefully prepared cheese platter, although it is often exceptional in the opinion of the specialist in the art of cooking.

In some French regions such restaurants promote local products, among which are cheeses. This is the case for *Munster* in the *fermes-auberges* in the Vosges.[15] Tourism has largely contributed to the appreciation and in this way to the selling of regional cheese from the Alps, the Pyrenees and Massif Central, in the same way as it has done for wines that were until now little known outside the country.

The success often met by the majority of French cheeses in different circles has led to promotion in symposia and in international congresses organising wine and cheese parties, where there is an opportunity to enjoy the products of different regions, although they are not always processed according to the previously-mentioned rules.

During the last twenty years the producers of industrial and cottage cheeses have been helped by some more or less swiftly adopted new techniques.

For the younger consumer and perhaps for the least expert, the range of fresh products has largely extended, due to new flavours with exotic fruit (Kiwi, maracuja) and the adaptation to new technical processes, like ultrafiltration. Young cheeses and fully matured cheeses are raised to high savoury levels and get the desired label of guaranteed cheese (in French: *Appellation d'Origine Contrôlée*: *A.O.C.*). In the period between 1951–52 the Convention of Stresa was approved and signed by several European countries, extending the guarantees to food products outside France. The European Economic Community has recently in 1991 admitted the notion of a geographical guaranteed appellation for food products. French dairy training has a high standard and managers from these schools, as well as engineers from the higher Agricultural Colleges, are much in demand. In these circumstances it is not surprising that the increase in the consumption of cheese has not slowed down. A part of this increase can be explained by the usual products that are daily consumed in restaurants of businesses, canteens and fast-food places. Cheeses of good quality, cottage or industrial cheeses are nowadays much in demand in spite of the higher price, and thanks to the general growth of the standard of living. A growth in a standard of living would be accompanied by progress in the consumer's taste so that he should be able to distinguish differently produced cheeses or food products in general and turn for his daily consumption to quality cheeses, that were formerly either served only on festive occasions, or reserved for the rich and the connoisseur.

**Notes**

1  Bonnain-Moerdijk (1975).
2  Thouvenot (1987).
3  Delfosse (1987).
4  Gaudefroy (1987).
5  Gilbank (1987).
6  Pitte (1987).
7  Vivier (1987).
8  Pinard (1988), p. 58.
9  Peltre (1987).
10  Thouvenot (1987).
11  Garnier (1987).
12  Courtine (1987), p. 116.
13  Vidal (1987).
14  Le Liboux (1984), p. 23.
15  Dietrich (1987).

**Literature**

Bonnain-Moerdijk, Rolande, 'L'Alimentation paysanne en France 1850 et 1936'. *Études Rurales*, no. 58 (April–June 1975), pp. 29–49.

Courtine, Robert J., *Les fromages*. Larousse 1987, 2nd ed., pp. 255.

Delfosse, Clairee, 'Une richesse locale menacée: la production de Brie dans la région de Meaux à la fin du XIXème siècle', in *Histoire et Géographie des Fromages*, Université de Caen 1987, pp. 43–52.

Dietrich, Geneviève, 'Le Munster. Paysages et systèmes d'élevage', in *Histoire et Géographie des Fromages*, Université de Caen, pp. 67–77.

Le Liboux, Jean-Luc, *Nouveau Guide des Fromages en France*. Rennes, Ouest France ed. 1984, 185pp.

Garnier, Bernard, 'Paris et les fromages frais au XIXè siècle. Un demi-siècle de vente en gros aux halles', in *Histoire et Géographie des Fromages*, Université de Caen, pp. 123–135.

Gaudefroy, Ghislain, 'Le fromage de Neufchâtel. Note historique', in *Histoire et Géographie des Fromages*, Université de Caen, pp. 137–144.

Gilbank, Gérard, D'une production de survie à une production commerciale. L'histoire du 'Crottin de Chavignol', in *Historie et Géographie des Fromages*, Université de Caen, pp. 151–156.

Peltre, Jean, 'Un pionnier de l'industrie fromagère: le département de la Meuse', in *Histoire et Géographie de Fromages*, Université de Caen, pp. 201–207.

Pinard, Jacques, *Les industries alimentaires dans le monde*. Masson 1988, 216pp.

Pitte, Jean-Robert, 'Une lecture ordonnée de la carte des fromages traditionnels en France', in *Histoire et Géographie des Fromages*, Université de Caen, pp. 201–207.

Thouvenot, Claude, 'Fromages de 'pauvres' et fromages de 'riches'. L'exemple de la France', in *Histoire et Géographie des Fromages*, Université de Caen, pp. 209–221.

Vidal, Christianne, 'Le fromage de Roquefort et l'évolution récente de la production laitière dans la Lozère', in *Histoire et Géographie des Fromages*, Université de Caen, pp. 223–230.

Vivier, Michel, 'Production traditionnelle et système agricole. Le cas des fromages et de la fromagée du Perche', in *Histoire et Géographie des Fromages*, Université de Caen, pp. 231–242.

Divers. *Alimentation et régions*. Études réunies par J. Peltre et C. Thouvenot d'un Collogue sur le thème 'Cuisines, régimes alimentaires et espaces régionaux'. Presses Universitaires de Nancy, 1989, 524pp.

We gratefully record our thanks to Professor P. Laborde of the University of Bordeaux III for information provided on ewe's milk cheese in the Atlantic Pyrenees.

# II

# FROM ELITE CONSUMPTION TO MASS CONSUMPTION. THE CASE OF CHOCOLATE IN BELGIUM

*Peter Scholliers*

Till the end of the 19th century, chocolate was a very expensive product, consumed exclusively by rich people. Quite suddenly, around 1900, the price of chocolate diminished appreciably, and more and more people could start enjoying it. So, within the time-span of a few years, chocolate shifted from an elitist consumption item to a product that was on its way to become mass-consumed. In this respect, various questions can be asked. For instance, what were the causes of the rapid fall of chocolate prices and when did working-class families start to consume chocolate? Such questions, limited to the subject, refer to more general problems with regard to processes of introduction and spread of consumption goods, and to the formation of the modern diet and way of life.

Belgium offers a good example of the changes with regard to food consumption since the country was open to many foreign influences. This paper aims at considering the emergence and development of Belgian chocolate producers and, more in particular, the move from a luxury consumption item towards a current foodstuff of the modern Belgian diet.

## Fine Belgian chocolates

The first Belgian chocolatiers appeared at the end of the 17th century.[1] These were small with very limited production, and only using human energy. The city of Brussels played an important role, being the capital of the Southern Netherlands where the demand for luxury goods was high. Cocoa, sold as a beverage, was very much appreciated by the court and the haute bourgeoisie, thus testifying to a genuine 'chocolatomania'.[2] In Brussels, steam power was introduced in 1835 for the manufacturing of slabs of chocolate. The 'Almanach du Commerce' of 1841 listed 50 'confiseurs, chocolatiers et patissiers', among which were Claret ('Fabricant de chocolats fins et hygiéniques') and Cordier ('Confiseur du Roi').[3] The industrial census of 1846 reported that Brussels had 61 confectioners, employing 177 workers and two steam engines of 2 H.P. each. The capital represented 14% of all Belgian chocolatiers and confiseurs, but 30% of total employment. Next to the two

Brussels steam engines, a third one (of 14 H.P.) had been installed in Tournai (province of Hainault). It was not until the late 1850s that the Brussels chocolate trade underwent a (modest) mechanization process. Between 1858 and 1864 seven steam engines, totalling 22 H.P., were installed. A second 'wave' of mechanization occurred in the 1870s, when six engines (totalling 24 H.P.) were introduced.[4] The 13 new engines averaged 3.5 H.P., clearly indicating technological inferiority with regard to producers in some other Belgian cities. The 'Almanach du Commerce' of 1871 mentioned 48 choco-latiers in Brussels, among which were Joosten ('usine à vapeur') and Schreurs frères ('usine à vapeur modèle, gros et exportation').[5]

The industrial censuses of 1896 and 1910 show an intensified mechaniza-tion, and further expansion and decentralization. The chocolate manufac-turers had left the city of Brussels for the suburbs, while producers in other Belgian cities outgrew the Brussels ones. The average number of workers in the Belgian factories reached 14.6 in 1896 and 30.4 in 1910, whereas the engines averaged 12.9 H.P in 1896 and 21.2 in 1910. Of course, these figures are still low compared to some other industries, and even within the food industry, the mechanization of the chocolate factories remained rather modest. Yet, the average hides spectacular developments (see an example below). Moreover, the pace of growth was important. Between 1896 and 1910, the growth rate of the average H.P. was low in sugar refineries (+ 7 per cent), flour mills (+ 15 per cent) or margarine factories (-11 per cent), while a growth of 65 per cent in the average H.P. was reached in the chocolate factories.[6] This indicates a rapid and fundamental change in the production process of chocolate factories in the 1890s and 1900s.

The Côte d'Or factory in the Brussels suburb Anderlecht is a good example of changes occurring in the industry.[7] Ch.Neuhaus started a small choco-laterie in 1870. Business seemed to flourish and in 1885 a steam engine of 25 H.P. was installed, which was quite important in this trade during that period. In 1889, the Neuhaus factory was bought by J. Bieswal for 200,000 gold francs. Although the entreprise was being mechanized, the production was still artisanal. 'A la fin du 19e siècle la fabrication tant du chocolat que de la confiserie était encore en partie artisanale et manuelle', as P. Bieswal put it. Due to expropriations for building the Gare du Nord, Bieswal moved to Anderlecht in 1899 where he shared the hall of an old flour mill with the confiseur L. Michiels. Documents of the sale of 1889 and the expropriation of 1899 permit comparison of the factory's equipment at an interval of ten years: there were many more engines, machines and semi-automated tools in 1899 than ten years earlier.[8] P. Bieswal noted that 'on constate déjà l'apparition de nouvelles machines: machines à nettoyer le cacao et armoire frigorifique ainsi que (. . .)des petites machines pour la confiserie'. Many of these machines had been introduced recently in the international chocolate manufacture. How-ever, P. Bieswal mentioned that the machines which revolutionized the production process, the 'conches', were only installed in 1906.[9]

This was due to the fact that the purchase of such machines was quite expensive. Bieswal and Michiels decided to fuse their firms into the 'Société Anonyme Alimenta', to erect new buildings, to raise the company's capital (to 400,000 francs in 1906 and 600,000 francs in 1908) and to install new steam engines in 1908 (65 H.P.), 1911 (25 H.P.) and 1913 (250 H.P.). In 1930, a powerful engine of 1,000 H.P. was used. This rapid expansion required a growing number of employees from some 50 in the 1850s, to 100 in 1913, 230 in the 1920s, and finally 350 in 1930.[10]

So, the turn of the century was a decisive period when it was decided to enter fully into the path of mechanization. Côte d'Or was not the only Belgian firm which did so: for instance, Victoria s.a. started in 1896 (with 800 employees and 1,000 H.P.), Jacques s.a. also started in 1896 (using 200 H.P.), while several firms modernized in the 1900s (such as the Chocolaterie Ruelle or the Chocolaterie Grétry).[11] According to the 'Annuaire du Commerce' of 1901, the Brussels area had 61 chocolatiers (against 48 in 1871).

The Belgian chocolate producers intensified their mechanization efforts around 1900 in order to respond to increased competition. Indeed, Germany, France, England, the Netherlands and Switzerland imported a growing quantity of chocolate into Belgium (untaxed). In their turn, producers in these countries probably intensified their mechanization efforts in order to respond to price increases of cocoa beans and to wage rises in the 1870s. The increased production capacity required new markets. The Belgians were forced to follow the mechanization process, albeit with arrears of some years. However, around 1900 the Belgians benefited from this since they were able to use much of the latest technology.

The special position of the Belgian chocolate producers can be noticed when prices are considered. According to Belgian trade statistics, the price of Belgian and imported chocolate ran fully parallel throughout the 19th century till 1896. Between 1895–99 and 1900–05, the wholesale price of domestically produced chocolate fell by 20 per cent, whereas the price of imported chocolate diminished by only 12 per cent.[12] Belgian chocolate remained at a lower price level till the great war. The largest price differential was reached in 1912, when Belgian chocolate cost 25 per cent less than the imported. This price development was quite remarkable since it contrasted with that of imported cocoa beans: although the raw material became cheaper in the 1890s, it did not experience such marked price diminution. Thus, it can be assumed that the Belgian price decline was the result of the mechanization effort, which probably was more intense in this country than in most of the surrounding countries during that period. An additional factor might have played a role. The introduction of new technology allowed the recruitment of an increasing number of (young) women coming from rural areas. In 1846, 5 per cent of the work force was female, in 1896 this rose to 34 per cent, in 1910 to 38 per cent and in 1926 to 47 per cent. The Cote d'Or factory e.g., situated next to the Gare du Midi since 1899, could largely employ workers commuting daily from the Flemish countryside.[13] Also, union membership was weak. Undoubtedly, all this helped to save on the wage bill.

## Price of Belgian and imported chocolate

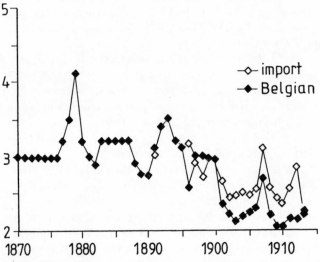

*Source:* D. Degrève (1982), p.469–70.

As a consequence of these various changes, Belgium's chocolatiers were able to improve their position on the international market. Indeed, between 1890 and 1910 the exported quantity of chocolate grew by 3170 per cent, whereas the imported quantity rose by 130 per cent.[14] In 1900, an official report noted that 'malgré les progrès réalisés, cette industrie parvient difficilement à se créer des debouchés à l'étranger(. . .). C'est que nos fabricants se trouvent en présence de la forte concurrence qui leur est faite au dehors'.[15] In 1900, Belgium exported little to France, the U.K., the Netherlands and Germany. In 1904 however, an author wrote: 'L'exportation des chocolats de fabrication belge est aujourd'hui très importante'.[16] In 1910, chocolate was shipped to at least 17 different countries, amongst which were the direct competitors (Germany, the U.K., France, Holland and Switzerland, accounting for 29 per cent of total export), far-away competitors (the U.S.A. and Canada, accounting for 4 per cent of export), but above all new markets in Northern Africa and Turkey (accounting for 59 per cent of the total Belgian export!).[17] This can be considered as a real success, since it was precisely this latter market which was the subject of harsh competition between the European producers.

The growth of Belgium's chocolate producers can also be observed from the appreciable increase in the consumption of cocoa beans. Between 1894 and 1906, the world's consumption of cacao beans rose by 140 per cent;

Belgium's needs increased by 300 per cent, which was below the growth of the cocoa bean consumption of Germany (+320 per cent) and the U.S.A. (+370 per cent), but above the growth of all other producing countries (Austria-Hungary +280 per cent; Switzerland +205 per cent; U.K. +100 per cent; France +55 per cent; Holland +15 per cent).[18] But of course, the part of Belgium in total consumption of cocoa beans was still very modest: it amounted to 1.5 per cent in 1896 and to 2.5 per cent in 1906. After the war, the country succeeded in maintaining this share of about 2.5 per cent.[19]

Belgium's chocolate confectioners did particularly well around 1900. Mechanization caused a fall in the production cost, and together with the diminution of the price of the raw material, this caused a marked decline in the selling price.

### A genuine treat for children and adults . . . of all classes?

Till the 1890s, chocolate remained quite expensive. An advertisement in the 'Annuaire du Commerce' of 1891 mentioned a price of 2.50 francs for half a kilo of imported 'bon ordinaire' chocolate; Belgian chocolate must have been cheaper, say by 25 per cent. An unskilled bricklayer in Brussels earning 0.32 francs per hour, had to work for five to eight hours to buy half a kilo of chocolate. This, of course, was far beyond his means. The most expensive chocolate in the advertisement, the 'chocolat vanille extra', was worth 5.0 francs for 500 g.

The report of 1900, mentioned above, noted that consumption of chocolate had started to increase during the previous years: '(. . .) le chocolat, il y quelques années à peine, était considéré comme un aliment de luxe, est devenu un article de consommation beaucoup plus courant'. Does this mean that all classes of (Belgian) society started to enjoy the consumption of chocolate around 1900? Most probably, there was only a limited democratization of this consumption at first: the price diminution at the end of the century allowed the middle classes to start drinking and eating regularly this delicacy.

In the years previous to the war of 1914, working-class families did also start to consume chocolate. This can be observed from the results of a large-scale inquiry into food habits of Belgian working-class families in 1910. Whereas no chocolate consumption was reported in the 1891 budget inquiry, the 1910 inquiry showed an average consumption of 182 g per year and per consumption unit ('quet').[20] Probably, this meant the eating of some chocolate on special occasions such as the feast of St Nicholas or an anniversary. This is confirmed by literary sources, and one can find many references dealing with working-class chocolate consumption on special occasions. Just to give two examples from prominent Flemish writers: C. Buysse, describing a wedding in a Flemish village in 1905, mentioned that the guests were given currant buns with hot cocoa; S. Streuvels, describing school children in front of a bakery just before the St. Nicholas feast, mentioned the many desirable sweets amongst which were chocolate cigars.[21] Without great difficulty, more such references can be found in novels.

It is possible to follow the chocolate consumption of working-class families after the first World War, thanks to large-scale budget inquiries in 1921 and 1928–1929. In 1921, per year and per 'quet' 390 g of chocolate were consumed[22], and 1928–1929 650 g were eaten.[23] This was a growth of 114 per cent between 1910 and 1921, and of 67 per cent between 1921 and 1928. These figures show that chocolate had been introduced into the working-class diet just before the war, and that it had become more popular in the 1920s. One can assume that by then the 'special treat' of chocolate on the occasion of feasts had disappeared, and that chocolate became an everyday delicacy for the working class, including children and adults.[24]

The inquiry of 1928–1929 shows that within the working class, there was a direct relationship between income levels and consumption of chocolate and sweets in general. Indeed, the expenditure item 'confiture, sirop et chocolat' grew according to the increase in the family income[25], and the highest income group spent twice the amount of money on sweets as the lowest income group.

The budget enquiries give information on the consumption of families of white-collar workers. In 1921, their consumption of chocolate reached 534 g per year and per 'quet', against 390 g for working-class people, a difference of 36 per cent. In 1928–1929, the white-collar families consumed 717 g of chocolate per year and per 'quet', which was only 9 per cent more than working-class families. The chocolate consumption of working-class people obviously increased faster than that of the white-collar families in the 1920s. Yet, incomes of the latter families remained higher.

Seemingly, particularly working-class people had a marked preference for chocolate in the 1920s. This preference was maintained from the 1920s onwards, up to the 1970s. According to budget enquiries, working-class families caught up with the chocolate consumption of families of white-collar workers, independent workers, and employers from the late 1940s.[26]

Contemporaries had noticed the increased consumption of chocolate by the working class in the 1920s. In 'Le Sucre', a corporation's journal, it was written in November 1923: 'Avant la guerre, le chocolat était considéré comme un aliment de luxe, aujourd'hui il n'en est plus ainsi. Comme alimentation, chez l'ouvrier, cette friandise a pris une extension considérable; il n'y a pas un ménage qui n'en consomme, pour ainsi dire, journellement'.[27] A Belgian representative on the international conference of chocolate confectioners in Antwerp in 1930, said: 'Le chocolat et le cacao sont consommés d'une manière courante par toutes les classes de la société et spécialement par la masse des travailleurs'. He added that working-class people consumed chocolate 'non comme une friandise mais comme un élément important faisant partie intégrale de l'alimentation habituelle'.[28] He may have exaggerated (since he was pleading for the abolition of the 'taxe de luxe' of 6 per cent applied in 1921), but the fact remains that he was able to refer to augmented consumption by working-class people.

There are several factors which explain the particular interest in chocolate of the working class. First, the price development played an important role, or rather, the real price of chocolate.[29] The mechanization led to diminishing production costs and lower retail prices. Together, the average wage rose. So, the real price of chocolate diminished. This can be observed from the simple comparison of the price of chocolate per kilo and the hourly wage of a Brussels unskilled bricklayer.[30] In 1914, the real price of chocolate equalled 1.90 hours of work, and after an initial increase to 2.50 hours in 1919, it fell to 1.50 in 1920 and 1.60 in 1921. This meant an actual price decrease of some 20 per cent compared to the pre-war level. Although chocolate became more expensive in the second half of the 1920s (especially in 1926, with 3.00 hours of work for one kilo, when the Belgian franc devalued), the real price diminished in 1929 (to 1.70 hours). During the crisis years of the 1930s, this price fell even more (averaging 1.35 hours), reaching a level that was some 30 per cent below the pre-war one.[31] After the second World War, the price of chocolate remained at this rather low level.[32]

Chocolate was highly considered (after all, it had been a luxury product for centuries), and the sudden fall in the real price incited people to start consuming this food item. Still, other factors played a role. One of these was the fact that the energy value of chocolate was very high: in less than no time, a huge quantity of energy (for a relatively low price) could be taken in. It was noted in a popular cookbook, published in 1949, that 'chocolate has a very high caloric value, it gives high dynamic force and it is very digestible'[33], which was a generally accepted opinion. Could a slab of chocolate be considered as the predecessor of fast food?

Also, the cookbook enumerated other qualities of chocolate: 'cocoa is very healthy and not somniferous, nor does it cause heart palpitations'. This refers to a debate between supporters and opponents of chocolate, which goes back to the introduction of cocoa. In the 17th century chemists were selling cocoa as a medicine and in the early 19th century, factories advertised their chocolate as being 'hygiénique'. Chocolate confectioners became highly interested in the results of dietetic research. At the international conference of chocolate confectioners in Antwerp in 1930 for instance, the French professor of Medicine, H. Labbé, presented a survey of the scientific research of chocolate in the 19th and 20th centuries (concluding that chocolate consumption should be increased).[34] The fact that chocolate had been declared 'healthy' by many researchers was not without signifi-cance: it made socially acceptable the eating of chocolate by the young and the old, as long as 'normal' portions were not exceeded. This contrasted with the general opinion with regard to coffee, alcohol or tobacco which more and more were considered to be not very healthy.

This was good news for those who were fond of sweets. Many people simply enjoyed eating chocolate. In fact, consuming chocolate was one aspect of the global rising interest in eating sweetened food. The inter-war years could be characterized as the 'sugar years', because from that period consumption of sugar sky-rocketed in all European countries. So chocolate consumption was but one variable of this newly emerging interest.

Without doubt, there were class differences with regard to both the quantity and the quality of the consumed sweets. There are no data available on qualitatively differentiated consumption before the 1970s; the budget enquiry of 1978–1979 shows that the working class purchased the cheapest possible chocolate (and sweets in general), or the lowest quality.[35] Assuming that a similar relationship existed from the first World War, it can be suggested that, from then on, groups with high incomes continued eating cake, 'pralines', luxury chocolates and other expensive products, whereas working-class people chose the ordinary chocolate which became cheaper. So, while the richer classes had coffee or tea with 'patisserie', 'pralines' or other luxuries, the working-class families had their coffee with a piece of chocolate. Chocolate was not only eaten as a snack, but also as the working-class's everyday titbit.

Of course, the confectioners used in their advertisements the results of scientific research into characteristics of chocolate. This leads me to the last, but certainly not least factor in explaining the particular success of chocolate with the working class from the 1920s. Chocolate was a standardized product, which could be promoted and advertized throughout the country and indeed, throughout the world. Before 1914, simple advertisements were published in newspapers, but after the war, campaigns became much more sophisticated. It suffices to look at magazines of the period after 1918. Just to give one example: during the second World War, the 'Secours d'Hiver' helped in organizing food aid in Belgian cities; this institution published a monthly journal, and in December of 1942, a special issue with many advertisements was published.[36] Out of the 52 advertisements with regard to food and drinks, 12 concerned chocolate (or 23 per cent). All important brands were present (Côte d'Or, Victoria, Cibon, Kwatta, Martougin, Meyers, Van Loo . . .) often with impressive lay-out (using more than plain text, with drawings and an eye-catching font).

Advertising campaigns were not limited to publicity in papers and magazines. Producers quite often distributed free chocolate. Two examples can be given: the co-operative store, 'Limburgsche Cooperatie', distributed 25,000 slabs of chocolate in January 1922, in order to promote their own-produced product;[37] 'Côte d'Or' did the same on the occasion of the Brussels world fair of 1935.[38] Indeed, much was done in order to sell to as many people as possible.

## Concluding remarks

This, of course, was (and is) the quintessence of industrial capitalism, and chocolate proved to be an excellent product to achieve this purpose. In fact, the case of chocolate production and consumption is excellent in showing the introduction and spread of a food item in the modern diet, presenting interrelations between technology, management, marketing, science, retailing, state regulation, consumption and human wants, or in short: demand and supply sides.

So, the eager acceptance of chocolate by the public in general and the working class in particular, can be explained by a multitude of factors. Of decisive importance was the mechanization process which intensified in Belgium in the 1890s. The cost of production and the retail price fell. This was the prime condition for the spread of chocolate. With the significant rise in the output, much was done to increase the sale: advertising campaigns (in newspapers, by distributing free samples, and using doctors' opinions on the characteristics of chocolate), diversification and specialisation of the product, premiums (such as prints)[37], etcetera. Both the international and the domestic market were aimed at, and Belgian confectioners succeeded in improving their export position.

As for the demand side, various factors can further explain the chocolate's success story: the increase in the average wage, the 'penchant' for sweets in general and chocolate in particular (being a luxury product for decades), the high energy which could be consumed and digested rapidly, the functions of chocolate as both a simple snack and a tasteful titbit, and the general acceptance by all age groups. In general, chocolate was introduced in three stages: before the war of 1914, it was eaten by a wide public on special occasions; in the early 1920s, it was consumed on a more regular basis; and from the late 1920s onwards, chocolate had become a daily foodstuff.

In many respects, chocolate can be considered as a model for many other (food and non-food) products of which the production was industrialized and the products commercialized in the course of the 20th century.

## Notes

1  Henne & Wauters (1968), II, p. 577.
2  Degryse (1989) and Libert (1995) comment on the Belgian development; see also Toussaint-Samat (1987), pp. 422–425 on France.
3  Almanach (1841), p. 427.
4  Eeckhout, van den (1980), III, p. 35.
5  Almanach (1871), p. 541. Only chocolate factories were listed ('confiseurs' and 'patissiers' were excluded).
6  Recensement 1896, I, p. 60 and Recensement 1910, V, pp. 236–237.
7  Scholliers (1991), pp. 12–13. Part of this article was based on the (written)

testimony of P. Bieswal (June 1980).

8   Scholliers (1991), p. 12.
9   For changes in the production process, see Fritsch (1910), Knapp (1920), and Whymper (1921).
10  Scholliers, (1991), p. 12.
11  Journal de la chocolaterie (January 1931), p. 3: 'L'industrie de la chocolaterie et de la confiserie en Belgique'.
12  Degrève (1982), pp. 469–470.
13  Scholliers (1991), pp. 12 and 17.
14  Tableau général (1891), p. 11, 60; (1911), p. 88.
15  Exposé (s.d.), III, p. 331.
16  Prost (1904), p. 134–5.
17  Tableau général (1911), pp. 88–89.
18  Fritsch (1910), pp. 39–40.
19  Knapp (1920), p. 186.
20  Enquête (1922), p. 694.
21  Buysse (1974), p. 52; Streuvels (original: 1907), quoted in Ghesquiere (1989), p. 164.
22  Enquête (1922), p. 694.
23  Julin (1934), p. 530, published the expenditures on chocolate (and no quantities); sums were converted into consumed quantities by Jacquemyns (1950), p. 72.
24  The budget inquiries do not give information on the distribution of food between the members of the family. Yet, according to a literary source (Streuvels, 1972, p. 594), sweets were increasingly consumed by grown-ups after 1918.
25  Julin (1934), p. 531. The lowest income group spent 2.09 francs per 'quet' and per 'quinzaine' on these food products, the second spent 3.31 francs, the third 4.07 francs, and the highest income group spent 4.37 francs on sweets.
26  1947–1848: workers: 1,160 grams/year/'quet', white-collar workers: 1,180 g (Jacquemyns (1950), p. 72) 1978–1979: workers: 3,670 g; white-collar workers; 3,680 g; liberal professions: 3.450 g; employers; 4,030 g (Gezinsbudgetonderzoek (1984), p. 21 and 29).
27  Le Sucre (November 1923), p. 7 ('Des chocolateries').
28  Congrès international (1930), vol. II, p. 332.
29  The 'real price': the amount of time needed by an unskilled worker to buy a product. The 'real price' actually expresses the cost of a product in hours of work.
30  The price is taken from the 'Prix Courants' of the Brussels co-operative store 'Union Economique'.
31  'Les prix de vente ont été abaissés et une grande satisfaction s'est manifestée parmi les acheteurs' testifies to this (Journal de la chocolaterie, April 1931, p. 3).

32  Jacquemyns (1950), p. 72.
33  De keuken (1949), p. 177 (translated from the Dutch).
34  Labbe (1930), p. 217.
35  Gezinsbudgetenquête (1984), p. 21 and 29.
36  Bulletin officiel (1942).
37  Manuscript 'Limburgsche Cooperatie. Verslag vergadering, 24 december 1921' (collection of author).
38  The Côte d'Or factory published a pamphlet on this occasion, including many pictures of the factory in Anderlecht and the stand at the exhibition; see Côte d'Or (1935).
39  See e.g. Hoebanx (1992).

## Literature

*Almanach du Commerce ou indicateur de la Belgique* (Brussels, 1841; Brussels, 1871).

Annuaire du commerce. *Liste des habitants de Bruxelles* (Brussels, 1891; Brussels. 1901).

Bourgaux, A., *Quatre siècles d'histoire du cacao et du chocolat* (Brussels, 1935).

*Bulletin officiel du comité exécutif central du Secours d'Hiver* (Brussels, 1942).

Buysse, Cyriel, 'Het leven van Rozeken van Dalen'. The life of R. van Dalen, in *Verzameld werk* (Brussels, 1974), pp. 4–301 (original: 1905).

*Congrès international des fabricants de chocolat et de cacao.* Anvers 1930. (Brussels, 1930), 2 vols.

Côte d'Or. *Hoe in 1935 goede chocolade wordt gemaakt.* [How good chocolate is made in 1935] (Brussels, 1935).

Degrève, Daniel, *Le commerce extérieur de la Belgique 1830–1913–1939* (Brussels, 1982).

Degryse, Karel, 'Thee-, koffie- en cacaoverbruik tijdens de vroege 18e eeuw in de Zuidelijke Nederlanden'. [Consumption of tea, coffee and cocoa in early 18th-century Southern Netherlands]. *Archiefkunde*, 4 (1989), pp. 75–80.

Eeckhout, van den, Patricia, *Determinanten van het 19e eeuwse sociaal-economisch leven te Brussel.* [Determining factors of 19th-century socio-economic life in Brussels]. (Brussels, unpublished Ph.D, 1980).

'Enquête sur la nature et le coût de l'alimentation des classes laborieuses', *Revenue du Travail* (mai 1922), pp. 690–696.

*Exposé de la situation du Royaume de 1876 à 1900* (Brussels, s.d.).

Fritsch, J., *Fabrication du chocolat d'après les procédés les plus recents* (Paris, 1910).

*Gezinsbudgetonderzoek 1978–1979.* [Household budget inquiry] (Brussels, 1984), vol. 3.

Ghesquiere, Rita, *Van Nicolaas van Myra tot Sinterklaas.* [From Nicolaas of Myra to Saint-Nicolas] (Leuven Amsersfoort, 1989).

Henne A. & Wauters A., *Histoire de la ville de Bruxelles* (Brussels, 1968), 2 vols.

Jacquemyns, Guillaume, *L'alimentation dans les budgets familiaux 1947–1948* (Brussels, 1950).

Hoebanx, Michel, 'Chocolat et publicité. L'histoire en chromos', *Les Cahiers de la Fonderie*, 11 (1991), pp. 52–55.

*Journal de la chocolaterie, biscuiterie et confiserie* (Tervuren, 1923–1939).

Julin, Armand, 'Résultats principaux d'une enquête sur les budgets d'ouvriers et d'employés en Belgique, 1928–1929'. *Bulletin de l'Institut International de Statistique*, XXVIII-2 (1934), pp. 516–559.

*De keuken in ieders bereik.* [Cooking for everyone] (Tournai, 1949).

Knapp, A.W., *Cocoa and chocolate. Their history from plantation to consumer* (London, 1920).

Labbe Henri, 'Le cacao et le chocolat au point de vue alimentaire et hygiénique', in *Congrès international* (Antwerp, 1930).

Libert, Marc, 'Fressen und Saufen. De tussendoortjes van Charles-Alexander van Lorreinen'. [The in-betweens of Charles-Alexandre of Lorraine] *Tijdschrift voor Sociale Geschiedenis* (1995), forthcoming.

Prost E., *La Belgique agricole, industrielle et commerciale* (Liège-Paris, 1904).

*Recensement général des industries et des métiers au 31 octobre 1896* (Brussels, 1900–1903).

*Recensement de l'industrie et du commerce au 31 décembre 1910* (Brussels, 1913–1921).

Scholliers, Peter, 'Chocolat, machines, travail et salaires vers 1900', in *Les Cahiers de la Fonderie*, no. 11 (1991), pp. 9–17.

Streuvels, Stijn, 'Land en leven in Vlaanderen' [Land and life in Flanders], in: *Volledig werk* (Brugge, 1972), pp. 500–517 (original: 1923).

*Le sucre* (Revue mensuelle de la corporation des representants des usines belges chocolateries, biscuiteries et confiseries) (Brussels, 1920–1925).

*Tableau général du commerce avec les pays étrangers pendant l'année 1890.* (Brussels, 1891). Published annually.

Toussaint-Samat, Maguelonne, *Histoire naturelle et morale de la nourriture* (Paris, 1987).

Whymper, R., *Cocoa and chocolate. Their chemistry and manufacture* (London, 1921).

# 12

# INDUSTRIALIZATION AND FOOD CONSUMPTION IN UNITED ITALY

*Francesco Chiapparino*

The purpose of this review is to show some of the main trends in Italian food consumption since the unification of Italy in 1861. The most difficult aspect of this issue is the uncertainty of official statistics in both national accounts and food availability. These are presented in the following pages, taking account of their most recent revisions.[1]

Furthermore, only the 'material' aspects of food consumption have been considered, leaving what Vovelle calls the 'third level', the evolution of connected mentalities and symbolic representations, in the background.[2]

## Food consumption and patterns of Italian development

The low level of private consumption is one of the points most agreed upon by the students of the first century of Italian unitary history. It was considered by the postwar season of social and economic historiography either as the main consequence of the 'nonrevolution' of the national unification in the countryside,[3] or, alternatively and more optimistically, as the painful but necessary condition of 'primary accumulation'.[4] The extremely poor standard of living of the largest part of the nation remained a central assumption, also in more recent and articulated viewpoints. Since Gerschenkron's contribution onward,[5] it has been more and more organically framed in the terms of a late industrialization process (Table 1). Prevalently located in the North-West regions and largely supported by the State demand and custom protections, this process would have been mainly orientated toward labour saving manufactures, producing infrastructural, strategic and investment goods. The basis and, at the same, consequence of this pattern of growth is a permanent abundance of labour-force, especially in the other non-leading sectors, in the vast areas of backward agriculture, and, broadly speaking, in consumer goods' production. This type of development device benefits on the one hand from a large availability of cheap labour, while on the other, because of the small entity of the monetary wages pool, is unable to promote a larger generalized dynamism of domestic demand. The lack of huge sectorial interdependences and a 'low consumption equilibrium'[6] would therefore be the result of the partial, imperfect modernization of Italian society.

*Table 1:* GNP per capita in some Western European countries and in Italian macroregions (Italy = 100)

|  | U.K. | Germany | France | Belgium | Netherl. | Italy North | North -West | North East + Centre | South |
|---|---|---|---|---|---|---|---|---|---|
| 1870 | 216 | 107 | 130 | 172 | 171 |  |  |  |  |
| 1890 | 252 | 132 | 150 | 204 | 197 |  |  |  |  |
| 1913 | 193 | 125 | 131 | 156 | 152 | 136 | 100 |  | 75 |
| 1929 | 180 | 125 | 154 | 262 | 185 |  |  |  |  |
| 1938 | 191 | 154 | 177 | 147 | 159 |  |  |  |  |
| 1950 | 200 | 118 | 147 | 150 | 167 | 157 | 96 |  | 64 |
| 1973 | 117 | 118 | 120 | 110 | 120 |  |  |  |  |
| 1989 | 104 | 108 | 107 | 99 | 98 (1988:) 129 | 107 |  |  | 68 |

*Sources:* Maddison (1991), Appendix A and B; Italian areas: Zamagni (1990) p. 57

Apart from a late growth of GNP per capita, Italy presents an even more stagnating trend of private consumption. As such, Engel's law seems not to have operated on the macro aggregate level as a whole until the end of the 19th century, and not to have produced a structural alteration of its composition before the interwar period[7] (Table 2).

*Table 2:* Growth and structure of private consumption in Italy (three-year averages, lit. 1938 and index 100 = 1861-63)

|  | Available GNP per capita | | Private consumption per capita | | Composition of priv. cons. (%) Household. Food and clothes | | Others |
|---|---|---|---|---|---|---|---|
| 1861–63 | 1978 | 100 | 1795 | 100 | 68.6 | 22.3 | 9.1 |
| 1896–98 | 1944 | 98 | 1759 | 98 | 67.7 | 18.9 | 13.4 |
| 1912–14 | 2665 | 135 | 2167 | 121 | 65.9 | 17.0 | 17.1 |
| 1920–22 | 2850 | 144 | 2358 | 131 | 67.9 | 19.1 | 13.0 |
| 1937–39 | 3556 | 180 | 2625 | 146 | 54.4 | 26.1 | 19.5 |
| 1949–51 | 3267 | 165 | 2713 | 151 | 59.4 | 18.0 | 22.6 |
| 1959–61 | 5339 | 270 | 3983 | 222 | 47.2 | 22.6 | 30.2 |
| 1970–72 | 11150 | 564 | 7625 | 425 | 37.4 | 22.8 | 39.8 |
| 1983–85 | 14717 | 744 | 10466 | 583 | 29.2 | 23.0 | 47.8 |

*Sources:* Ercolani, pp. 412, 422–432; Istat (1986) pp. 154, 174, 316 ff.

More particularly, it is only around the sixties that a large part of Italians leave the traditional triad of 'bread, soups and legumes', becoming familiar with dietary modernisation, and move into the 'civilization of white bread', significantly increasing their meat consumption.[8]

## Low consumption equilibrium in the countryside

To have a comprehensive idea of the Italian diet, one must first look at the nourishment of the rural population, set in a large variety of cultural environments and production systems (large ownership with farm-hands, small- and shareholding, tenancy), but all homogeneously affected by very low standards of living. Italian agriculture employed more than 60% of the active population until the turn of the century, and 50% still at the eve of World War II. It was characterized by large under-employment, widespread use of marginal lands and a weak market structure. Exceptions were the heart of the Po valley, and limited areas of the Mediterranean garden and some other specialized cultivations.

These backward conditions became even worse after the national unification, due to unfavourable economic policies and a general delay in economic and social development. Then, at the end of the century, the Great Depression left many with no alternative other than emigration. It was paradoxically this, rather than internal progress, that induced through remittances or repatriations and diminishing rural overpopulation, the biggest dietary changes, at least in the case of many Southern regions.[9]

Apart from this, however, available data on the accounts of peasant families[10] indicate that food expenses generally ranged from the national average (ca.68%) to over 80% of the incomes during the last three decades of the 19th century. Yet cases in which this item covered even larger parts of the family's assets were not unusual.

Furthermore, the composition of this consumption was generally poor although broadly varying according to local traditions, cultural framework and prosperity of the family. It is therefore possible to mention only certain common characteristics of the rural Italian diet.

A first notable aspect was the 'meat hunger'[11], the virtual non existence of meat in the diet, while cheese and milk were consumed only by the more affluent. According to a study in the 1880s, for instance, the meat available in urban centres came out at double the amount of the national average (about 13 kg p.c. in a year), and was at least five times higher than in the countryside. These proportions were confirmed by research carried out in the 1910s and 1920s, which on the other side estimated a national yearly average of meat consumption as stagnating around 13 and 18 kg.[12] If a comparatively low use of meat can be considered peculiar to the Mediterranean diet, it was however almost totally lacking in the peasants' diet, where this foodstuff was used only for feasts and special occasions.[13] To a certain extent therefore, the deficiency of animal proteins, an insufficient contribution of fats and other typical remarks about the traditional Italian diet had to be referred mainly to the countryside and only marginally to the urban population.

The basis of the country's nourishment was made up of inferior cereals and legumes until recently.[14] Variously mixed together and with minimal amounts of vegetables and fats, they represented the largest source of sustenance for most of the peasants, especially during the Great Depression, when wheat became more and more only a cash crop.[15] An 1870s' picture of the varied geography of peasants' consumption[16] shows legumes, especially beans, broad beans and lupins, as generally used in the *Mezzogiorno*. Yet in the poorest parts of the South even wild fruits sometimes represented bread substitutes, obviously provoking a large imbalance in the peasants' diet[17]. More diffused problems from this point of view, however, were caused in North and Central Italy by maize monophagism, which in the last decades of the 19th century induced a great insurgence of pellagra.[18] Maize was also widely used in Campania (Naples) and in Tuscany, where it was integrated with legumes and also potatoes and chestnuts. Wheat bread was the basic foodstuff in Sicily alone, although also in this case it was very far from white bread, containing mostly bran. Rice, barley, rye, millet and even acorns were also widely used in breadmaking. Even very typical Italian products, like olive oil, found a limited use in the peasant diet, being mostly considered a cash crop, whereas wine was often replaced, especially in North and Central Italy, by its second-choice and water-fermented surrogate, *vinello*.

*Table 3:* Daily consumption in Italy of nourishment substances, calories, and shares of those of animal origin.

|  | Proteins gr. | % anim. | Fats gr. | % anim. | Carbohy-drates (gr.) | Calories No. | % anim. |
|---|---|---|---|---|---|---|---|
| 1921–30 | 97.5 | 21.7 | 67.1 | 42.3 | 444.7 | 2834 | 12.8 |
| 1931–40 | 93.0 | 23.9 | 59.9 | 48.6 | 418.2 | 2641 | 14.2 |
| 1941–50 | 74.7 | 22.6 | 43.1 | 50.1 | 359.1 | 2171 | 13.1 |
| 1951–60 | 71.4 | 35.6 | 60.5 | 44.8 | 384.1 | 2418 | 15.7 |
| 1961–70 | 85.4 | 43.4 | 89.2 | 39.7 | 423.1 | 2897 | 17.6 |
| 1971–80 | 96.5 | 48.3 | 113.9 | 39.2 | 445.3 | 3259 | 19.6 |
| 1983–85 | 109.3 | 52.4 | 126.8 | 48.1 | 429.8 | 3190 | 25.9 |

*Source:* Istat (1985), p. 184

This set of conditions remain basically the same during the first half of the 20th century, although mainly in the 1900s–1910s localized progress is not to be undervalued [19]). Apart from this an overall improvement, due to increased availability of foods like wheat or poultry, must also be considered. A qualitative growth of agriculture as well as the connected standard of living, was however stopped by the fascist policy toward the sector. This meant, mainly, a restoration of archaic social-economic relationships, growth of overpopulation and regression of intensive cultivation in favour of cereal self sufficency.[20]

Such a blocking of rural development during the interwar period is largely testified to by recent studies on subsistence productions.[21] On the one hand, these estimations reappraise the incidence of domestic-consumption from the traditional figure of 33% and more of the total national consumption, to 20–

25%. On the other hand, however, they stress the substantial stability of this share from the last decades of the 19th century to the 1930s[22], suggesting such a limited sphere of natural economy to be the result of much older processes of mercantilization, probably dating even to the late Middle Ages or early modern period. Moreover, this calculation expressly excludes the whole range of very local transactions. And these latter had to be largely prevailing if, for exemple, in 1872 only 585 of the 74,764 Italian mills produced flour for strictly non-local needs.[23]

Actually undernourishment, a low standard of living and strained market relations disappeared only through the 'rural exodus' after World War II. But at that time, urbanization significantly meant a global refusal of country life and home-made or self-produced foodstuffs.[24]

## Development at the beginning of the 20th century

A strong contrast between rural poverty and the magnificence of the town or, better, of urban *élites*[25] had been an Italian peculiarity since the late Middle Ages. In the fifty years after unification it was, however, possible to speak only of the welfare of restricted groups of higher classes.

Popular consumption in the towns did not differ, essentially, from those of the countryside, although the degree of self-sufficency was of course much lower. Workers' diet was generally poor in proteins, coming almost exclusively from legumes and cereals and rarely from cheese, sausages or cold cuts. Bread was largely made with bran and inferior cereals, wine was often replaced by *vinello* or was simply lacking.[26]

Moreover, urban lower classes were affected by the depression of the end of the 19th century as much as were those in the country. In Milan, inhabitants using no meat at all grew from ⅓ of the total population in 1879 to over 45% in 1899.[27] Per capita consumption of meat in the largest Italian town of Naples decreased by half in the same time span. Wine consumption decreased from over 100 litres a year in the late 1870s to 78 in the 1890s, whereas wheat bread and pasta were widely replaced by maize and low quality cereals.[28]

Nevertheless urban demand showed some dynamism, expecially when, at the turn of the century, Italy benefited from the expansion of international economy. Groups of middle class and, on a very small scale, worker aristocracies began to appear during the *Belle Epoque* alongside the traditional urban *élites*. If in the 1870s–1880s the pioneer of the Italian preserves industry, Francesco Cirio, still had to sell ¾ of his vegetables trade from *Mezzogiorno* abroad (mainly in Central Europe),[29] in the first two decades of this century the North-West regions and a few other big urban centres began to represent markets importing non-traditional consumer goods and manufactured foodstuffs.

The Italian food manufacture was, and would remain till this latest post-war era, of three main kinds.[30] The first large group was the backward and traditional productions. They remained at a very primitive technical and enterpreneurial level, serving a local market only and constituting the largest part of food handicraft or rural industries. In this section the largest part of the above-mentioned milling sector was included, as well as of other basic branches, like wine, olive oil, fish productions, pasta and bread making.[31]

Another set of manufactures, or also of single firms within these latter sectors, were assuming modern industrial characteristics, working either for the foreign demand or for the strengthened but developing North-West and urban domestic markets. The growth of foreign outlets was now also supported by growing emigrant colonies. Their demand for canned tomatoes, pasta, and hard cheese amounted to the traditional Italian exports of luxury specialities, like grana cheese, citrus fruits,[32] or marsala wines.[33] In the case of domestic middle class consumption, on the other hand, its growth also very often meant the appearance of trained foreign competitors, backed by much larger home outlets and by more mature commercialization techniques. So, at least until the war, branches like confectionery (chocolate, biscuits, etc.), meat extracts, luxury cheese, beer, condensed milk and soups were partially controlled by foreign exporters or by their Italian affiliates. Nevertheless, it was competing in these export- or urban market-orientated sectors that a first core of national enterpreneurial experiences reached industrial dimensions in the first quarter of this century. Among them, apart from the Cirio company (vegetable preserves and trade) or some *Chianti* producers,[34] whose establishment already dated from the 19th century, Bertolli (olive oil, cheese, wine),[35] Buitoni (pasta, chocolate),[36] Cinzano (vermouth wine), Polenghi and other cheese manufactures (often cooperatives) as well as spirits and special wine producers[37] of Northen Italy are to be mentioned.

A third area of the food industry was finally represented almost exclusively by sugar and was much closer, in the pattern of development, to the heavy sectors than to the rest of the Italian consumer goods branches. Strongly protected and subsidised by the State since 1883, the sugar manufactures grew rapidly as a highly concentrated oligopoly, with overproduction problems as early as 1907. What is paradigmatic in the case of this sector is the place of sugar consumption. As a matter of fact, sugar protectionism has always assured high profits to producers, rich tax revenues to the Treasury and a very low level of sugar consumption in the country.[38]

### The interwar period

The war was a breakpoint for food standards as well as for many other aspects of social and economic life.[39] For large rural masses military service represented also the first contact with a new way to eat food, largely caloric and, above all, including meat.[40] It would play a strong role immediately after the conflict, when the period of workers' and peasants' struggles widely influenced the redistributive effects of inflation, increasing the popular purchasing power and provoking a short outburst of consumption.[41]

Although the echoes of this small boom kept on till the middle of the 1920s, the fascist victory totally reversed the trend.

Affecting the remuneration of both industrial and rural work and founding its consent on relative improvements in middle class revenues, fascist policy again set the traditional accumulation device based on low living standards and support to big business in strategic and investment goods. From the viewpoint of consumption, these deflation measures of the late 1920s and autarchy in the 1930s reached the goal of reabsorbing, or at least controlling, the surplus of consumer goods' importations. Such a deficit of trade balance punctually appears in periods of high home demand for consumer goods and is mainly due to the structural weakness of the domestic production in this sector.

Therefore, during the interwar period constraints on the living standard of the popular classes produced a decrease of food consumption per capita. At the same time, however, the social policy of the regime, preserving the purchasing power of the middle classes, stimulated the first onsets of a modern consumer society – although asphyxiatingly narrowed to limited urban *élites*. Consumeristic fever by department stores, mass advertisement and leisure consumption remained out of most people's reach.[42] It assumed respectively either the poorer forms of factory stores[43] and standard price shops,[44] or those of means of consent manipulation, like autarchy propaganda and firm institutions organizing workers' free-time.[45]

Apart from the peculiar workings of Engel's law, these trends also explain the evolution of the food industry during the interwar period. In the above-mentioned second group of the branch, those manufactures mainly based on export outlets were badly affected by deflation policies in the late 1920s. The only productions with good chances were those working for luxurious home markets and able to replace imports without suffering too much from the autarchy at the same time. In this context, the case of the confectionery industry can present some means of interest. A big concern, the SA Unica, was created in 1924 with the aim of modernizing the branch introducing mass production and consumption. Six years later, it could be partially saved thanks to State intervention and low quality chocolate orders for public institutions or factory shops. On the other hand, the crisis was much easier to overcome for middle-size firms, strictly interconnected through syndicate agreements and strongly orientated towards luxury urban markets. And later in the 1930s, during the autarchy, the small production volumes and good government relationships allowed them also to obviate the severe restrictions of cocoa import.[46]

## The modernization of the Italian diet after World War II

It was only after World War II that the traditional dietary pattern, as well as the general social and economic conditions of the country, changed radically. Since the first half of the 1950s, once the reconstruction was over, Italy went

145

through a period of intense development. The yearly growth rate of GNP was on average 6% in 1953–63, about 5% during the following decade, 3.7% in 1973–80 and, after the recession of 1981–83 (+0.6%), around 3% in the late 1980s.[47] In spite of low starting points, which emphasized the first stages of growth, this trend deeply modernized Italian society.[48] The initial period of development continued to be characterized by a limited dynamism of private consumption, unequal income distribution and an export-led pattern of growth.[49] In the the 1960s however industrial employment had substantially grown, rural overpopulation as well as emigration flows were disappearing, and the traditional abundance of cheap labour began to run out. Then, a wide range of labour conflicts and social claims induced a larger distribution of purchasing power, permanently breaking the low consumption equilibrium.

These tendencies are reflected by food consumption as well as by other components of private demand. The first decade after the conflict was characterized by the recovery of the pre-war standard of living and by narrowed advancements. From the late 1950s the main indicators began to grow intensively. Actually, only in the following decade were the highest consumption levels of the interwar period largely overcome. The time span between 1958 and 1973 saw the strongest slope in the share of food consumption on the global private demand and the widest quantitative increase in caloric availability. Thanks to a growth of over 36%, Italy passed from the lowest position except for Portugal, among West European countries with less than 2500 daily calories per capita, to about 3300, a figure perfectly on the average of contemporary European standards.[50] The dynamic of carbohydrates, which constitute the base of the Italian popular diet, was similar, being characterized by its largest growth from the end of the 1950s to the turning point around 1974. The dietary contributions of fats and proteins, on the contrary, developed more slowly, continuing until the 1980s.

Although the economic boom of the 1960s induced huge increases in consumption of a wide range of goods, like vegetables, citrus and exotic fruits, fish, sugar and coffee, the main aspect of this dietary revolution was the widespread appearence of meat on the Italian table. At the beginning of 1970s, consumption per capita was over 3.5 times more than twenty years before, that is about 60kg compared to an average of 17kg – not substantially different from those of the first decades of the century. At the same time, milk consumption increased by 50% (from 48kg. to 72) and cheese almost doubled (from 6 to 11kg). This wide demand for animal foodstuff, however, if on one hand it did not cover the differences between Mediterranean and Nordic diets, on the other it induced strong deficits in the Italian trade balance. In 1965 zootechnical imports represented 60% of food imports and about 15% of the total Italian purchases abroad.[51] Such an imbalance is significant of the difficulties in the Italian primary sector to keep up with the development of the country's demand patterns[52] and has been obviated only very partially in the last decades.[53] Between 1965 and 1985 meat consumption passed from 2.1 to 4.4 million metric tonnes and imports from 0.29 to 1.01.

The case was different for manufacturing branches. Development of the food industry followed consumption levels. During all the first stages of the 'economic miracle', from 1953 to 1965, its production index increased by 77.8%, that is about half of the whole secondary sector. In 1966–70 the growth was similar, respectively 26.3 and 27.6%. Development was higher in food sectors in the following years ( + 31% in the 1970s, 14.8% for basic food sectors and + 29.1% for sugar, beverages and others in the 1980s) than in the rest of the manufacturing sectors (respectively + 26% and +13.7%).[54] The characteristics of development have also changed since mid-1970. During the previous two decades, growth concerned mainly new productions, particularly innovative for the Italian diet and with marked industrial attributes, such as confectionery, soft drinks, baby food, frozen and dehydrated products. In the last fifteen years industrialization has also looked at old and traditionally backward branches, like milk and its derivates, wine, olive oil, cold cuts and sausages or coffee.[55] Mechanization and concentration in big firms have invested the largest part of food productions in this way. This type of evolution, however, has not obviated structural deficiencies in the Italian agro-alimentary system. Consequently, especially in South and Central Italy, distribution networks are still largely based on small retailers and therefore too expensive. The integration between the manufacturing and agricultural sector is marginal, often hindering a convenient valorization of resources. The financial and managerial weakness of the national groups has led, in these latest years, to the incorporation of the largest part of the food industry into foreign multinationals[56].

During the last decade, food consumption has continued to change, although by now much less dynamically than other expenditure items. Rather than quantitative aspects, the recent evolution has regarded an improvement in the composition of the diet. Since the middle of the 1970s, the share of carbohydrate contributions has constantly decreased (from 455.9 gr.per capita a day in 1974 to 424.3 in 1984), as have calories (from 3,331 cal. to 3,168), whereas percentages of proteins, fats and animal foods have kept on growing. So, in one sense, it is only in the 1980s that the Italian diet has definitively reached modern patterns, losing its traditional nourishment imbalance and nevertheless, as the last table shows, maintaining many original characteristics, typical of a Mediterranean diet. It is still based on a wide use of bread and pasta, of fresh vegetables and fruits (instead of the traditional dried ones), the prevalence of olive oil in composition butter and margarine, or wine – yet declining from the late 1960s – to beer. Such a traditional dietary pattern on the other hand, obviously deprived of the imbalances of the past, has been in most recent times revalued. It seems to suit well the contemporary refusal of hypercaloric or hyperproteic diets, as well as many of the health and ecological anxieties typical of mature nourishment regimes[57].

*Table 4:* Some indicators of food consumption in the West European countries 1988–1989 (Kg. p. c./year)

|  | UK | Nl | GFR | Fr | Gr | Sp | Port | Dk | Irl | It |
|---|---|---|---|---|---|---|---|---|---|---|
| Cereals | 79 | 51 | 75 | 79 | 104 | 73 | 90 | 65 | 91 | 112 |
| Potatoes | 109 | 86 | 72 | 73 | 87 | 97 | 94 | 65 | 142 | 39 |
| Vegetab. | 65 |  | 83 | 124 | 167 | 182 |  |  |  | 225 |
| Sugar | 40 | 36 | 33 | 34 | 33 | 24 | 28 | 37 | 37 | 27 |
| Meat | 77 | 87 | 104 | 109 | 77 | 93 | 65 | 104 | 93 | 86 |
| Milk & fr. derivates | 128 | 131 | 93 | 101 | 54 | 110 | 86 | 147 | 186 | 75 |
| Butter fats | 5 | 4 | 8 | 9 | 2 | 1 | 1 | 7 | 7 | 3 |
| Wine (l) | 12 | 14 | 26 | 73 | 33 | 46 | 53 | 21 | 4 | 70 |

*Source:* Eurostat (1991), pp. 224–225

**Notes**

1  For criticism of official statistics of Istat (1958) and Barberi (1961) see Toniolo (1988), p. 12ff.; Zamagni (1990), p. 52; Somogyi (1973), p. 877ff.; Federico (1982). Revisions of those data are provided by Ercolani (1978) and Istat (1986).
2  Vovelle (1979), p. 53 and 59ff.
3  The origin of this perspective is in Gramsci (1975), pp. 93ff. and 124ff. After World War II it was organically developed by Sereni (1968), part. pp. 26–41. See also Dal Pane (1963).
4  Romeo (1963), pp. 45–51, 111ff.
5  Gerschenkron (1974), pp. 71–114.
6  Bonelli (1978), p. 1224; Federico (1980), p. 450ff.; Farina (1976); Cafagna (1971).
7  Pettenati (1978), p. 325.
8  Van Bath (1972), p. 8; Braudel (1982), p. 81ff., 114, 175–178; Sabbatucci Severini, Toniolo (1981), p. 25.
9  Bevilacqua (1981).
10  Somogyi (1959), pp. 136ff.
11  For general aspects of meat consumption, see Harris (1990).
12  Niceforo, p. 97ff. and 188ff.
13  See, e.g., Teti (1976) pp. 222ff., pp. 276–79.
14  Faccioli (1973), pp. 1024–1029.
15  Giglioli (1903), p. 9ff; Bachi (1926), p. 24.
16  Raseri (1879), pp. 39–45.
17  Bodio (1879), pp. 182, 186, 193.
18  Corbino (1934), p. 97 and, among the other recent studies, Finzi (1982) and De Bernardi (1984).
19  Cafagna (1980), pp. 224–226.
20  Tattara (1978); Cohen (1976).

21. See in general on this point, Romano, Tucci (1983); Federico (1984; 1985; 1987).
22. Federico (1986), pp. 163ff.
23. Aliberti (1977), pp. 347–350, Caizzi (1975), p. 102ff.
24. Barberis (1983).
25. Romano (1989), p. 293–298.
26. Merli (1976), 439ff.
27. Zaninelli (1974), pp. 39–40.
28. Balletta (1986), p. 742.
29. Caizzi (1975), pp. 112–118.
30. For a first, comprehensive outlook about food manufacture see Confindustria (1929); Zamagni (1980), pp. 95–101.
31. Lanino (1917), pp. 141–148, 176–187, 213–224.
32. Lupo (1990).
33. Candela (1986); Barone (1991); Assoc. Marsalese St Patria (1987).
34. Biagioli (1980), pp. 83–86.
35. Segreto (1986).
36. Gallo (1990).
37. Cirio, Rapetti (1986).
38. Zamagni (1978), pp. 78–87; Bianchi Tonizzi (1988), p. 241ff. Caizzi (1965), pp. 404–406; Sabbatucci Severini (1982).
39. For the food policy during World War I see Dentoni (1987).
40. Bachi (1926), p. 453.
41. Zamagni (1980 and 1983); about the effective impoverishment of the middle class standard of life see also Sabbatucci Severini, Toniolo (1981), p. 37.
42. Venè (1988).
43. Romano (1983).
44. Zamagni (1981), Amatori (1989).
45. De Grazia (1981).
46. Chiapparino (1990).
47. Zamagni (1990), p. 423–26.
48. See for this proposal the general analysis of a foreign observer in Ginsborg (1989), II, p. 325ff.
49. Graziani (1979), pp. 53ff., Castronovo (1975), p. 409.
50. For the relative position of Italian consumption in West Europe in the late 1950s see Yates (1962), for data of 1970s and those following, Istat (1986), pp. 182–5.
51. Somogyi (1966), pp. 61ff., 72–77.
52. Castronovo (1975), p. 485–486, speaks of an 'abdication of Italian agriculture to the needs of the domestic market'.
53. Casati (1990), p. 150.
54. Castronovo, (1980), statistical appendix; Istat (1988), p. 377; Istat (1991), p. 363.
55. Sicca (1977), pp. 39–55; Bertelé, Brioschi (1981), pp. 161ff, 226ff.

56. Sicca (1977), pp. 7–32, 85ff.; see further the case of Buitoni-Perugina-Sme in Buitoni (1992).
57. Insor (1984); Riva (1985); Scaravelli, Beltramini (1987) Censis (1990), p. 23ff., part. p. 28; Ismea (1991), pp. 75–77;

**Literature**

Aliberti, G., 'Fra tradizione e rinnovamento: l'industria molitoria dopo l'Unità'. [Between tradition and renewal: The mill industry after Unification], in G. Mori (ed.), *L'industrializzazione in Italia (1861–1900)*. [Industrialization in Italy (1861–1900)] (Bologna 1977), pp. 347–364.

Amatori, F., *Proprietà e direzione. La Rinascente 1917–1969.* [Ownership and management. The Rinascente 1917–1969] (Milano 1989).

Associazione Marsalese per la Storia Patria, *Benjamin Ingham nella Sicilia dell'Ottocento*. [B.I. in 19th century Sicily] (Marsala 1987).

Bachi, R., *L'alimentazione e la politica annonaria in Italia*. [Nutrition and provision policy in Italy] (Bari 1926).

Barberi, B., *I consumi nel primo secolo dell'Unità d'Italia, 1861–1960*. [Consumption in the first century of united Italy] (Milano 1961).

Barberis, C., 'L'autoconsumo in Italia' [Domestic consumption in Italy], in *Storia d'Italia*, Annali VI, *Economia naturale, economia monetaria*. [History of Italy, Natural economy, monetary economy] (Torino 1983), pp. 743–774.

Barone, G., 'Il tramonto dei Florio' [The setting of the Florio]. *Meridiana*, 11–12 (1991), pp. 15–46.

Bertelè, U., Brioschi, F., *L'economia agro-alimentare italiana*. [The Italian agro-alimentary economy] (Bologna 1981).

Bevilacqua, P., 'Emigrazione transoceanica e mutamenti dell'alimentazione contadina calabrese fra Otto e Novecento'. [Overseas emigration and changes in the Calabrian peasant diet between the 19th and 20th century]. *Quaderni storici*, 47 (1981), pp. 520–555.

Biagioli, G., 'Vicende e fortuna di Ricasoli imprenditore'. [Life and successes of Ricasoli entrepreneur], in *Agricoltura e società nella Maremma grossetana dell '800* [Agriculture and society in Maremma, area of Grosseto, during the 19th century] (Firenze 1908), pp. 77–102.

Bianchi Tonizzi, M.E., 'L'industria dello zucchero in Italia dal blocco continentale alla vigilia della Grande Guerra (1807–1914). [The sugar industry in Italy from the Napoleonic age to the eve of World War I]. *Annali di storia dell 'impresa*, 4 (1988), pp. 211–278.

Bodio, L., 'Sui contratti agrari e sulle condizioni materiali di vita dei contadini in diverse regioni d'Italia'. [On the agrarian contacts and the material life conditions of peasants in various Italian regions]. *Annali di statistica*, II, 8 (1879), pp. 125–206.

Bolletta, F., 'Commercio e dazi di consumo a Napoli nella seconda metà del XIX secolo'. [Trade and city consumptions duties in Naples during the second half of the 19th century], in *Mercati e consumi*. [Markets and consumption] (Bologna 1986), pp. 729–742.

Bonelli, F., 'Il capitalismo italiano. Linee generali d'interpretazione'. [Italian capitalism: General outlines of interpretation], in *Storia d'Italia*, Annali I, *Dal feudalesimo al capitalismo*. [History of Italy, From feudalism to capitalism] (Torino 1978), pp. 1195–1255.

Braudel, F., *Le strutture del quotidiano* (Torino 1982). [*Civilisation matérielle, économie et capitalisme (XVe-XVIIIe siècle). Les structures du quotidien: le possible et l'impossible* (Paris 1979)].

Buitoni, B., *Pasta e cioccolato. Una storia imprenditoriale.* [Pasta and chocolate. An enterpreneurial history] (Perugia 1992).

Cafagna, L., 'Intorno alle origini del dualismo economico in Italia'. [The origins of economic dualism in Italy], in *Scritti in memoria di Leopoldo Cassese* (Napoli 1971), II, pp. 99–136.

Cafagna, L., 'La rivoluzione industriale in Italia (1830–1914)'. [The Industrial Revolution in Italy (1830–1914)], in C.M. Cipolla (ed.), *Storia economica d'Europa [The Fontana Economic History of Europe* (Brighton 1971)] (Torino 1980), IV, pp. 207–246.

Caizzi, B., *Storia dell'industria italiana dal XVIII secolo ai giorni nostri.* [History of Italian industry from 18th century to present day] (Torino 1965).

Caizzi, B., *Il commercio* [Trade] (Torino 1975).

Candela, S., *I Florio* [The Florio] (Palermo 1986).

Casati, D., 'Mercato dei prodotti agricoli'. [Market of agriculture production], in C. Colombi, M. Domenichini, *Attorno al piatto. Contributi per un' analisi del problema alimentare.* [Around the dish. Contributions to an analysis of food problems] (Milano 1990), pp. 133–166.

Castronovo, V., 'La storia economica'. [Economic history], in *Storia d'Italia* [History of Italy] (Torino 1975), IV, 1, pp. 3–506.

Castronovo, V., *L'industria italiana dall'ottocento a oggi.* [Italian industry from the 19th century to today] (Milano 1982 [1980]).

Censis, *Consumi* 1990. [Consumption 1990] (Milano 1990).

Chiapparino, F., 'Il tentativo di concentrazione dell'industria dolciaria italiana negli anni Venti: Gualino e l'Unica (1924–1934)'. [The attempt at concentration of the confectionery industry during the twenties: Gualino and the Unica]. *Annali di storia dell'impresa*, 5–6 (1989–1990), pp. 323–374.

Cirio, P., Rapetti, V., 'Alle origini dello spumante italiano: l'industria enologica di Canelli (fine '800–1939)'. [At the origins of Italian sparkling wine: The oenological manufacture in Canelli (end of 1800s–1939)], in *Mercati e consumi.* [Markets and consumption] (Bologna 1986), pp. 213–226

Cohen, J.S., 'Rapporti agricoltura-industria e sviluppo agricolo'. [Agriculture/industry relations and agriculture development], in G. Toniolo (ed.), *L'economia italiana del periodo fascista.* [The Italian economy during the fascist period] (Bologna 1976), pp. 379–408.

Confindustria [Confederazione Generale Fascista dell'Industria Italiana], *L'industria italiana* [The Italian industry] (Roma 1929).

Corbino, E., *Annali dell'economia italiana*, IV, *1891–1900*. [Yearbooks of Italian economy] (Città di Castello 1934).

Dal Pane, 'Alcuni studi recenti e la teoria di Marx'. [Some recent studies and Marx's theory], in A. Caracciolo (ed.), *La formazione dell'Italia industriale*. [The making of industrial Italy] (Bari 1963[1962]), pp. 101–111.

De Bernardi, A., *Il mal della rosa. Denutrizione e pellagra nelle campagne italiane fra '800 e '900*. [The 'rose-sickness'. Undernourishment and pellagra in the Italian countryside between the 19th and 20th century] (Milano 1984).

De Grazia, V., *Consenso e cultura di massa nell'Italia fascista*. [Consent and mass culture in fascist Italy] (Bari 1981).

Dentoni, M.C., 'Questione alimentare e "questione sociale" durante la prima guerra mondiale in Italia'. [Food and social problems during World War I in Italy]. *Società e storia*, 37(1987), pp. 607–636.

Ercolani, P., 'Documentazione statistica di base'. [Basic statistical materials], in G. Fuà (ed.), *Lo sviluppo economico in Italia*. [Economic development in Italy] (Milano 1978[3]), III, pp. 380–460.

Eurostat, *Eurostatistics* (Luxembourg 1991).

Faccioli, E., 'La cucina' [Cooking], in *Storia d'Italia*, V, *I documenti*. [History of Italy] (Torino 1973), 1, pp. 981–1030.

Farina, F., 'Modelli interpretativi e caratteri del capitalismo italiano'. [Interpretative patterns and characteristics of Italian capitalism]. *Quaderni storici*, 32(1976), pp. 487–514.

Federico, G., 'Di un nuovo modello dell'industrializzazione italiana'. [On a new pattern of Italian industrialization]. *Società e storia*, 8(1980), pp. 433–455.

Federico, G., 'Per una valutazione critica delle statistiche della produzione agricola italiana dopo l'Unità (1860–1913)'. [For a critical evaluation of the statistics of Italian agricultural production after Unification]. *Società e storia*, 15(1982), pp. 87–130.

Federico, G., 'Azienda contadina e autoconsumo fra antropologia ed econometria: considerazioni metodologiche'. [Farming and subsistence production between anthropology and econometry: Methodological considerations]. *Rivista di storia economica*, I (1984), 2, pp. 222–268.

Federico, G., 'Autoconsumo e mercantilizzazione: spunti per una discussione'. [Subsistence production and mercantilization: points for a discussion]. *Società e storia*, 27 (1985), pp. 197–212.

Federico, G., 'Mercantilizzazione e sviluppo economico in Italia (1860–1940)'. [Mercantilization and economic development in Italy]. *Rivista di storia economica*, III (1986), 2, pp. 149–186.

Federico, G., 'Contadini e mercato: tattiche di sopravvivenza'. [Peasants and market: Survival tactics], *Società e storia*, 38(1987), pp. 877–913.

Finzi, R., 'Quando e perché fu sconfitta la pellagra in Italia'. [When and why pellagra was defeated in Italy], in M.L. Beltri, A. Gigli Marchetti (eds.), *Salute e classi la voratrici in Italia dall 'Unità al fascismo*. [Health and working classes in Italy from unification to fascism] (Milano 1982), pp. 319–429.

Gallo, G., 'Dagli esordi alla seconda guerra mondiale'. [From the beginning to World War II], in Id., '*Sulla bocca di tutti'. Buitoni e Perugina, una storia in breve*. ['On everyone's lips'. Buitoni and Perugina, a short history] (Perugia 1990), pp. 9–32.

Gerschenkron, A., *Il problema storico dell'arretratezza economica*. [*Economic Backwardness in Historical Perspective: A Book of Essays* (Cambridge, Mass., 1962)] (Torino 1974).

Giglioli, I., *Malessere agrario ed alimentare in Italia*. [Agrarian and food malaise in Italy] (Portici 1903).

Ginsborg, P., *Storia d'Italia dal dopoguerra a oggi*. [History of Italy from the postwar period to present day] (Torino 1989).

Gramsci, A., *Il Risorgimento*, (Roma 1975).

Graziani, A., (Ed.), *L'economia italiana dal 1945 a oggi*. [Italian economy from 1945 to present day] (Bologna 1979).

Harris, M., *Buono da mangiare. Enigmi del gusto e consuetudini alimentari* (Torino 1990). [Good to Eat. Riddles of Food and Culture]. (New York 1985)

INSOR [Istituto Nazionale di Sociologia Rurale], *Gastronomia e societa:* [Gastronomy and society] (Milano 1984).

ISMEA [Istituto Studi Ricerche e Informazioni sul Mercato Agricolo], *Gli italiani e l'educazione alimentare*. [Italians and nutrition education] (Roma 1991).

ISTAT [Istituto Centrale di Statistica], *Sommario di statistiche storiche italiane 1861–1955*. [Summary of Italian historical statistics 1861–1855] (Roma 1958).

ISTAT, *Sommario di statistiche storiche 1926–1985* (Roma 1986).

ISTAT, *Annuario statistico italiano 1988*. [Italian statistical yearbook 1988] (Roma 1988).

ISTAT, *Annuario statistico italiano 1991* (Roma 1991).

Lanino, P., *La nuova Italia industriale*. [The new industrial Italy] (Roma 1917), III, 'Industrie chimiche, alimentari e agricole'. [Chemical, food and agricultural industries].

Lenti, L., 'I consumi degli italiani negli ultimi cent' anni'. [Italian consumption in the last hundred years]. *Rivista di politica economica*, III, 9(1958), pp. 1235–1248.

Lupo, S., *Il giardino degli aranci. Il mondo degli agrumi nella storia del Mezzogiorno*. [The garden of oranges. The world of citrus fruits in the history of the Mezzogiorno] (Venezia 1990).

Maddison, A., *Dynamic Forces in Capitalist Development. A Long-Run Comparative View* (Oxford/New York, 1991).

Merli, S., *Proletariato di fabbrica e capitalismo industriale*. [Factory proletariat and industrial capitalism] (Firenze 1976).

Niceforo, A., 'Dati statistici sull'alimentazione della popolazione italiana'. [Statistical data on the nutrition of the Italian population], in *Documenti per lo studio della alimentazione della popolazione italiana nell'ultimo cinquantennio* [Documents for the study of Italian population's nutrition in the last fifty years] (Napoli 1933), pp. 79–265.

Pettenati, P., 'Alcune relazioni tra i consumi e lo sviluppo'. [Some relations between consumption and development], in G. Fuà (Ed.). *Lo sviluppo economico in Italia*. [Economic development in Italy] (Milano 1978[3]), pp. 317–336.

Raseri, E., 'Alimenti e bevande prevalenti nell'alimentazione dei poveri e in quella dei ricchi'. [Food and beverages prevailing in the diet of the poor and in that of rich]. *Annali di statistica*, II, 8(1879), pp. 37–96.

Riva, M., 'Novità dell'appetito. Dalla fame arretrata alla grande abbuffata: evoluzione dei consumi alimentari e della razione dietetica degli italiani'. [Novelties of appetite. From outstanding hunger to overabundance: Evolution of Italian food consumption and dietetic rations], in *La gola*, 4, 27 (Jan. 1985), pp. 4–6.

Romano, R., Tucci, U., 'Premessa'. [Introduction], in *Storia d'Italia*, Annali VI, *Economia naturale, economia monetaria*. [History of Italy, Natural economy, monetary economy] (Torino 1983), pp. XIX-XXXIII.

Romano, R., 'Una tipologia economica'. [An economic typology], in *Storia d'Italia*, I, *I caratteri originali*. [History of Italy. The original characteristics] (Torino 1989[2]), I, pp. 256–304.

Romeo, R., *Risorgimento e capitalismo*. [Risorgimento and capitalism] (Bari 1963[1959]).

Sabbatucci Severini, P., 'Bieticoltura e industria saccarifera nelle Marche: uno sviluppo mancato'. [Beet cultivation and sugar industry in the Marche Region: a non-development], in R. Paci (ed.), *Scritti storici in memoria di Enzo Piscitelli* (Padova 1982), pp. 379–426.

Sabbatucci Severini, P., Toniolo, G., 'Aspetti macroeconomici del problema della povertà in Italia, 1860–1963'. [Macro-economic aspects of the problem of poverty in Italy, 1860–1963], in *Ricerche di storia sociale e religiosa*, 19–20 (1981), pp. 7–55.

Scaravelli, E., Beltramini De'Casati, G.M., *L'alimentazione mediterranea*. [Mediterranean diet] (Milano 1987).

Segreto, L., 'I Bertolli. Appunti per la storia di una dinastia industriale'. [The Bertolli. Notes for the history of an economic dynasty]. *Lucca. Bollettino economico*, 4–5 (1986), pp. 22–27.

Sereni, E., *Il capitalismo nelle campagne*. [Capitalism in the countryside] (Torino 1968 [1947]).

Sicca L., *L'industria alimentare in Italia*. [Food industry in Italy] (Bologna 1977).

Somogyi, G., *La bilancia alimentare dell'Italia*. [The balance of trade in the Italian food industry] (Bologna 1966).

Somogyi, S., 'Cento anni di bilanci familiari in Italia (1857–1956)'. [One hundred years of family budgets in Italy (1857–1956)], in *Annali dell'Istituto Giangiacomo Feltrinelli*, 2(1959), pp. 121–263.

Somogyi, S., 'L'alimentazione nell'Italia unita'. [Nutrition in united Italy], in *Storia d'Italia*, V, I documenti (Torino 1973), I, pp. 841–887.

Tattara, G., 'La battaglia del grano'. [The wheat battle], in G. Toniolo (ed.). *L'economia italiana 1861–1940* [Italian economy 1861–1940] (Roma-Bari 1978), pp. 337–380.

Teti, V., *Il pane, la beffa e la festa*. [The bread, the mockery, and the feast] (Rimini-Firenze 1976).

Toniolo, G., *Storia economica dell 'Italia liberale, 1850–1918.* [Economic history in liberal Italy, 1850–1918] (Bologna 1988).

Van Bath, S., *Storia agraria dell'Europa occidentale (500–1850)* [*De agrarische geschiedenis van West-Europa (*500–1850*)* (Utrecht-Antwerpen 1962)] (Torino 1972).

Venè, G.F., *Mille lire al mese. Vita quotidiana della famiglia nell'Italia fascista.* [One thousand lire a month. The everyday life of the family in fascist Italy] (Milano 1988).

Vovelle, M., 'Storia e lunga durata' [Histoire et longue durée], in J.Le Goff(Ed.), *La nuova storia [La nouvelle histoire* (Paris 1979)] (Milano 1983[2]), pp. 47–80.

Yates, P.L., 'Alimentation, boissons et tabac', in J.F. Dewhurst, *Besoins et moyens de l'Europe* (Paris 1962), pp. 145–164.

Zamagni, V., *Industrializzazione e squilibri regionali in Italia.* [Industrialization and regional imbalances in Italy] (Bologna 1978).

Zamagni, V., 'Distribuzione del reddito e classi sociali nell'Italia tra le due guerre'. [Income distribution and social classes in interwar Italy], *Annali dell'Istituto Giangiacomo Feltrinelli*, 20(1979/80), pp. 17–50.

Zamagni, V., *La distribuzione commerciale in Italia tra le due guerre* [Commercial distribution in interwar Italy] (Milano 1981).

Zamagni, V., 'Le alterazioni nella distribuzione del reddito in Italia nell'immediato dopoguerra (1919–1922)'. [Alterations in income distribution in Italy in the immediate postwar period (1919–1922)], in P. Hertner, G. Mori (eds.), *La transizione dall'economia di guerra all'economia di pace in Italia e in Germania dopo la prima guerra mondiale.* [The transition from warfare economy to peacetime economy in Italy and Germany after the First World War] (Bologna 1983), pp. 509–532.

Zamagni, V., *Dalla periferia al centro. La seconda rinascita economica dell'Italia, 1861–1981.* [From outskirts to the centre. The second economic renaissance of Italy, 1861–1981] (Bologna 1990).

Zaninelli, S., *I consumi a Milano nell'Ottocento.* [The Consumption in Milan during the 19th century] (Roma 1974).

# 13

# FROM FAMINE TO WELFARE: FOOD PATTERNS IN FINLAND DURING THE PAST HUNDRED YEARS

*Marjatta Hietala*

## Introduction

Three important aspects have to be taken into account when examining the diet and nutrition of the Finnish population: the geographical location and the climate of the country as well as the late industrialization process. In the middle of the 19th century Finland was more agrarian than many other European countries during their pre-industrial periods. There were famine years during the latter part of the 19th century. At the end of the last century there were many attempts to develop cattle raising, whereas grain was imported from abroad. When Finland gained her independence, the import of wheat from Russia ceased and there was a shortage of food in 1918.

During the 1920s and 1930s the belief in agricultural self-sufficiency was strong. Agricultural activities and landownership were highly valued. The land settlement legislation of 1922, Lex Kallio, resulted in the formation of small-holdings, giving the former landless population a possibility to obtain additional domains of farming land. This was achieved by turning forests and marsh land into fields. These activities were encouraged by the state, and as late as in the 1950s special prizes were awarded for creating new farm land. After the war, during the 1940s, the Government policy was to settle also the most northern and eastern parts of the country. The number of smallholdings increased.

Industrial change took place in the 1960s and the country became urbanized. From 1960 onwards, when all war reparations had been paid, one could see rapid growth in all fields and sectors. During 1980–1986 the annual growth of Gross National Product was 2,7 per cent, one of the fastest in Europe.

## The Great Famine Years

During the last centuries there have been several bad harvests and shortages of food. The most serious famine years were 1866–1868. Then approximately

270,000 inhabitants died of famine and epidemics, especially of typhus. The overall mortality rate was over ten per cent and in some areas even higher. The total population was 1,843,000. Epidemic diseases touched nearly every citizen in the countryside. By European standards this was a rather late catastrophe.[1]

The famine years 1867–68 did not come as a surprise. Actually, there had been several bad years with poor harvests in the 1860s. In 1867 the summer came one month too late. The spring had been long and cold and the spring sowing was about a month late in all parts of the country. In the night between the 4th and 5th of September, 1867, the temperature fell to below zero degrees Celsius and damaged rye, barley, oats and potatoes in nearly all parts of the country. The only exception was the southern coast area. The descriptions of that frost night have a special significance in the folklore of Finland. 'I remember well how in the famine years large masses of beggars went from house to house. It was sad because one had to give them bread even though one was short of it oneself.'[2]

The poor harvest meant unemployment because farm labourers and their families were paid in food. People in the central and eastern parts of the country suffered most, and especially the lowest social classes (tenant farmers, farm labourers) were hit hard by the famine.

The famine years 1867–1868 contain many paradoxes on the official level (as far as the attitudes of the Government are concerned): grain was exported to Sweden, but the Government was only able to import foreign grain valued at 6,5 million marks. On the other hand the Government took a loan of 28 million marks for railway constructions.

The Government was incapable of organizing the aid and its policies were either weak or wrong. Neither were the farmers eager to organize aid. People were asked to pick mushrooms and use bark as a substitute ingredient in bread. Bark mixed with rye flour tasted good and was quite nourishing. The process of making bark bread was a complicated one since the raw material could only be collected at a certain time of the year. Using bark was a common custom in the Northern European regions until this century.[3]

There were no large political protest movements or food riots during the Famine Years. After the Famine Years the next poor crop was reaped in 1902. It was followed by a general strike.

**Earliest studies**

From the 1870s onwards, the Government, municipalities and private organizations invested money in the promoting of agriculture and cattle raising. Cattle breeding, however, was not as vulnerable; even during the bad years, enough hay and fodder were available to feed the cattle.[4] From the 1890s onwards, special farming, gardening and cattle raising consultants were hired.[5] Agricultural schools and farming institutes were established.

After the famine years medical doctors began to pay attention to the diet of the population and the quality of food. For their popular magazines they wrote articles in which they promoted the importance of hygiene and the availability of food. Also the Lutheran clergy was active in promoting a healthy and clean diet. The priests encouraged people to hire dairymaids in order to improve the quality of milk.

Konrad Relander, the district surgeon in Haapajärvi, described the quality of butter as follows: 'When I came to Haapavesi in 1887, I could not find a mistress who could make butter of good quality. Now (i.e. in 1892) I can see that there has been a change for the better. Now I do not have any difficulties in finding butter which tastes good. The explanation for this development is the fact, that there is a dairymaid working in Haapavesi. For this we must thank the Reverend J. Pöyhönen who with his enthusiasm has broken the resistance of the farmers.'

One of the first studies which dealt with the diet of the population is the study carried out by the above-mentioned district surgeon Konrad Relander from Haapajärvi[6]. Over one hundred years ago, in 1892, he published a survey on health and housing. He found a close relationship between the standard of health and that of hygiene, and paid attention to housing, cleanliness, hygiene and diet.

Relander's study is based on his own experiences of 13 years in the area, as well as on a detailed questionnaire in which he asked questions about housing, ventilation, light conditions, and sleeping conditions in the houses. He also made questions about meals and diets. He paid attention to the quality of soil on which the houses were built. He asked detailed questions about the sizes of windows. As a starting point he used the standards based on the recommendations of the association 'Der deutsche Verein für öffentliche Gesundheitspflege' approved in Strassburg in 1889. The average proportion of the floor area to the area taken by windows was 1:12. He found out that the farm yards were separated from the main buildings, the wells were far away from the compost heaps and the milk-houses were in shaded places and the means of storage for food were quite clean.

About the daily meals in Haapajärvi in 1892 Relander received the following information: During the winter season and on Sundays people had three meals, but during the spring and summer seasons four daily meals were served. In winter breakfast was eaten at six to seven o'clock, lunch was served at twelve to one, and dinner at eight to nine, whereas in the summertime breakfast was eaten at six to seven (and porridge at nine to ten), lunch was taken at four to five, and dinner at nine to ten.

The diet was based mostly on grain products, milk products (butter, homemade cheese), meat and fish. The most common types of food were smoked meat, salted fish and porridges made of rye, oats, barley and lingonberries. In this northern region milk was available during most of the year (with the exceptions of October, November, December, and January). One of the most important food items was turnip. People used turnips in various ways. Nowadays we would say that turnips were used as substitutes for potatoes. Relander does not make any reference to the use of potatoes.[7]

Finnish research on the food and nutrition of the population can be divided into studies on the quality and sufficiency of food and studies on the living costs. Both types of study, which have been sponsored by the Government and committees for nutrition appointed by the Government, have clearly tried to direct the consumption of food in the desired direction.

In 1905–1907 Sigfried Sundström made the first study on the sufficiency of the food among the agricultural population. The study covered 18 farming families from different parts of the country, a total of 103 persons. According to the study, the daily energy intake of an adult male was approximately 4000 calories. For females, the figure was 2700–2800 calories, and for children of 2–3 years 1000 calories. As Table 1 indicates, the diet of a male consisted of 15% proteins, 21% fats, and 64% carbohydrates. Sundström emphasized that the intake of fats was low and that the diet was based too much on the use of dried food.[8]

On the basis of Sundström's findings, Robert Tigerstedt made a study and defined chemically, in 1910, the calcium, magnesium, and phospor contents of the diet. He concluded that there was a good deal of these elements in the diet because of the abundant use of milk. Tigerstedt also recommended margarine as a substitute for butter. The first margarine factory started to operate in 1911.

In 1912–13 Tigerstedt conducted a study of 20 families belonging to different social groups. The study covered 130 persons whose daily food was weighed on seven days. In order to find out any seasonal variation the study was repeated for one part of the group after 4–5 months. The results showed that the daily energy intake for males was 3069–4089 calories. For children it was 1344–2432 calories. Among females the figure was as low as 1667–3161 calories per day. The share of proteins in the total energy intake was 12.2–18.2%, that of carbohydrates 38.7.%, and fats 8.5–43.5%. The intake of fats was considered to be too low, especially in the diet of women and children. During the 1920s Carl Tigerstedt developed a special guide-book for school meals in which he promoted the use of vegetables. A private organisation, Mannerheimin Lastensuojeluliitto, was active in distributing the books. At the beginning of the 1930s, the same organisation, under the leadership of the famous pediatrician Arvo Ylppö, developed on the basis of Norwegian experience a healthy breakfast (in Finland known by the name of Oslo breakfast). It included vegetables and sandwiches and it was easy to prepare without special kitchen utensils. This innovation was not very successful at schools and children protested at vegetables which they regarded as 'the food of cows'.[9]

*Table 1:* The percentage of different foodstuffs in Finland as the source of energy according to different studies

| Foodstuff | 1 Sundström in 1905–07 % | 2 Tigerstedt 1915 % | 3 Committee 1936–37 % | 4 Hjelt 1912 % | 5 Roine 1954 % |
|---|---|---|---|---|---|
| Grain and grain products | 51 | 40 | 43 | 40 | 34 |
| Potato | 10 | 27 | 9.6 | 10 | 6,5 |
| Other vegetables | – | 2.5 | 1.3 | 1,2 | 1 |
| Fruit and berries | | 0.5 | 0.6 | .. | 1.5 |
| Sugar | 4 | 4 | 6.1 | 7.5 | 10.5 |
| Margarine | – | – | 2.4 | – | 3 |
| Butter | 7.5 | 4 | 7.5 | | |
| Other Milk products | 18 | 15.5 | 19.2 | 24.5 | 20 |
| Meat and meat products | 8 | 5 | 9.3 | 5.5 | 7.5 |
| Fish | 1.5 | 1.5 | 0.9 | 0.5 | 1.2 |
| Eggs | – | 0 | 0.2 | 0.3 | 1.4 |

*Source:*  Sundström (1908), Tigerstedt (1915), Virtanen & Turpeinen (1940), Hjelt (1912) and Roine (1954)

**The Committee for Nutrition of the Population**

In 1936 the Finnish Government appointed a special Committee for Nutrition of the Population. In 1936–1937, the Committee ordered a study of the diet of the low-income rural population. It was concluded that 51% of the studied families (288 persons) received less energy than they needed. The situation of 21% of these families was very poor. The reasons for this were economic. However, the greatest problem was not in the availability of food but in the quality of the consumed food (see Table 1 column 3). The most important nutritional element which was lacking from the diet was vitamin A. Also the diet lacked calcium. The greatest seasonal variations occurred in the availability of vitamin A and ascorbic acid. In its report the Committee emphasized the importance of vitamins and minerals in the future.[10] The method recommended by the Committee was to develop adult education for nutritional enlightment. Adult education centres were activated to organize study and discussion groups in which the topic was the person's own responsibility for his or her diet. The Finnish educators chose the same book for a basic material as their Nordic colleagues did, namely 'Terveellinen ravinto' by Juliana Sobraa-Bay.[11]

**Social statistical studies**

Table 1 column 4 is based on Vera Hjelt's study from 1912 in which she calculated the living expenses in various families. Later researchers have managed to create, on the basis of her results, data which are comparable with earlier studies. It seems that Hjelt's study gives bigger proportions for

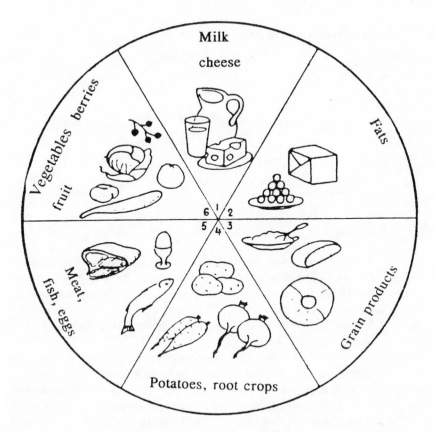

*Figure 1:* Foodstuffs in daily nutrition recommended in an instruction book for young people.
*Source:* Virtanen & Roine (1951)

meat, meat products and potatoes as sources of energy.[12] The trend has been that people consume more sugar and fat.

In 1950–1951 Professor Roine found out in his research that 54.5% of all energy came from carbohydrates, 34% from fat and 12% from protein. At that time it was emphasized that the amount of fats in diets was proportionally too large. Column 6 in table 1 shows that consumption of fats (both butter and margarine) has increased.[13]

In spite of this Roine was willing to recommend to students at the secondary schools that 50–100 g fat per day was enough. He wrote the book together with the famous Nobel Prize winner A.I. Virtanen.[14] In the final chapter of the book they concluded that the main food items that the Finns used were rye bread, milk, turnips (source of vitamin C) and later potatoes and they believed that these food items would be the most suitable basis for the diet in the future as well.[15]

*Table 2:* Consumption of selected food commodities in Finland

| per inhabitant | 1938 | 1970 | 1980 | 1991 |
|---|---|---|---|---|
| Fluid milk products (litres) | 292 | 261 | 263[1] | 215[1] |
| Butter (kg) | 11.0 | 14.0 | 12.2 | 7.5 |
| Margarine (kg) | 3.8 | 7.4 | 7.9 | 7.8 |
| Cheese (kg) | 1.1 | 4.5 | 7.2 | 12.8 |
| Wheat (kg) | 75.5 | 65.3 | 59.6 | 57.3 |
| Rye (kg) | 69.2 | 26.0 | 21.2 | 17.6 |
| Meat (kg) | 34.3 | 42.9 | 58.9 | 64.2 |
| Coffee (kg) | 7.3 | 9.8[2] | 10.3[2] | 10.0[2] |
| Sugar (kg) | 34.9 | 45.1 | 36.8 | 34 |

1. Incl. butter in butter-oil mixtures
2. Sales of roasted coffee
*Source:* Finland in Figures 1992, Helsinki 1992, p. 21.

The Nutrition Department of the University of Helsinki was established during the 1960s. The National Nutrition Board funded a project on Nutrient Intake of Finns in 1967 – 1969, and the follow up survey was made during 1973–1976. This study was carried out in connection with the Mobile Clinic activities of the Finnish National Pensions Institute.[16] The main results of the study were:

–The consumption of cereal products had decreased about 50 per cent from the beginning of the century and the proportion of rye to wheat changed from 4:1 to 3:4. The consumption of potatoes had decreased more than 50 per cent and that of fish about 65 per cent during the last 60 years.

–The consumption of milk products had decreased a little during this century but not markedly in the 1960s and the consumption of cheese had increased since the 1940s.

–The consumption of fats, vegetables, meat products, eggs and sugar had steadily increased. The use of vegetables had began to increase in the 1930s and since then the consumption of various vegetables had grown by about 40 per cent. In the 1950s the consumption of fruits and berries had doubled.

–The consumption of meat products had increased, and the total meat consumption had increased heavily during the 1960s (especially the consumption of sausages).

–The usage of sugar had been about 12 grams daily per person at the beginning of the century but increased to 70 grams per day in the late 1960s. At that time the average daily protein intake for men had been 106 grams and that for women 76 grams.

At the end of the 1960s the average daily energy value of the diet of men was 3150 kcal (13 MJ) and of that of women 2300 kcal (9.6 MJ). According to FAO studies in 1970–1971 the average daily energy value was 2940 kcal. The contribution of fats has increased from 64 g per day in 1905–07 to 120 g per day in 1964. The contribution of carbohydrates and proteins decreased.

While in 1905 people consumed carbohydrates approx. 446 grams per day, in the 1960s the consumption was approx. 375 g per day.

According to FAO studies the amount of protein decreased from 109 g per day in 1905 to 90 g per day during the 1960s.[17]

In Table 2 is shown the latest information on the consumption of selected commodities per inhabitant compared with that of earlier decades. Of various commodities the consumption of cheese has increased rapidly and the consumption of grain products has decreased, especially the consumption of rye.

## Food industry

In 1860 about 4 per cent of the country's population was employed in industry, in 1900 the percentage was 11 and in 1960 it was 31 per cent. At the end of the last century the growth rate of the food, beverage and tobacco industry was the fastest. In 1910–1913 the employment rate in the food, beverage and tobacco industry was 13.3 per cent (cf. the percentage rate of manufacture of wood, cork, furniture, which was 24.6) of all the industrial employment. Between the wars the share of the food, beverage and tobacco industry was 15 per cent of the gross domestic product.[18] The development was so vigorous that before the Second World War Finnish domestic markets were dominated by products of the domestic tobacco industry as well as the sugar and margarine industry. On the other hand, it took two decades before the Finnish mill industry was compatible with the increase of the crop, and the import of grain ended.[19] In 1989, only 11 per cent of the Finns were employed in food manufacture. The main products of food manufacturing were meat, vegetables and fish. The second largest group of food manufacture products was that of bakery products.[20]

At the turn of the century, the sugar industry was one of the most important fields of industry. At first imported cane sugar was used as raw material, but from 1897 onwards Russian beet sugar – due to lower customs duties – was the most important raw material for the Finnish food industry. Before the First World War the customs duties favoured domestic production. At the beginning of this century a cartel for the sugar industry was created and during the 1920s and 1930s it was based more and more on domestic beet sugar as raw material.[21] Even though the sugar industry centralized at the turn of the century, it took two decades before the same trend was to be found with dairies. The number of private or cooperative dairies was up to the 1930s over 600. It can be explained by the dispersed settlement structure and the long distances between villages and towns. The development has followed the same trend toward centralized industry in all groups of the food industry.

Valio, a firm that produces milk products, is a clear example of a centralized company which has aimed to control the whole production chain of the dairy industry. It founded its own chemo-bacteriological laboratory where innovative research was conducted throughout the 1920s. This research work influenced clearly the quality of the food. Chemist A.I. Virtanen developed the AIV salt and the production method of AIV fodder. These innovations improved the production structure of the Finnish farm industry and opened a route to the world market for products like butter and cheese. In the 1930s Professor Virtanen focused his research on the bio-chemistry of vitamins.[22] Valio has almost managed to monopolize the dairy market till now. It has fully used the possibilities of marketing and participated actively in publishing dietary manuals and cookery books.

In Finland, the state has exercised strict authority in supervising the quality of food. In the 1950s and 1960s, the State Technical Research Centre had several research projects on the quality and preservation of food. Freezing and vacuum packing became popular. The research focused especially on the vitamin contents and methods for preserving the flavour of frozen products.[23] The relatively high percentage of women in the labour market has increased the popularity of frozen foods. Various kinds of frozen foods, especially berries and mushrooms, belong to the staple diet of every Finn.

### Differences between Eastern and Western Finland

One of the most challenging questions has been the difference in mortality rates in the western part of the country and the eastern part of the country. Could it be explained by the differences in the diets in eastern and western Finland?

During the 1950s there were studies on seasonal variations in the diet of the rural population in selected areas of eastern and western Finland. Maija Pekkarinen's study concerned 83 families in 1956, 40 families in 1957, and 60 new families in 1959. The survey took about three weeks in every season, and the recording period in every household a week each time. The food consumption was measured by accurate weighing.

The results show that in both areas and during the various seasons, 30–40% of the total energy was derived from cereals, 9–15% from butter, 20–24% from other milk products, 9–11% from sugar, 5–8% from meat and meat products, 3–5% from margarine, 5–7% from potatoes, 0.2–3% from other vegetables, 1–4% from fruit and berries, 0.3–2% from fish and 0.6–2% from eggs. The consumption of grain products, butter, milk and fish was higher in eastern than in western Finland, whereas more vegetables, fruit, berries, margarine, cheese and eggs were consumed in the west. This has resulted in a high rate of heart diseases in eastern Finland.[24]

These differences prevail up to the present, in spite of the efforts by heart surgeons to increase the proportion of vegetables in the diet. The latest studies reveal also that the lack of wine in the Finnish diet might contribute to the high rate of heart diseases.

## Conclusions

The Finnish diet has been affected by the particularly hard climate. People have been at the mercy of nature. Good potato and grain crops have been of great importance to the Finns. The bad memories of famine years were alive in people's minds for decades. The last famine year occurred in 1867–1868 and then diseases killed nearly 300,000 Finns. Finland was not self sufficient in grain before her independence in 1917, but after that year there was a strong will to achieve self sufficiency. Due to land reform policy, by which the number of independent landowners was increased, and the clearing of land, supported by the state, the arable land area became larger to the extent that today self sufficiency has been achieved in milk production (see Table 3) as well as in rye production in the late fifties. Now we have overproduction in all agricultural products.

*Table 3:* Self sufficiency in agricultural products in Finland

|              | 1950 | 1955 | 1960 | 1965 | 1970 | 1975 | 1980 | 1985 | 1990 |
|--------------|------|------|------|------|------|------|------|------|------|
| Milk (fat)   | –    | –    | 121  | 115  | 115  | 127  | 138  | 128  | 150  |
| Milk (liquid)| –    | –    | 115  | 113  | 111  | 123  | 130  | 129  | 133  |
| Pork         | 100  | 95   | 94   | 101  | 110  | 101  | 120  | 110  | 114  |
| Beef         | 100  | 100  | 91   | 93   | 110  | 98   | 102  | 121  | 109  |
| Eggs         | 105  | 106  | 123  | 124  | 136  | 153  | 140  | 162  | 138  |
| Rye          | 84   | 56   | 103  | 110  | 86   | 63   | 110  | 66   | 267  |
| Wheat        | 60   | 40   | 65   | 92   | 105  | 182  | 110  | 136  | 199  |

*Source:* Leppälä (1992)

Due to the state's strong agricultural policy the Finns have been accustomed to use milk products. The amount of fats in food was high till the Second World War. The consumption of butter increased from four kilos per person per year in 1860 to 14 kilos in the late 1950s. Figures that contained recommendations of proportions of different nutrients in food were sent to schools from the 1950s onwards (see Fig. 1). The importance of the use of vegetables in food has been systematically emphasized during the time of Finnish independence. Different organizations giving instructions have taken this information to homes since the 1870s. People have been encouraged to cultivate and use root crops and vegetables that were known to contain valuable vitamins and micronutrients. Finnish nutritionists know well the results from the newest research work. The efforts to change the eating habits have been stronger particularly after the Second World War as international research work has proved the connection between the quality of food (especially fats) and the high mortality rate of the Finns in heart diseases.

**Notes**

1 Turpeinen (1986), pp. 22, 231–237.
2 Häkkinen (1992), pp. 149–165.
3 Ibid., pp. 159–160.
4 Vihola (1991), pp. 379–380.
5 *Report of the economic situation in Finland 1871–1875, Official Statistics of Finland II:5.*
6 Relander (1892), pp. 12–27.
7 Ibid., pp. 85–99.
8 Sundström (1908).
9 Tigerstedt (1916).
10 Korppi-Tommola (1990), p. 70.
11 Virtanen and Turpeinen (1940), pp. 64–126.
12 Heikel (1941) and Sobraa-Bay (1940).
13 Hjelt (1912).
14 *Study of Living Expenses 1928*, SVT XXXXII, V, 14 A, and Roine (1954).
15 Virtanen and Roine (1956).
16 Ibid., pp. 92–93.
17 Koskinen (1974).
18 Ibid., pp. 15–20.
19 Hjerppe et al. (1976), p. 208.
20 *Suomen Taloushistoria 2* (1982), pp. 251–253.
21 *Finnish Statistical Yearbook 1992* (1992), p. 145.
22 *Suomen Taloushistoria 2* (1982), p. 80.
23 Michelsen (1993), pp. 51–58.
24 Ibid., pp. 246–247.
25 Pekkarinen (1962), pp. 151–152.

**Literature**

*Finnish Statistical Yearbook* (Helsinki, 1992).
Heikel, Armas, *Ravinto-oppi* (Helsinki, 1941).
Hjelt, Vera, *Tutkimus ammattityöläisten toimeentuloehdoista Suomessa 1908– 1909* (Helsinki, 1912).
Hjerppe, Reino, Riitta Hjerppe, Kauko Mannermaa, O.E. Niitamo and Kaarlo Siltari, 'Industry and Industrial Handicraft in Finland 1900–1965'. *Studies on Finland's economic growth VII* (Helsinki, 1976).
Häkkinen, Antti, 'On Attitudes and Living Strategies in the Finnish Countryside in the Years of Famine 1867–1868', in Antti Häkkinen (ed.), *Just a Sack of Potatoes?* (Helsinki, 1992).
Korppi-Tommola, Aura, *Terve lapsi – kansan huomen. Mannerheimin lasten- suojeluliitto yhteiskunnan rakentajana 1920–1990* (Helsinki, 1990).
Koskinen, Esko H., *Suomalaisten ruoankäyttö ja ravinnonsaanti vuosina 1967–1969* (Helsinki, 1974).

Leppäla, Juhani, *Ravintotaseen mukainen ruoka-aineiden tilastointi Suomessa* (Helsinki, 1992).

Michelsen, Karl-Erik, *Valtio, teknologia, tutkimus. VTT ja kansallisen tutkimusjärjestelmän kehitys* (Helsinki, 1993).

Pekkarinen, Maija, *Tutkimuksia maalaisväestön ravinnosta eräissä Itä- ja Länsi-Suomen pitäjissä* (Hämeenlinna, 1962).

Relander, Konrad, *Terveyshoidollisia Tutkimuksia Haapajärven Lääkäpiiristä I, Terveyteen vaikuttavien olosuhteiden ja tapojen ynnä yleisen terveyskannan valaisemiseksi Haapaveden kunnassa* (Diss.) (Kuopio, 1892).

*Report of the economic situation in Finland 1871–1875*, Official Statistics of Finland II:5.

Roine, Paavo, 'Työläis- ja toimenhaltijaperheiden ravinnon riittävyys Suomessa vuosina 1850–1951'. *Sosiaalinen Aikakauskirja, 48* (Helsinki, 1954).

Sobraa-Bay, Juliana, *Terveellinen Ravinto* (Porvoo, 1940), (first edition, Spis Dig Frisk).

*Study of Living Expenses 1928*, SVT XXXXII, V, 14 A.

*Suomen Taloushistoria 2, Teollistuva Suomi* (Helsinki, 1982).

Sundström, Sigfried, *Untersuchungen über die Ernährung der Landsbevölkerung in Finnland* (Helsinki, 1908).

Tigerstedt, Carl, 'Untersuchungen über die Nahrungszufuhr des Menschen in ihrer Abhängigkeit von Alter, Geschlecht und Beruf'. *Skandinavische Archiv der Physiologie, 34* (Helsinki, 1916).

Turpeinen, Oiva, *Nälkä vai tauti tappoi. Kauhunvuodet 1866–1868*, Societas Historica Finlandiae, Historiallisia Tutkimuksia, 136 (Helsinki, 1986).

Vihola, Teppo, *Leipäviljasta lypsykarjaan. Maatalouden tuotantosuunnan muutos Suomessa 1870-luvulta ensimmäisen maailmansodan vuosiin*, Societas Historica Finlandiae, Historiallisia Tutkimuksia, 159 (Helsinki, 1991).

Virtanen, A.I. and Paavo Roine, *Ihminen ja Ravinto* (Helsinki, 1956).

Virtanen, A.I. and O. Turpeinen, 'Tutkimus suhteellisen vähävaraisen väestön ravinnosta Suomessa 1936–1937'. *Komiteanmietintö, No 5* [Report of Committee no. 5] (Helsinki 1940).

# 14

# ECONOMICS OF SHORTAGE: CONDITIONS OF THE FOOD 'MARKET' IN THE CASE OF HUNGARY

## Eszter Kisbán

Standing on the Eastern periphery of regions that pioneered the socio-economic development of the modern age in Europe, Hungary, with a population of 10 millions, and a population density of 115/km², was still a primarily agrarian country with an underdeveloped industry at the mid-20th century. The decline in the proportion of the agricultural population, broadly coincides with the growth of urbanization, industry and services. The country had always been able to feed itself, and from the late Middle Ages, its leading exports were unprocessed agricultural commodities in large quantities. Food shortages were not unknown; these were not due to insufficient agrarian potential but had a social character.

*Table 1:* Agricultural population as a percentage of the total population in Hungary

| 1869 | 1880 | 1890 | 1910 | 1920 | 1945 | 1968 | 1990 |
|------|------|------|------|------|------|------|------|
| 75 | 73 | 71 | 62 | 56 | 49 | 30 | 14 |

*Sources:* Pach (1978), p. 427, 432; Berend – Ránki (1972), p. 184, 263; *Census returns* (1990), p. 31.

An organic economic development was interrupted by the coming of an imported totalitarian political system and its economic policy after the Second World War. At the expense of exports, the new social policy promised the availability of basic foods for everybody, and succeeded in this in the long run. But the economic policy caused tremendous trouble in domestic food production at the early stages, and, for lack of real marketing, could not get rid of symptoms of permanent shortages in the realm of food at later stages either.

## The economic system 1948–1989

Agriculture, industry and markets had still not recovered from wartime losses, when radical economic changes began to lead towards a socialist economic system.[1] The completely centrally directed economic system, which was being introduced by force to Hungary from 1948/49 onwards, had been developed in the USSR under totally different socio-economic circumstances from the late 1920s. Both the totalitarian philosophy itself and the targetted economic system required the nationalization of production and trade in Hungary. This was quickly and radically carried through. Only agriculture was omitted, because it was politically expedient to win over the agricultural population.

Economic historians make a twofold division of the period of controlled economy in Hungary on the basis of the dominant methods of economic direction: 'command economy' in the earlier decades, and an improved 'controlled economy' after 1968. As it quickly turned out that the system did not work efficiently, there was criticism from economists already in the first period; this was usually suppressed, but sometimes broke through, and did lead to improvements at some points in the system. From 1953, agriculture was the first area to benefit in this respect.

The classical socialist command economy not only wanted to plan the whole economic circle – namely, providing the producers with financial investment (for which capital was always lacking), energy, materials, man-power, deciding on the range of products to come to the market, controlling purchasing power and meantime eliminating the real market, real costs, real prices and real trade – but was also controlling all these by direct commands through a hierarchical bureaucracy that stretched from the National Planning Office down to the single person. Anyone unable to fulfil the plan, for reasons outside his control, might lose his life.

From the mid-1950s, partial improvements in the economic system appeared increasingly, but dogmatic politics kept on causing set-backs – a factor which did not cease after the 1960s either. Such improvements, however, re-introduced training in some mechanisms, providing experience which eased the way back to a market economy in the 1990s.

The domestic price-system was separated from world-market prices in August 1946, when a new currency (the forint) was introduced after a postwar hyper-inflation. It was presumed that the agricultural prices in Hungary, an agricultural country, could be regulated for a short time outside world-market influences by Government decisions, especially since just then there was no marketable agricultural export surplus. These presumed short-term measures were very soon integrated into the new socialist economic policy, in which, in relation to the whole economic scale, sale prices bore then no relation to costs, and foreign trade prices no relation to domestic prices. A chance to improve the system was greatly helped by improving trading opportunities for Hungary in the world market during the 1960s. The 1968 'new economic mechanism' brought with it a new philosophy of direction. This replaced the system of compulsory plan directives by indirect economic regulators to influence firms' activities, introduced something like market links amongst the participants in the economic theatre, granted more independence and some degree of involvement for the participants and also widely re-established domestic market prices, even if they were still strongly controlled and heavily subsidized. The 1979 price reform began for the first time to link domestic prices again with the world market. From the early 1980s onwards, combinations of state ownership and small private businesses were encouraged, and prestige again began to be given to individual enterprises. The increasing number of reform steps towards a market economy could, however, not change the essence of the system, without the proper political structure for such a change.

After this happened in 1990, the last three years have been hard years of transition towards a functioning market economy, and there will be many more such hard years to come. After the shortages of the socialist economy, there is already an increased offer of food and consumer goods, but the consumer is hit by severe impoverishment, by unemployment (11% in January 1993), and by such high inflation – all of which had been unknown since 1946, and with which the social security system is not yet able to cope adequately.

## An 'Economics of Shortage'

Consumption statistics show that the supply of basic foods progressively increased during the second half of the 20th century over the long run. This could raise the illusion that there hardly had been shortages in the supply of provisions in Hungary. This illusion is partly right and partly wrong. It is true that the Hungarian food policy differed from that of some other socialist countries, where, up to the late 1980s, there periodically appeared, for extended periods, food shops with rows of empty shelves. The impression of a good supply in Hungary is still false, because one of the permanent central problems of a socialist economy is shortages. This is not a specific Hungarian phenomenon, but it is in Hungary that economists were allowed to demonstrate the all-pervading character of the shortage-symptom; they described it empirically, and analysed it using mathematical means. Occasional shortages can also occur in market economies, but in the socialist economy, shortage cannot be eliminated because certain features of the social conditions and the economic mechanism perpetually recreate or regenerate shortage. The precise functioning can be found in János Kornai's two famous, substantial volumes in English on the 'Economics of Shortage'.[2]

As shortage was the main problem of the economy, so it was also for the pre-1990 food and diet: shortage in production, shortcomings in the allocation and provision of supply between producer and consumer, shortage in terms of quantity, variety and quality, with changing intensity as time went on. The consumer had to be content simply with having enough food to eat. Often he had no other choice than to substitute another commodity, or to put up with the fact that the pre-war variety never seemed to be returning; that food innovations observed West of the Iron Curtain during travel possibilities which opened out after the 1960s, though still in a very limited way, would not reach Hungary soon; and that the domestic production of labour-saving convenience foods and household devices would grow only slowly. At household level, such shortage, queueing, and enforced substitution of commodities was the main long-term food-related problem of the period.

The standard of living, though tending to rise, remained low throughout the period, but people could afford to buy enough food. The allocation of household resources to food was 44 % and 35.3 % in the two main sections of society in 1960 and the proportion dropped to 32 % and 25.7 % respectively by 1983 (when it was 43.4% in the least and 24.6 % for the most privileged subsections).[3]

## Changing targets and the food supply

The security and range of the national food supply received changing digits in the hierarchy of economic targets during the relevant decades.

Interrupting post-war reconstruction and balanced stabilisation, the incoming socialist political system launched a new economic target, the goal being an ambitious, unrealistically rapid industrialization. Within five years, the Hungarian economy had to be changed from the agricultural-industrial stage to a primarily industrial status, to a 'country of iron and steel'. Capital accumulation highly surpassed the growth of national income and was primarily spent on mining and metallurgy. At the same time, a national economic self-sufficiency in almost all branches of production was targetted, taking into account the raw material resources of the member states of the Council of Mutual Economic Assistance when necessary. This development had to be financed at the expense of agriculture and of the standard of living. The policy was terminated as soon as a change in power relations in the USSR gave an opportunity.

Prospects for public supply began to change in 1953, with food as the primary concern. As time went on, the goals of the economic policy changed sharply several times but the stable supply of basic food increasingly stabilized. The first target was bread, the second sugar, than came fat and meat. Milk was rated lower and also proved to be a harder task to carry through. Although the 'food market' improved greatly, a markedly better range of offerings in food and consumers' goods set in only during the 1980s. Expanding the range in such commodities was now a political target to gain public sympathy. Heavy foreign loans were not sufficiently used for modernization of the industry but were abundantly spent on the standard of living.

**Production**

The elimination of a market economy and the exclusion of food imports minimized the role of trading in the dietary realm. The main question for the supply became that of how the agriculture and the food industries were allowed to perform. I have to exclude the development of food exports here but it has to be said that after painful periods of decline, the relatively early turn for the better again in agriculture was initiated by the domestic hunger for food while the country's hunger for hard currency initiated the later introduction of new technologies to the food industries and to the manufacture of food related household equipment. However restricted the way in which such innovations could come in, at the everyday level they represented the closest link to market economies within the dietary realm for the Hungarian consumer.

*Agriculture*

Pre-war Hungarian agriculture badly needed modernization. Only threshing was fully mechanised, while manual labour and animal draught, a low level of use of fertilizers, and underdeveloped food-processing dominated in other cases.

Priority after the War was not given to the quickest possible reconstruction of War damage but to radical reform in land ownership. (Fields were not sown in winter/spring 1944/1945, and there was a strong decline in live-stock and machinery.)

Between 1945 and the present, there have been five main, contradictory waves aimed at changing administratively the size of farming units, ownership, and individual or collective forms of farming. There were state farms all the time, but the crucial domain of production remained the individual/collective holding.

Motivated by administration of social justice, a democratically elected coalition government decided on and implemented a nearly all-embracing radical land reform for the benefit of agricultural labourers and the smallest landholders in 1945. Formerly, 72.5 % of landed properties averaged less than 1 ha. All holdings above 100 or 200 holds (1 hold = 0.57 ha) were expropriated and reallocated. This measure eliminated the institution of large estates of medieval origin. (Estates of over 1000 holds comprised 30 % of the land before the reform, with an average size of 4300 holds each.) The land reform created an agriculture on the basis of very small farming units. Time was not given for them to stabilize.[4]

Socialist policy started to 'collectivise' the agriculture already in 1948. Smallholders were to place their land at the disposal of new collective farms and amalgamate into the working of the unified, large fields. This was most disappointing for new holders of land. Better-off peasants, as 'class enemies', were not invited to join the cooperatives at that stage, nor were the trained managers of former large estates. Thus the emerging cooperatives lacked managerial experience in large-scale farming.[5] Because of poor economic performance and political tension, forced collectivisation of agriculture, aiming at 100 % elimination of individual farming, was discontinued between 1953 and 1959. 40 % of the members returned to individual farming which in this period held control of 78 % of all arable land.[6]

In the second wave between 1959 and 1961 the total collectivisation was completed, with the difference that experienced farmers were now appreciated and state subsidies began to go to collective farming. The early principle of one-village one-collective-farm was later replaced by the target of economic size, and the fields of several villages could be farmed as one unit. Agricultural engineers managed the large farms increasingly. Alongside the emerging large units, members of the cooperatives were allowed to keep 1 ha as household plots for individual farming. There were individual dramas and even tragedies, poor economic performances in the early stages, but later production rose continuously. Even if some cooperatives, mostly in a geographically poor environment, fared badly, most of the land was used profitably and agriculture allowed for large exports by the time of the next radical change.

In 1990, the incoming democratic political system decided to administer justice again in the domain of ownership and to offer free choice about the form of farming. All cooperatives have to declare their dissolution. Co-operative farming may be reorganized with farmers who wish to continue in that way. At the same time, everybody who was expropriated or was forced to place his holding at the disposal of the state or cooperatives at whatever period after the war, will now be compensated in a very complicated way. (Compensation excludes the estates with over 1000 holds before 1945.) It cannot yet be seen what size of farming units will emerge as dominating for future Hungarian agriculture, nor when agriculture – now in decline – will revive.

The goal of considerable mechanisation of agriculture was not even set before 1957. The first target was the grain-harvest. This was done up to 57% by the scythe in 1960, then mechanised up to 93% by 1970. Machinery was adapted to large farming units.[7]

Decision making about production had been taken away from agriculture by the end of the 1940s. The National Planning Office calculated the size of the sowing area for each product, the number of livestock the country demanded for domestic supply and possible exports. The figures were then bureaucratically broken down from the national level to the single farming units themselves. For field cultivation these directives were know as the 'sowing plan'. Such plans every so often ordered the cultivation of plants for which the soil of a farm was not suitable. Agricultural units were instructed through the local administration and were not given the chance to disobey.

Up to 1953 it was also centrally decided on which day (not weather permitting!) the major tasks in agriculture should begin and end. Daily reports to the main centre were required from everywhere on the progress of the plans. The hated concept of the 'sowing plan' was eliminated in 1956 but continued in the form of strong suggestions of such control, and only after 1966 was it reduced to bread-grain alone. Decision making on farming was later increasingly returned to the cooperatives.

The post-war limitation of marketing for the sake of public supply continued as an integral part of the socialist economy. In the late 1940s three channels were specified for agricultural products. These were 'compulsory delivery' to the state at a symbolic price; sale to state organs at specified low prices, and free marketing. The first two channels included nearly every agricultural product. Compulsory delivery and taxation in kind provided for 74% of the national grain store in 1950, compulsory delivery alone for 73% of all agricultural products in such concentration in 1952, while not enough product was allowed to remain to feed the producers themselves. In practice only products which had always been rarities were admitted to the free market. Only 1% of grain went there in 1952–53.[8] Compulsory delivery meant that the producer had to deliver a fixed quota of his products to the state at pennies only. In principle, the quota should not have endangered seed-corn, breeding stock and home consumption, but in view of the character of requisition, it very often did. Collection of the quotas was implemented by local authorities with rude force in order to carry out the local share of the central plans. After 1956, compulsory delivery was replaced by the building up of stocks through the buying up through state organs of agricultural products at a specified low price. Instead of using administrative commands, those prices became the means of directing agricultural production. The prices now recognised the basic costs of production, in order to motivate sufficient supply, the satisfaction of the demand of the food industries, and to ensure state exports as well. This change in the agriculture was the pioneering step towards the not yet officially announced 'new economic mechanism'. Soon the agricultural producer was allowed to choose between national purchasing agencies and could bargain for a somewhat better price in contractual procurement. They could also build up a small share in the actual food processing.

With such specific problems, and also heavy common burdens to carry, agricultural performance was very poor until the mid-1960s. Animal husbandry suffered most. From the 1960s onwards the strongholds of animal husbandry became the household farming plots of members of the cooperatives. Such plots specialized also in market-gardening of labour intensive vegetables. Animal products and such vegetables always paid best. Grain and fodder predominated on the large fields of the cooperatives. During the 1970–80s, cooperatives introduced complete large-scale systems for breeding chicken, producing eggs, and also for growing maize as fodder. At the same time, private market-gardening began to grow vegetables out of season, paprikas and tomatoes in plastic-covered green-houses. Agriculture, at last, was once again steadily performing well.

## Food industry

The main driving force towards modernization of the food industry in Hungary has always been the world market. In the region of the country which provided the main exports, cattle, from the late Middle Ages, a wheat monoculture developed from the mid-19th century, taking advantage of industrialization in Western Europe. This was soon followed by the building up of the first large-scale food-related industry, modern market-milling, which became the main Hungarian industry.[9] The rural population, however, used small mills up till the mid-20th century. When the possibility of flour export diminished by the turn of the century, an export-orientated sugar industry was ready to take its place (the domestic average per capita consumption of sugar in 1900 was only 4 kg a year per head).[10] Between the Wars, a canning industry began to develop, also with an export orientation, producing in particular tomato conserves; even urban middle-class households, however, were still doing their own preserving.

In the mid-20th century, not only the part of the population that lived by agriculture, but also other rural and even urban elements practised the baking of bread, the preservation of fat, meat, milk, vegetables (sauerkraut, paprika), fruit and the making of noodles as domestic skills. In 1910, for example, only 15% of all Hungarian settlements had a baker; in the others there was no demand at all for ready-made bread.[11] This situation did not change to any great degree until the middle of the century. At the beginning of the War, the larger cities were not yet served by bread-factories, but by several small bakeries. As a consequence of the War, then of nationalization and the persecution of small craftsmen, the food industry collapsed, and the reconstruction took place on a concentrated, large-scale basis. The preferences here were also bread, sugar, fat, meat and milk, and brewing probably escalated unexpectedly. The reconstruction of the sugar industry was given preference, in order to satisfy the demand for calories; this task was more easy to promote than the provision of fat. Between 1934–38 the national average of sugar consumption was 10.5 kg only per year, in 1954 24.2 kg. The low level of milk production especially hindered the development of the milk industry. The consumption of milk and milk products regained the very low pre-war level by 1967 only (just over 100 l. of milk per annum). Brewing had already been concentrated in a few large breweries before the War. Only after the War did the reconstructed brewing industry turn to the domestic market. In this wine-growing country, in 1934–38 the average annual beer intake per head was only 3.1 l., but consumption was in practice only an urban phenomenon.[12] In 1960, intake stood at 36.8 l. per head. Manufacturing of another cereal food, noodles, a traditional basic food in the dietary system, became important after the War when women were increasingly sent out to work.

The introduction of modern technologies into the food industry began from the 1960s, when there again first opened up the possibility of export markets to the West, when the product could come close to Western quality. Packaging technology always lagged far behind the quality of the products. The domestic consumer profited, but with some delays, from the results of modernization, but never up to the level of demand.

Whilst carrying the burden of the economic policy and its mechanisms, the food industry was able to respond, especially badly, to the demands upon it between 1944–1968. At that time, the number of consumers not living from agriculture grew by 20%, and as a new factor, even the agricultural sector from time to time needed to purchase bread and fresh meat. At such a critical period, the food industry, like any other producer, instead of having a market orientation, was under the obligation of supplying provisions. In spite of central planning, the food industry often was in trouble from lack of raw resources, for it could not get quickly at the existing domestic agricultural products that were allocated to it through bureaucratic channels. At the early stage of command economy, the food industries were not being helped by proper allocation of supplies, but efforts were made to improve them by the imposition of death sentences. In September 1950 the crime against public supply of the chief executives of the National Meat Concern was heard before a 'workers' court'. The two main defendants were sentenced to death. The sentence was carried out on the same day.[13]

During the post-war decades, production of food and consumer goods was carried out at a level affordable by everyone, but at a low standard of quality. The main target was quantity. Such variety as existed before the War was lost, and the quality deteriorated seriously. This decline, and especially the attitudes developed by such a policy in the long run, have had a continuing influence up to the present day, although there was considerable development later.

The food policy put stress on the priorities of the former urban demand. One example is wheaten bread. Formerly, in many parts of the country, a light-coloured rye-bread was traditional. In the 1960s, over half the bread production was of 'white' wheaten bread (with 10–15% of rye in it, out of necessity); over a third was made of pure wheat flour ('fine-white' so called). Only a little rye-bread was made for the delicatessen shops in the capital.[14] The first post-war innovation in variety came onto the bread market in the 1970s. This was the first dark-looking bread to have appeared in Hungary for centuries, as the only contribution of the occupying Soviet army to the Hungarian food industry.[15] It was marketed in small quantities as a delicacy in the capital, mainly, although the source of inspiration for it was not revealed. Forms of bread in wider variety, including non-traditional additions which had been very fashionable in the West of Europe, only came onto the market after the mid-1980s. This was at a time when the demand for bread had declined seriously, and the producer became interested in sales again. Amongst meat products, top quality salami remained a good export commodity, and was therefore in short supply on the national market nearly throughout the socialist period. The Hungarian food industry started to offer deep-frozen commodities and convenience foods much later than Western producers, and the amount on offer increased only slowly.

Taking milk as an example of packaging, the replacement of bottles by plastic bags for more than two decades was not an unmixed pleasure, because of the poor quality of the bags. But because milk could not be marketed abroad anyway, the greatly desired milk cartons only appeared in 1991, when environmentalists were already querying their benefits.

For all sections of the food industry, a real reviving interest in domestic sales has slowly been becoming the outstanding driving force again, but only after the mid-1980s.

*Household equipment*

For long, even less investment went into the manufacturing of food-related consumer goods than into the food industries. The first in sequence was the iron cooking ranges both for those who were leaving the countryside and for those who stayed. Gas- and electric cookers replaced them in manufacturing later.

Refrigerators were not officially seen as a primary necessity. A single, export-orientated, domestic manufacturing plant served the market between the 1960s and the mid-1980s, in addition to poorer quality imports from the USSR in low numbers. In different types of households in 1960, 0–4 refrigerators were found per 100 households. In 1970 the figures run between 11–62, in 1980, 84–101, and in 1983, 91–114.

Deep-freezes in 1983 varied 0–7 in number per 100 households of different types, a lower figure than that for cars, although the latter were considered (alongside housing), as the most serious shortage for the public.[16] Up to 1989, people were queueing in front of the only domestic producer's own shop on the first day of the year in order to be amongst those for whom delivery of a deep-freeze or a particular kind of refrigerator would be assured during the year. When the Government made a mistake in the late 1980s and opened three possibilities for a few months – namely, the buying of limited amounts of hard currency, permission to travel to the West and a low import tax for tourists at the same time – then families travelled in tens of thousands to Austria to buy great numbers of inexpensive Jugoslav deep-freezes and refrigerators. The whole family was needed to qualify for taking advantage of all favours, so some aged grandparents died of exhaustion, accidents happened through the overloading of cars with goods, Austrian sellers profited and the instalment repayment of national debts was jeopardized.

Microwave-cookers were not available before the mid-1980s and started to appear in Soviet-made heavy variants at first.

## Distribution: allocation and marketing

The wholesale and retail trade alike were nationalized after the War, and only the keepers of small family shops had to be frightened into giving up private enterprise. The agricultural product was channeled by the state to industrial plants and the products of the food industry into the trading shops, all according to 'plans of allocation of provision'. Products moved hierarchically through many more steps than were rational. The complicated and changing network has not been properly studied yet.

Instead of real marketing, the wholesale and retail trade had the 'obligation of supplying' the public properly as did the food industries. Wholesale enterprises were spread through the country, served large regions, and specialized in groups of commodities. The retailers' orders travelled a long route through several intermediaries, many of them without a telephone in the earlier stages. The route of the product to the shop was not shorter either. The shop manager could only hope that an order would be carried out on time and would not be short in quantity. To get the supply, shops had to fraternize with the supplier and give regular tips to the carrier. If the supply did not arrive, there was no way of easy immediate substitution. Shops would indicate public demand for better quality or for variety to the supplier in vain, as long as the food industries were not ready to respond or not yet interested in doing so. No wonder that the morale of the especially badly paid shop-personnel quickly deteriorated and did not recover fully until the present day, when real trading has begun again.

To build up a new network of foodshops after nationalization, two chains of food stores were early established to serve the whole country, in the place of individual shops which formerly dominated. The Közért chain (1948, the acronym means 'for the public') served urban, and another chain the rural areas.[17] Later a parallel urban chain of foodshops was established, called Delicatessen, but in fact it was a sligthly better quality general foodshop. Then fruit and vegetables together developed their own urban chain of shops. This was practically the whole network of foodshops for more than 30 years. Providing all of them with the necessary cooling capacity could not even be completed within that timespan. Open market places and covered market buildings remained in operation for fresh agricultural products. After the 1960s they looked increasingly good as the countryside had more and more to offer in them.

The last measures of post-war rationing ended ceremonially in August 1949. However, rationing had to be reintroduced for sugar, flour, fat, meat and finally for bread in 1951. This again ended in December of that year.[18] The appearance of the shelves of urban shops may be gauged from these facts. Rural shops fared worse always. Sometimes strange surrogates had to be offered for sale in the shops during the 1950s, for example South-American frozen beef, imported against the principle, and never seen before in the country, so serious was the absolute shortage of meat.

From the late 1970s, food supply in the shops became, in quantity and quality, though still not in variety, so adequate, that Austrians from near the border started to shop for food regularly in nearby Hungarian cities, mainly meat, eggs, and milk products. With the heavily subsidized Hungarian prices it has, though decreasingly, been good value for them.

Most imported and some domestic commodities did not reappear in the shops after 1948 for a long time. Such was veal. Why eat veal when a calf would become a grown-up animal and give more meat? – said the food policy literally at an early stage. Later the absence of veal just continued up to 1992. Alongside several foreign spices and coffee, the supply of tropical fruit was short as well (see Table 3). In the oral history of the 1950s, there are brilliant narratives about the lack especially of oranges. Later bananas became the most desired of such commodities.

As long as the sale of food was not real marketing but just allocation and distribution, haunted by shortage, there was not much sense in advertising, nor was it much practised either. Advertising is now just beginning. The few earlier pioneering steps would be worth looking at.

During the present transition, many large old industrial plants, including those of food industries, went into receivership after 1990. This led to shortages of supply even in everyday foods. West European businesses have been quick to fill such gaps. The top executive of Budapest's largest, new supermarket tells in January 1993 that 65% of their turnover was Hungarian, and 35% was of West European products during the previous 10 months. Prices of imported commodities are up to 30% higher there than those for domestic commodities of the same kind, but the price difference usually includes differences in quality as well. The shop, which is in an industrial district, flourishes.[19] Such a welcome explains why so many Western companies accepted invitations to a special food-show in Budapest in 1992, the first for more than fifty years.

**Consumption and diet**

The year by year statistics of those commodities of concern to the Government during the last fifty years, not only show the trend of development in the long run, but also reflect well the disorder in the supply that has been previously referred to. Recently, consequential and serious cuts in the subsidisation of consumer prices for food products have run from 1988 onwards, while real wages have not kept up with them. The milk industry, for example, gave the information in January 1993 that consumption had dropped from the nearly 200 litres per capita a year average in 1987 to 130–140 litres at the present.[20] To the statistics that follow, it should be added that fish has always been an unimportant commodity (its share was 0.7 kg in 1934–38 and 2.8 kg in 1989); the milk includes liquid and manufactured milk; cereals include grain flour and rice, where rice is not a basic commodity (its consumption figures were 2.3 kg in 1934–38 and 4.5 kg in 1989).[21]

*Table 2:* Annual per capita food consumption (kg) and daily calorie-intake in Hungary 1934–1990

| year | meat, meat products, fish | milk | eggs (piece) | fat | cereals | sugar | potatoes | nutritive material kJ/day |
|------|------|------|------|------|------|------|------|------|
| 1934–1938 | 33,9 | 101,9 | 93 | 17,0 | 147,0 | 10,5 | 130,0 | 11 221 |
| 1950 | 34,9 | 99,0 | 85 | 18,7 | 142,1 | 16,3 | 108,7 | 11 317 |
| 1960 | 49,1 | 114,0 | 160 | 23,5 | 136,2 | 26,6 | 97,6 | 12 301 |
| 1970 | 60,4 | 109,6 | 247 | 27,7 | 128,2 | 33,5 | 75,1 | 12 971 |
| 1980 | 73,9 | 166,2 | 317 | 30,5 | 115,2 | 37,9 | 61,2 | 13 486 |
| 1990 | 75,8 | 169,9 | 389 | 38,6 | 110,4 | 38,2 | 61,0 | 14 164 |

*Source:* Statistical Yearbook (1990), p. 15, (1991), p. 14.

Out of the total meat/processed meat/poultry consumption from 1934–38 to 1989, the proportion of carcass pork rose from 45% to 55.3%, that of beef dropped from 17% to 9.7%, and poultry rose from 25% to 28.2%. It would be an urgent task to see the development of the use of milk products alongside liquid milk, but sufficient statistical data for that have not yet been processed.

Vegetables and home-grown fruit are commodities, the production of which central planning was least able to control in the long run. The development of their consumption, along with beer and wine, coffee and tropical fruit, completes the picture of the structure of supply and of the diet. For 1934–38 the consumption figure for vegetables and fruit is available in a combined figure only, and it was 95 kg.

*Table 3:* Annual per capita food consumption (kg) in Hungary 1950–1990

| year | vegetables | fruit | domestic fruit | tropical fruit | coffee | beer litres | wine litres |
|------|------|------|------|------|------|------|------|
| 1950 | – | – | – | – | 0.1 | 8.3 | 33.0 |
| 1960 | 84.1 | 55.3 | 53.5 | 1.8 | 0.1 | 36.8 | 29.9 |
| 1970 | 83.2 | 72.5 | 66.5 | 6.0 | 1.6 | 59.4 | 37.7 |
| 1980 | 79.6 | 74.9 | 65.9 | 9.0 | 2.9 | 86.0 | 34.8 |
| 1989 | 82.2 | 77.5 | 66.7 | 10.8 | 2.6 | 104.0 | 22.8 |
| 1990 | 85 | 70 | – | – | 2.2 | 106.9 | 23.9 |

*Sources:* Statistical Yearbook (1985), p. 246, (1990), p. 216.

Lack of space prevents discussion of the details of consumption development, changes and turning points in the trends, the variety underlying the main groups of commodities, nutritional status, the relationship to real income, and a comparison with the development of European regions that operated within the framework of a market economy. Some important trends of such regions appeared in Hungary also, but with a time gap, and others will still come.

Leaving aside price-wage relations, conditions of persistent shortage would themselves explain why the nutritional consciousness of the people stayed underdeveloped. The availability of daily calories again reached in

1950 what had been the national average of 2800 in 1934–38, and thereafter never fell below that figure. Before the War, there were serious deficiences even in calories amongst some groups of the working classes, but after that there was a balancing out throughout all levels of society. Official dietetics found that the 3000 calories which were reached in 1955 were ideal in terms of energy-intake for that time. When calorie-intake reached 3200 daily for a single year in 1956, the risks of an excessive diet began to be pointed to. Such warnings never ceased but they have failed to catch the primary concern of the population. In nutritional terms it has been suggested that calorie-intake should never have risen above the daily 3000 average and should preferably decrease as time went on,[22] whereas the actual figure passed the daily 3200 calories permanently in 1968 and stood at 3550 in 1990.

The development of diet, and people's ambitions and attitudes towards it, were, in the socialist economic setting, basically influenced by the actual supply offered to them and thus by the autarchy of the supply which was marked by a disturbed domestic agriculture, an underdeveloped food industry, and inefficient 'marketing'. The psychology of shortage, and the low rate of innovations offered to the households, made people concentrate on what they were familiar with in foodstuffs and in ways of preparation of dishes, and also the composition of meals. This is not 'tradition' in the ethnological meaning of the word but forced traditionalism. For simplicity, however, I shall refer to such elements as traditional ones. All the elements I call traditional were known and used in the country before the War. For many items there was strong social stratification in their use, fluctuating between no and frequent occurrences. After the War, the most important change in the national diet has been a levelling out. New generations were interested in making up for quantity and variety. They were increasingly able to achieve these ends, and to become familiar with forms of food which had been there before but which their forefathers could not afford or would not as yet want to eat. These people felt such development to be an achievement. Others, who had to cook and eat within their old frameworks, now tightened, had to concentrate their ambition on the invention of how to find the basic traditional foodstuffs most quickly and easily under the conditions of short, irregular supply.

The one and only statistically representative national dietary inquiry, which specified all daily meals together with their dishes, refers to the year 1958–59. It already reports significant changes as against pre-war patterns in the organisation of family daily meals as well as the shifting frequency of the preparation of different foods. The change was towards urban habits. I shall give three examples. Not only those who had recently left agriculture, but also those who remained in it, changed the sequence of meals during the day, reshaped the composition of breakfast, and noticeably rearranged the ways of preparing meat. Previously the agricultural population excercised an only two-meals-a-day sequence during the winter half of the year, not out of poverty but as a tradition from the Middle Ages. In that system, the meals were in the mid-morning and the afternoon, but not at midday. It had now been changed into the urban breakfast-midday dinner-evening meal sequence. Previously no hot morning drink or coffee had gained much of a foothold in everyday rural diet, whereas is 1958/59, 80 % of agricultural households had a breakfast drink and 55 % of such drinks was white coffee (surrogate). (The rates for non-agricultural households were 96 % for a breakfast drink, of which 41 % was always white coffee.) The Wiener-Schnitzel preparation of meat, which became fashionable in the country in the early 19th century, was still only a rare element of highly festive cooking with the agricultural population before the War. The rate of its preparation (although from pork instead of veal) amongst all meat dishes had risen to over 10 % by 1958–59 amongst those who stayed in agriculture while the same quota was nearly 21 % amongst the non-agricultural population (pottage cookery with vegetables excluded in both cases).[23]

Much regional variety has been lost since the War. An example was rye-bread, since for decades even the growing of rye nearly disappeared entirely. Rural maize-dishes have been stigmatized as poor man's food and as being out of date, and have retired from their weekly occurrence to being, at most, a dish of nostalgia once a year. There are many more such examples. The revitalisation movement has as yet hardly begun.

Post-war novelties (as against 'traditional' elements) in foodstuffs, cooking, dishes and menus, i.e. innovations, would have been my preferred topic for this volume. Their rate of occurrence in the diet is still so low that in contrast to EC statistics,[24] official Hungarian food statistics have not yet included them as items with names.

Space prevents enumeration of which innovations have reached Hungary at all, of how their first occurrence has spread over the period, and of what their social stratification is like at the present date.

The only example I shall give, is based on a recent case study in an urban settlement, and may indicate the urban situation in Hungary reasonably well, excluding the capital.[25] Rural areas would be even more traditional. The town of Tatabánya is a country seat with 77,000 inhabitants, 65 km west of Budapest. In 1920, it was only a small colony of 8,500 inhabitants, which grew because of coal-mining. As a mining community and a new administrative centre, it became a priviliged place in the second half of the century. A sample taken there of eating habits, still in progress, is small as yet. It includes the meals of 21 children aged 10, from different social backgrounds, listed during one week in autumn 1992. At the present stage of the project I am unable to compare the number of traditional dishes which predominated, with the number of post-war new dishes, but I can tell in what percentage of all meals new items are included (alone or alongside traditional food and drink), as well as what these new items are. As meals during the day, breakfast, morning snack, dinner, afternoon snack and evening meals occured, though not everybody had all of these. The number of meals on which statistics could be based numbered 589, though the total recorded was greater. Of the 589, only 55 meals (i.e 9 % of all meals), included a food, dish or drink, which was new in Hungary in the second half of the 20th century. All the other items were available and used in the country before the Second Word War (not necessarily amongst the predecessors of these children).

In order of frequency of occurrence, the new items are: cola, fruit-juice, pizza, wholemeal rolls, a certain sparkling light drink (then heavily advertised), muesli, yoghurt, kefir, hamburgers, patisson, tonic and courgette.[26] Their individual occurrence in the sample is very low. Cola was most frequent, in 2.2 % of the 589 meals, and courgette the least frequent, at 0.16 %. There is another new phenomenon in the sample, as yet not numerically defined, and that is the eating of bread with margarine instead of bread with butter. The time range of the domestic availability of these new items varies but, in most cases, the beginnings fall within the last 20 years. So the range of innovations is very limited, and the rate of spread low. Compared with the range and recent spread of post-war food innovations in Western Europe, such a sample may most strikingly indicate the difference in dietary development between regions with a market economy and those with even improved socialist economies in Europe.

As a post-war novelty, nearly every workplace and school has gradually provided a canteen, or at least a midday dinner. These could not set examples for the households in terms of better nutritional value, nor in variety of dishes. Neither did the catering industry as a whole, as long as financial conditions allowed wide social strata to eat out frequently up to the mid-1980s. It required great efforts to run the canteen-system not with snacks but with the old urban middle-class three course dinner at midday. That model was so strong that not even salad as an independent dish or course could come in. Dinner was intended to be the main meal of the day. There was no official attempt to postpone the nation's main daily meal to the evening in their own households.

Ethnic food restaurants, selling foreign dishes, first began to operate only in the 1980s. Neither the Mediterranean nor the Chinese establishments are any cheaper than Hungarian food in comparable categories. American-type fast food was pioneered by McDonald's at the same date. Fish and chips have not intruded as yet.

The 20th century trend, both in consumption, and in the whole diet, was for both social and regional differences to diminish. The trend is the same as in market economies but the level at which the levelling out took place differs greatly in choice, in variety and especially in the rate of innovations at the advent of the 1990s.

## Conclusions

The foodways' framework of recent centuries was set in Hungary, with a continuing effect, in the élite culture between 1690–1720. The innovations (sequence, hierarchy, and character of the daily meals; hot morning drink; soup as introductory course at the main meals; compulsory use of individual plate, spoon, and fork; round or oval tables instead of rectangular ones) spread in the social scale but, for special regional reasons affecting Hungary, took a long time to be adopted by the agricultural population who, in cultural manifestations, all shared a peasant way of life. This situation began to change about 1880 when peasants began to orientate towards a middle class, urban culture. But the clock has not turned fully round even by 1948, when there were still many vivid old forms of eating habits in the countryside. In the acceptance of staple foods too, there was a greater gulf between the agricultural population and the rest of society between 1690 and the mid-20th century than before and after. The 40 years of socialist economy, controlled market circumstances, an economics of shortage, narrowed the range available for food innovations. Even urban eating habits could not change much. This situation gave the rural population, already disturbed in their ways of life, the chance to complete a continuing process in closing the old social gap in eating habits by giving up forms of organisation of meals and use of foodstuffs which had been long outdated in urban culture. Together with the changes in the social structure, these developments resulted in considerable progress in the levelling out of Hungarian foodways. This trend is similar (though not in content) to the tendency for a social levelling out in European market economies at the same period.

## Notes

* I am greatly indebted to the Hungarian National Research Foundation (OTKA) for assistance with the present research (Programmes No. 3109, 4876).

1  For a comprehensive survey on the economic history, see Berend – Ránki (1985), pp. 177–316; further specification is available only in Hungarian, see Petö – Szakács (1985); the second volume of this work has not been completed.
2  Kornai (1980).
3  *Household statistics* (1983), pp. 21, 33.
4  Donáth (1980), pp. 51–170.
5  Donáth (1980), pp. 171–279.
6  Berend – Ránki (1985), pp. 221, 231.
7  Petö – Szakács (1985), p. 489.
8  Petö – Szakács (1985), pp. 133, 184, 201.
9  *Hungarian flour-milling industry* (1896).

10 Wiener (1902); Kisbán (1989b).
11 *Census 1910* (1913), pp. 2–917.
12 *Statistical Yearbook* (1964), p. 288.
13 Benda (1982), p. 1057.
14 Gasztonyi – Schneller (1963), pp. 248–278.
15 The name, Bakony-bread, referred to the Bakony Mountain area, one of the main strongholds of the Soviet army.
16 *Household statistics* (1983), pp. 20, 22, 119, 137.
17 Benda (1982), p. 1043.
18 Benda (1982), p. 1050; Petö – Szakács (1985), p. 219.
19 *Népszabadság*, January 26, 1993, p. 14.
20 Radio-interview, January 25, 1993.
21 For 1934–38 and 1989 figures, here and later, see *Statistical Yearbook* (1964), p. 288, (1990), p. 216.
22 Sós (1959).
23 *Dietary habits* (1960), pp. 12–15; Kisbán (1989a), p. 91.
24 Yoghourt, for example, has been named in EC statistics since 1980. *EEC Dairy Facts* (1987).
25 Szpevák (1992).
26 The vegetables patisson and courgette are *Cucurbita pepo L. convar. Patissoniana* and *Cucurbita pepo L. convar. Giromontiina*.

## Literature

Benda, Kálmán (ed.), *Magyarország történeti kronológiája.* [The chronology of Hungarian history] Vol. IV. 1944–1970. (Budapest, 1982).
Berend, T. Iván – Ránki, György, *A magyar gazdaság száz éve.* [Hundred years of Hungarian economy] (Budapest, *1972*).
Berend, T. Iván – Ránki, György, *The Hungarian Economy in the Twentieth Century* (London-Sydney, 1985).
[Census returns 1910] *A Magyar Szent Korona országainak 1910. évi népszámlálása. II. A népesség foglalkozása* (Budapest, 1913). (Magyar Statisztikai közlemények, Új sorozat, 48).
[Census returns 1990] *1990. évi népszámlálás. III. Összefoglaló adatok* (Budapest, 1992).
[Dietary habits in Hungarian households 1958–59] *Étrendi szokások a munkás-, alkalmazotti- és paraszti háztartásokban* (Budapest, 1960).
Donáth, Ferenc, *Reform and revolution. Transformation of Hungary's Agriculture 1945–1970* (Budapest, 1980).
*EEC Dairy Facts and Figures 1987* (Surrey, 198).
Gasztonyi, Kálmán – Schneller, Margit, *Sütöipar.* [The baking industry] (Budapest, 1963).
[Household statistics] Háztartásstatisztika (Budapest).
[Hungarian flour-milling industry in 1894] *Magyarország malomipara 1894-*

*ben* (Budapest, 1896). ( = Magyar Statisztikai Közlemények, Új folyam 14).

Kisbán, Eszter, *Népi kultúra, közkultúra, jelkép: a gulyás, pörkölt, paprikás.* [Goulash: a popular food item that became a national symbol] (Budapest, 1989a).

Kisbán, Eszter, 'Aufnahme des Zuckers in die bäuerliche Nahrungskultur in Ungarn'. *Az István Király Múzeum közleményei* A/29 (1989b), pp. 279–287.

Kornai, János, *Economics of Shortage*, Vol. A-B, (Amsterdam-New York-Oxford, 1980).

*Népszabadság* (a leading daily paper) (Budapest).

Pach, Zsigmond Pál (ed.), *Magyarország története tiz kötetben.* [The history of Hungary in ten volumes] Vol. 7. 1890–1918. (Budapest, 1978).

Petö, Iván – Szakács, Sándor, *A hazai gazdaság négy évtizedének története 1945–1985.* [The economic development of Hungary 1945–1985] Vol. I. 1945–1968, (Budapest, 1985).

[Statistical Yearbook] *Magyar Statisztikai Évkönyv* (Budapest)

Sós, József, *Népélelmezés.* [Nutrition in Hungary] (Budapest, 1959).

Szpevák, Éva, *Táplálkozás-vizsgálatok általános iskolás tanulók közt Tatabányán.* [Dietary studies amongst school children at Tatabánya] (Budapest, 1992). Student manuscript at the Dept. of European Ethnology at the University of Budapest.

Wiener, Moszkó, *A magyar czukoripar fejlödese.* [The development of the Hungarian sugar industry] Vol. I–II., (Budapest, 1902).

# 15

# FROM CORNER SHOP TO SUPERMARKET: THE REVOLUTION IN FOOD RETAILING IN BRITAIN, 1932–1992

## *Derek J. Oddy*

> God made the wicked Grocer
> For a mystery and a sign,
> That men might shun the awful shop
> And go to inns to dine.
> G.K. Chesterton, *Song against Grocers.*

Between 1932 and 1992, free trade and cheap food – two fundamental policies for Britain – were abandoned. Against this background, food retailing in Britain underwent a transformation from small scale businesses based on personal service to large scale enterprises engaged in selling a vast range of goods by complex computerized operations. This transformation of the food market in Britain was by no means a simple process, nor did it fit tidily within the dates chosen for this paper. By 1932, for instance, the corner shop was no longer the only food supplier available to British consumers. Indeed, at the very beginning of the century, the independent grocer's survival seemed in doubt. In an editorial called 'The Passing of the Grocer', *The Times* saw the small shop as being threatened by multiple-branch retailers and co-operative societies alike[1]. Even so, by their very numbers, small scale retail shops were still by far the commonest places in which the British bought their food. The corner shop varied considerably in scale and status: some, but not all, occupied large specialist premises; most were not exclusively food retail outlets. Moreover, businesses of any kind were far from permanent: the small shop was easy to open in the front room of any terraced house; it was even easier to close down. Nevertheless, the shop gave many a family the hope of social advancement and there were always thousands ready to take the risk. Early in the century, just prior to the First World War, it may well have been the case that Britain was over-supplied with food shops. Besides the countless small traders, estimates for 1910 suggest that there were 114 multiple-shop firms in the grocery and provisions trade selling through some 2870 branches between them. The meat trade encompassed 23 multiples with 3828 branches, the bread and flour confectionery trade included 21 firms with 451 branches while chocolate and sugar confectionery added another 10 firms with 308 branches. Milk supply involved 20 multiples with 324 branches[2]. Moreover, in 1913, the retail co-operative societies claimed almost 2.9M members in working-class areas of Britain[3]. Competition, if one can believe the trade press, had reached a point where the small retailer felt it was 'excessive' and 'unfair' to honourable tradesman. This state of affairs was the outcome of developments in the British economy during the nineteenth century which had fundamentally altered earlier patterns of retailing.

By the first decade of the twentieth century, Britain no longer depended upon local or even regional markets for many of its food materials. Instead, Britain relied on international trade for the provision of foodstuffs to an extent greater than any other country had ever done before[4]. This was the result of two closely interrelated factors: maritime power, which ensured overseas foods reaching Britain, and free trade policies, which gave imports free access to British domestic markets. The effect was to bring grain from North America and Australia, meat from the United States, South America and New Zealand, dairy produce from Europe, North America and New Zealand, and tropical produce, such as sugar, tea, coffee, rice and fruit, from the West Indies, West Africa, India, Ceylon (Sri Lanka) and so on. The growth of this commodity trade in the nineteenth century profoundly altered the organization of food retailing in Britain.

## Changing nature of the food marketing process

The customary structure of food markets had been for farmers to dispose of their produce via auctions or wholesale markets to a large number of retail outlets many of which were of a specialist nature, for example, butchers, dairymen or greengrocers[5]. While the food trade had originally been a relatively local enterprise, the growth of towns in the nineteenth century and the facilities provided by railways led to it becoming increasingly long distance in character from the 1860s onwards. Food processing also took place traditionally at the local level: sausages, pies, bread, biscuits and cakes were made by retailers. From the late nineteenth century the growth of specialist food processors and manufacturers began to change the balance of the market; in practice, by the 1930s, a considerable degree of market power had passed to food processors.

Imports of tea, bacon, and especially the new 'artificial' food – margarine – came to market in a way which began to blur the older distinctions between grocer and provision merchant. Providing outlets for these foodstuffs throughout the growing working-class urban areas of Britain during the late nineteenth and early twentieth centuries was the function of the multiple unit retailers. The aggressive marketing of foodstuffs by the multiple chains of retailers which grew up between the 1870s and the First World War –

Lipton's, International Tea Company, Home and Colonial Stores, Maypole Dairies, Pearks, and so on – caused a dramatic change in food-retailing practices.

Thus, by the 1930s, the retail market for food comprised three sectors: the retail co-operative societies backed by the Co-operative Wholesale Society (CWS); the multiples both in general foodstuffs and specialist trades such as meat (Dewhurst's), fish (Macfisheries) and bread (Bilslands of Glasgow); and the independent retailers ranging from Fortnum and Mason's in Piccadilly to the corner shops. These last were predominant by their very numbers, their claims to personal service, and their practice of delivering goods ordered by customers to their homes. Personal service had become the essential characteristic of the grocery trade in as far as it retained the notion that the grocer's original function had been to break bulk. The shopman's skill in merchandizing lay in cutting, slicing, weighing, and packing food exactly to the customer's order. The initial threat to the grocer and provision merchant's existence came from the standardization and pre-packaging of commodities such as tea, margarine and (but outside the food trade) soap. This gave an incentive to the wholesaler to control quality and to introduce product differentiation. The grocery trade became characterized by branded goods which were widely advertised in newspapers, on billboards, on railway stations, in theatres and, in the twentieth century, cinemas. The development of food technology in the nineteenth century for the manufacture of cakes, biscuits, breakfast cereals, pies, patent foods of varying kinds and soft drinks, created products for the food retailer in which the wholesaler's price became more significant than the skills of the shopman behind his counter. Indeed, with customers so concentrated into densely-inhabited urban areas, the retailer's risk was minimal. Thomas Lipton could open a store a month in the 1880s by putting down a week's rent on the premises and buying goods on a month's credit[6], a pattern not dissimilar to the growth of a modern retail chain, Kwik Save, in the 1960s[7].

The growth of multiples in the interwar years can be illustrated by noting the expansion of Sainsbury's, the market leader in food retailing in the 1990s. Like other multiples, Sainsbury's expanded after the First World War, opening at least three shops annually, particularly in the new suburban areas linked to London by the extension of the underground railway[8]. The number of branches increased from 123 in 1919 to 180 in 1929; by 1938 the firm had 244 outlets. None of this growth involved any new developments in retailing. The organization of the typical shop, which had developed before the outbreak of war in 1914, remained unchanged. In Sainsbury's shops there were six departments: groceries, bacon and hams, cooked meats, fresh meat, dairy products, and poultry, game and rabbits and, during the 1920s at least, the traditional trade of 'breaking bulk' was still important. Customers could expect to have their own containers filled with vinegar or mustard pickles; cheese and butter was still sold from the barrel and wrapped for each customer. Given the growing scale of the business, two developments of the interwar period were important for the change in retail techniques which came in the 1950s: first, from 1920 Sainsbury's began to sell 'own label' lines to match the growing tendency towards packaged goods which was occurring, and secondly, centralized packing at Blackfriars was introduced[9]. No multiple, though, could match the nationwide coverage of the co-operatives which, taken together operated 24,000 shops in 1939[10]. Despite their growth, price-cutting chains such as Tesco's and Pricerite's had only a regional coverage during the 1930s, and could make no impact at the national level[11].

The expanding role of food technology, and the introduction of food standards legislation from the late nineteenth century onwards, by imposing basic requirements of quality and cleanliness on food traders, gave market power to the food producers and wholesalers. During the early years of the twentieth century, the advertising of branded goods created national, or at least regional, reputations for a number of food processors. This trend was accentuated by mergers to generate more efficient firms. As market leaders in the food processing industry began to emerge, the extent to which they achieved product differentiation enabled them to exercise a degree of monopoly over their pricing policies and to dictate prices and quality standards.

By the 1930s, Associated Biscuit Manufacturers Ltd, United Biscuits Ltd, E H Nevill's, Garfield Weston, the British Sugar Corporation, Tate & Lyle Ltd, Unilever Ltd, and Vestey's were already important sources of supply for retailers. In bread, biscuits, sugar, chocolate confectionery, margarine and frozen meat the dominant position of a small number of firms had the effect of imposing rigidities upon the food market in much the same way as oligopolies developed generally in British industry during the interwar years. Nevertheless, the food market in the immediate years after the adoption of protection in 1932, was in a state of flux. Although food producers had gained the power to fix prices in a number of lines – particularly branded and processed foods – which made them expensive, the Import Duties Act of 1932 excluded food from the tariffs it introduced. Basic food materials continued to be imported unchecked. In addition, Britain experienced the dumping of foods such as bacon and dairy produce from several countries, notably Denmark and the Irish Free State, which tended to depress prices further in this sector of the market. Despite the government's attempt to raise food prices by the introduction of Marketing Boards for a number of home-produced foods – potatoes, pigs and milk, in particular – prices of basic food materials remained low up to 1939. This aided the expansion of the retail trade and facilitated the growth of price-cutting firms.

## Postwar Trends in Food Retailing

Self-service stores began to appear in UK in the early 1950s[12]. Although there have been claims that Romford Co-operative Society experimented with self-service in 1949 and that Portsmouth Co-operative Society had the first self-service store in Britain open by the late 1940s, the pioneering move is generally attributed to Sainsbury's. They adopted selfservice in their Croydon branch in July 1950 and opened their first supermarket in Lewisham some three years later. With a floor area of 7,500 sq ft (700m²) the Sainsbury's Lewisham branch was for some years the largest supermarket in Europe[13].

The success of self-service shops in the early 1950s was remarkable. Perhaps people whose food had been rationed for ten years were pleased to see food displayed and to be able to 'get their hands on it'. Initially, though, the development of supermarkets was slow, since building was still restricted by the postwar shortages of materials and the system of building licences. By the late 1950s, however, stores with floor areas of 11,000 sq ft (1022m²) were being built, though changes in retailing techniques remained limited as long as the multiples found it necessary to continue trading from small shops unsuitable for development as selfservice outlets. Tesco's, for example, through the acquisition of various regional traders in the 1960s, found themselves with many small shops having floor areas of no more than 3–4000 sq ft (270–370m²)[14]. The turning point in the development of larger units probably occurred in 1969 when Carrefour, the French retail chain, acquired planning permission for the development of the first of four hypermarkets. These stores, at Caerphilly near Cardiff, Telford, Eastleigh, and Minworth, were exceptional in that they were designed with 100,000 sq ft (9,290m²) floor areas and car parking spaces for 1000 cars.[15]

In response, the major British multiple retailers began building units within the range 10–25,000 sq ft (929–2323m²) during the 1970s and 1980s. By the early 1980s, the average floor area of British supermarkets was 13,900 sq ft (1291m²); later in the decade it had risen to around 20,000 sq ft (1858m²). For Tesco's, the decision to rationalize their outlets led to the closure between 1977 and 1983 of 371 supermarkets with an average floor area of only 3,700 sq ft (344m²) and their replacement by 97 superstores averaging 30,000 sq ft (2,787m²) floor area[16]. During the 1980s, as the concept of one-stop retailing developed, superstores and hypermarkets began to share the food trade with new lines of non-food merchandise. For example, Sainsbury's, a firm committed to food-retailing and previously resistant to diversification began to operate Savacentre hypermarkets jointly with British Home Stores. The largest of these in the 1980s was 89,000 sq ft (8,268m²) compared with Sainsbury's largest food superstore, Kempston on the south-western outskirts of Bedford, which had a floor area of 34,000 sq ft (3159m²).

The rationale for these moves was to benefit from economies of scale: the larger the unit the more the operating costs could be reduced both in terms of capital and labour. To achieve this required the adoption of a new policy of locating superstores on edge-of-town sites which, for its success, depended upon the expansion in private car ownership. By 1987, there were already 457 superstores with an average sales area of 38,250 sq ft ($3553m^2$) in operation. The leader in this trend was Tesco's with 124, followed by Asda with 92, Dee with 75, and Sainsbury's with 56[17].

Faced with the postwar growth of multiple retailers, the independent sector has been in long-term decline. This trend set in with the end of rationing. The process by which customers were compelled to register with a retailer was central to the scheme of food rationing in operation between 1940 and 1954. With the end of rationing, small retailers found that they could do nothing to retain customer loyalty in the face of newly-acquired freedom of choice. Overall, the total number of food retail outlets began to shrink, so that the growth in large units achieved by the expansion of the multiple retailers was offset by a decline in the total number of retail food outlets. The 1951 Census of Distribution indicated a total of 284,000 food shops: by 1979 this number had fallen to 121,000. While the brunt of this shrinkage was borne by the small scale retailer who operated one or perhaps two shops, the effect of the growth of multiple retailers also resulted in change for the cooperative societies: their market share declined from 15 per cent in 1970 to 11.6 per cent in 1985. The growth in concentration and the use of own-label brands within the food distributive trades generally has attracted the attention of the Monopolies and Mergers Commission (MMC). During the 1980s, Aldi, the German-owned multiple complained that it was discriminated against by its UK suppliers, though these charges were not substantiated by the Monopolies Commission[18].

## The purchasing power of the multiples

The balance of market power began to shift from the food processors and manufacturers to the multiple retailers during the 1950s. This was a direct consequence of the growth in sales volume resulting from the adoption of supermarkets. Retailers sought better margins from food manufacturers and began to develop own-label brands. During the 1960s, the growing power of the retail multiples broke down Resale Price Maintenance. Furthermore, the multiples began to press agricultural suppliers to adopt new production techniques and grading and packing procedures. The scale of their purchasing requirements meant they were successful in by-passing traditional wholesale markets and were able to develop their own distribution networks instead. The requirements imposed by multiples on their suppliers brought changes in technology which have extended product availability and reduced the seasonal nature of fresh produce[19].

In particular, the success of own-brand marketing enabled retailers to determine what profit margins on any particular line they were prepared to accept. The effect of this was to put pressure on suppliers to accept a reduction on their margins. Furthermore, the development of own-brand lines by Marks and Spencer and Sainsbury were seen by consumers as establishing quality standards. This has been taken up by Tesco, Safeway (Argyll), and Gateway. For example, Tesco's realized in 1978 that less than 20 per cent of their food was sold under their own labels, compared to 56 per cent of Sainsbury's[20]. The implications of own-label trading were not lost on other firms; the result was that the multiples' own-label share of packaged grocery turnover rose from 23 per cent in 1978 to 30 per cent in 1985.

The multiple retailers' command over the market has been reinforced by the concentration of buying power. This trend was apparent as early as 1970, when 600 buying organizations made up of retail-multiples, food wholesalers and the co-operative societies bought approximately 70 per cent of the goods sold retail in the grocery market. By 1975, 344 buyers (including 227 cooperatives) took 75 per cent of the grocery trade and, apart from the cooperatives, by the end of the 1970s, 90 buyers controlled two-thirds of the United Kingdom's grocery trade. By 1980, the total number of buying organizations had fallen to 275, while the proportion of the trade for which they bought had risen to 82 per cent of the grocery market. The six major multiples alone bought 43 per cent of the groceries sold in the United Kingdom.

During the twentieth century, the growth of food-retailing firms within British industry has been pronounced. Taking the fifty largest companies by capital valuation in 1905, only three firms could be found with major interests in food – Lever Brothers (ranked 24th), Huntley and Palmer (36th) and J & J Colman (43rd) – and they were all food manufacturers. By 1919, Lever Brothers ranked second and Liebig's and J Lyons were forty-third and forty-fourth. Maypole Dairy (ranked 25th) was the first food retailer in the largest fifty British companies. In 1948, after the Second World War, six companies – Unilever, Tate & Lyle, J Lyons, Rank's, United Dairies and Spillers – still principally food manufacturers or distributors, were among the leading fifty British firms by capital value.

Since then, the expansion of the food sector has been dramatic. In 1992, seven firms in the leading fifty are in food. Of these, Marks and Spencer (12th), J Sainsbury (17th), Tesco (30th) and Argyll (36th) are multiple retailers. Another multiple, Asda Group, ranks sixty-seventh within the one-hundred largest companies while the largest discounter, Kwik Save, is ninety-seventh. While such major food manufacturers as Unilever (15th), Allied-Lyons (27th) and Cadbury-Schweppes (39th) are still to be found in the largest fifty companies, the growth of the food retailers has been an outstanding feature in British industry.[21]

**New Retailing Techniques:**

Once the principle of self-service had been adopted during the 1950s, it spread into almost all aspects of food retailing. By the 1970s, even the single-unit retailer – the traditional corner shop – had abandoned counters in favour of wire baskets and 'check-out' style cash registers. Moreover, behind the facade of independence, voluntary associations had begun to develop as a defensive measure against the power of the multiples. Some of the advantages of bulk buying could be gained for the small shop by linking up with a large wholesale distributor. By the mid-1960s, a Dutch firm, Spar, had over 3,000 outlets and three German companies – Vege, Centra, and Vivo – had a further 7,500 shops in the United Kingdom tied to them for supplies. Corner shops sought other attractions such as trading stamps to stave off the multiples. By 1962, five years after its start, Green Shield claimed that 8,000 independent retailers were offering stamps to their customers.[22] This advantage was, however, short-lived. By adopting price-cutting policies in the late 1950s, the multiples came into conflict with Resale Price Maintenance. Trading stamps provided them with another weapon which could be used to reduce manufacturers' prices. Tesco's adopted Green Shield trading stamps in October 1963[23] and retained them until June 1977.

During the mid-1970s, food retailers faced rapid price inflation. In 1973, upon entering the European Community, the United Kingdom had been forced to abandon the cheap food policy which had been a basic tenet of domestic politics since 1860. The rise in food prices was rapid and pronounced. A second blow to the UK economy followed with the rise in oil prices from late 1973 onwards. This affected consumers' spending and the costs of all energy-intensive industries alike. As retail prices rose, the value of trading stamps was eroded and they began to lose their appeal for customers. Firms such as Tesco's, which had been built up by Jack Cohen on a price-cutting philosophy, found profits falling between 1973 and 1975. This forced Tesco's to evaluate their position in the cut-price sector of the market. Thus, when the decision to stop giving trading stamps was finally taken, it symbolized the end of Sir Jack Cohen's influence on the firm's policies.

The change in Tesco's which followed amounted to a metamorphosis for the company. Over the weekend of the Queen's Silver Jubilee celebrations, Tesco's closed all their stores from Saturday, 4 June to Thursday, 9 June 1977, re-opening in new trading colours and employing a much advertised new pricing policy, *Operation Check-Out*. Customer response was immediately enthusiastic and on such a scale that Tesco's wholesale and transport facilities came near to collapse in their efforts to supply goods to the shops. Their market share rose from 7.9 to 10.8 per cent, while that of all other major retailers fell, though Sainsbury's response, *Discount* 78, restored their lost share of the market.[24]

As the scale of the multiples grew, the development of management information control techniques and stock control systems became a pressing problem to ensure the rapid movement of goods from warehouse to stores and to safeguard the shelf-life of goods. Product coding and electronic scanning began to be used in the UK from 1972 onwards; during the 1970s, the Universal Product Code (UPC) was developed in the USA and this became extended by a system known as European Article Numbering (EAN). The expression of product numbers by bar codes and the subsequent introduction of laser scanners enabled product details of high volume-low value transactions to be read at the check-out without delaying the consumer. This system became widely used by the multiples during the 1970s.

## Electronic Point of Sale (EPOS)

Until the late 1960s, cash registers could record no more information than the price which the cashier 'rang up' on a roll of paper tape. In consequence there was an attempt to develop machines that could record more information; early versions used punched tape which could then be fed into a computer. The break-through came with the development of the ROM-driven terminal in the late 1970s and this system became general in the 1980s as the microcomputer was improved and its costs fell. By the 1980s, multiple retailers faced immense stock control problems. The major firms were operating 300 or more stores which commonly carried 16,000 stock lines. For the retailer, microcomputers solved sales analysis and stock control problems at a time when price competition was intense. However, the cost was significant: Tesco's, for example, spent £100M on new technology.[25] Retailers found additional sources of management information resulted from the installation of an EPOS system: turnover analysis led to assessment of profitability by merchandise lines; management of space became possible as the rate of sale of any line of merchandise could be measured against the retail space it occupied.

## Electronic Funds Transfer at Point of Sale (EFTPOS)

By the mid 1980s around 28 per cent of payments in UK supermarkets had become non-cash transactions. The development of credit sales of food depended upon the acceptance of credit cards by UK consumers. Credit cards were introduced into the UK in 1966 with the launch of Barclaycard. Access (MasterCard) followed in 1973. By 1986 more than 20M credit cards were in use in the UK, with Access having around 10M accounts, Barclaycard (Visa) a further 8.6M, plus other bankcards and travel cards such as Diners Club and American Express. In the late 1980s credit cards were used more in Britain than in any other European Community country. Food multiples therefore began to accept credit cards in the mid-1980s (except Sainsbury's, which held out against them until 1991). No food multiple has, as yet, issued its own retailer card, except for Marks and Spencer, which introduced its Chargecard in April 1985. By the late 1980s, however, all the major multiples accepted payment by Switch-cards which debited customers' current accounts at branches of the clearing banks.[26]

## The Retail Food Market Today

At the beginning of the 1990s, the multiple store retail chains had acquired a dominant position in food retailing. In 1991, the sales of 11 multiple chains amounted to 66 per cent of all retail grocery sales. Of these, the two leading multiples, J Sainsbury (16.1 per cent) and Tesco (14.6 per cent), between them have nearly 31 per cent of the market.[27] Safeway (Argyll), Asda and Gateway form a second group which shows no sign of narrowing the gap between themselves and the market leaders. The market share of the remainder is relatively marginal. The position of the market leaders is based on quality and each of them has acquired a considerable customer loyalty. While Sainsbury's had always claimed high quality for its goods, Tesco's underwent a dramatic conversion to quality and consumer concerns in the 1980s. With the launch of their 'Healthy Eating' campaign in 1985 and their environmental friendly promotions in 1989, Tesco's image was transformed from the 'pile it high, sell it cheap' philosophy which had been Jack Cohen's formula for growth.[28] At present, the position of the market leaders looks so unassailable that the retail clothing chain Littlewood's has abandoned its plans to enter food retailing via an association with Iceland Frozen Foods.[29] On the other hand, Marks and Spencer, also primarily a retail clothing multiple, has been very successful in food retailing at the quality end of the market. Moreover, specialist retailers have retained a place in the food retail market. In 1991, Gregg's sold 7.1 per cent of all bread and flour confectionery sales totalling £1345M, while JH Dewhurst's turnover amounted to 8.5 per cent of all butchers' sales in a market worth £2694M.[30]

Although price cutting by Sainsbury's was announced with much press publicity in January 1993, the likelihood of a price war between the leading multiples is remote at present, lest it damage margins. Leading multiples see more prospect of gaining market share by extending product ranges and developing facilities for one-stop shopping. Quality and range of goods has become the strategy adopted by the market leaders since the 1980s and price wars have no place in that scheme of things. The tendency towards 'one-stop shopping' has led the market leaders to introduce in-store bakeries, wet-fish counters, flowers and plants, coffee shops, cigarettes and tobacco, clothing and cash withdrawal facilities.[31] Sainsbury's and Tesco's sell petrol, oil and motorists' accessories, Sainsbury's has ventured into the do-it-yourself market, and Marks and Spencer has set up a financial services section which offers loans and operates unit trusts. Food retailers have ventured into some strange new territories in recent years; indeed, with Sunday opening increasing in the 1990s, despite its illegality in Britain, the superstore has given a new meaning to G.K. Chesterton's line: 'God made the wicked Grocer'![32]

**Notes:**

1 Winstanley, (1983) p. 39.
2 Fraser, Table 9.1 (based on J.B. Jefferys, *Retail Trading in Britain 1850–1950* Cambridge University Press, 1954).
3 Ibid., p. 124.
4 See the evidence presented before the Royal Commission on the Supply of Food and Raw Material in times of War, British Parliamentary Papers 1905 (Cd.2643) XXXIX.
5 Burns, McInerney and Swinbank (eds) (1983), p. 67.
6 Mathias, (1967), pp. 46–52, 98.
7 BBC Radio 4, 1 January 1993.
8 Boswell (1969), p. 44.
9 Ibid., p. 40
10 Powell, (1991) p. 32.
11 Ibid. pp. 32–44. Pricerite was jointly owned by Jack Cohen and Mick Kaye until 1956. Trading on his own account as Tesco, Cohen had over 100 small shops in London and the Home Counties by 1939.
12 Burns et al. (1983) p. 127.
13 Boswell, (1969) p. 61.
14 Powell (1991) p. 132.
15 Ibid., pp. 128–9.
16 Ibid., p. 197.
17 Institute of Grocery Distribution Research Services.
18 Sanghari et al. (1992), p. 8.
19 Burn et al. See p. 70 et seq. for the development of contract farming.
20 Powell (1991) p. 198.
21 See tables in Payne, 'Emergence of the Large-scale Company' and Hannah. (1983).
22 Powell (1991) p. 105.
22 Ibid., pp. 110–112.
23 Ibid., chs. 10–11.
24 Ibid., p. 190.
25 Switch transfers are not available at Marks and Spencer.
26 Sanghari et al., (1992) p. 6.
27 Powell, (1991) pp. 200–2.
28 *Sunday Times*, 31 January 1993.
29 Sanghari et al., (1992) pp. 6–7.
30 Since 1993, despite the efforts of financial journalists to dramatize its effects, the price war has been more of a 'phoney war' than a real one. The major multiple retailers have limited price-cutting mainly to their own-brand lines, though during 1994, however, some discounting chains have begun to cut not only own label but also tertiary brands, to the discomfort of the food manufacturers. Among the market leaders, J Sainsbury's profits increased by 16 per cent to £733M in 1993 and a

further 6 per cent to £738 in 1994. Share prices of the major retailers, Sainsbury, Tesco, Argyll and Asda have reversed their downward trend and risen significantly during 1994 as acceptance of lower margins has become general. Fear of costcutting discounters and warehouse clubs has receded and expansion through take-over bids has been resumed. In July 1994, Tesco out-bid J Sainsbury for the Scottish retail chain William Low. It was something of a pyrrhic victory. Sainsbury's bid forced Tesco to pay £100M more than it intended to acquire Low. While Tesco increased its market share as a result, it also acquired a number of small sites of the kind it disposed of in the 1980s. Sainsbury's still lacks a presence in Scotland, with only four stores open there in 1994. However, Sainsbury's has made significant expansion elsewhere and operates Shaw's, a supermarket chain of some 90 stores in the north-eastern United States. In October 1994, Sainsbury's obtained a substantial stake in Giant Food, a 159 strong supermarket chain centred around Washington, DC, and Baltimore. British food-retailing management techniques have entered a new phase in which major multiple retailers may become multinational companies!

31 By contrast to this trend, Tesco has even returned to the idea of the convenience of the corner shop. It has developed its Metro chain of small city-centre shops operating late-opening hours until 10pm.

32 The Sunday Trading Act, 1994, came into effect on 28 August 1994. Large stores are restricted to a maximum of six hours' opening, and restrictions on the hours during which alcohol may be sold remain in force. In the MetroCentre, Gateshead, which is Britain's largest indoor shopping area, Sunday opening on 28 August began with a religious service, inspired, perhaps, by St Matthew's Gospel, Book 22; verse 21: 'Render therefore unto Caesar the things which are Caesar's; and unto God the things that are God's.' Ironically, the Church Commissioners, who manage the Church of England's property, are the MetroCentre's landlords.

**Literature**

Beaumont, John, 'Trends in Food Retailing', in McFadyen, pp. 52–64.

Boswell, James (ed), *JS 100 The Story of Sainsbury's*, London, J Sainsbury Ltd, 1969.

Briggs, Asa, *Marks and Spencer 1884–1984*, London, Octopus Books, 1984.

Burns, Jim, John McInerney and Alan Swinbank (eds) *The Food Industry*, London, Heinemann, 1983.

Fraser, W Hamish, *The Coming of the Mass Market 1850–1914*, London, Macmillan, 1981.

Hannah, Leslie, *The Rise of the Corporate Economy*, London, Methuen, new edition, 1983.

Goldenberg, Nathan, *Thought for Food*, publisher not known, 1987(?).

McFadyen, Edward, (ed), *The Changing Face of British Retailing*, London, Newman, 1987.

Mathias, Peter, *Retailing Revolution*, London, Longmans, 1967.

Payne, Peter L, 'The emergence of the Large-scale Company in Great Britain, 1870–1914', *Economic History Review*, 2nd.Ser., Vol. XX, 3, December 1967, 519–42.

Perren, Richard, *The Meat Trade in Britain 1840–1914*, London, Routledge, 1978.

Powell, David, *Counter Revolution: The Tesco Story*, London, Grafton Books, 1991.

Sanghari, Nitri, Phil Smith and Geoff Wills, *The Retail Reference Book* 1992, Manchester, Centre for Business Research, Manchester Business School, 1992.

Stuyvenberg, J H van, (ed), *Margarine An Economic, Social and Scientific History* 1869–1969, Liverpool, Liverpool University Press, 1969.

Wilson, Charles, *The History of Unilever: A study of economic growth and social change*, 2 vols., London, Cassell, 1954.

Wilson, Charles, *Unilever 1945–1965: challenge and response in the post-war industrial revolution*, London, Cassell, 1968.

Winstanley, Michael J, *The Shopkeeper's World 1830–1914*, Manchester, Manchester University Press, 1983.

# 16

# RATIONALISATION AS A PERMANENT TASK

## THE GERMAN FOOD RETAIL TRADE IN THE TWENTIETH CENTURY

### Uwe Spiekermann

'Today the food trade is without a doubt the best-rationalised area of the market economy in Germany.'[1] Until the present it has not yet been clarified how this came about, and a search for precise data or a detailed chronology will not be successful. The aim of this study is to trace changes in the internal structure of the food retail trade in the 20th century. The development of business and turnover will be placed in the centre, and the changes in the business premises and in the assortment will be examined. In that way it seems possible to encircle the problem that is decisive for the cheap and continuous supply of the population with food and luxury food, i.e. the problem of internal rationalisation of this branch of economy.

### The establishment of the modern food trade

In comparison to the Western neighbouring countries the German food trade was a late starter. It was not until the German Kaiserreich that a modern, i.e. a distributional system adapted to the industrial market economy, was formed with a basic structure that would last until the early 1960s. The main characteristics at that time were:

1. The food trade grew on a scale far above the population growth and reached a number of firms in 1914 never to be regained later. The average number of employees per firm was only 1,6 persons in 1914, but had increased steadily since 1875 (Table 1).

Table 1: Firms and employees in the food trade in Germany 1875–1914

| Year | 1875 | 1882 | 1895 | 1907 | 1914 |
|---|---|---|---|---|---|
| Firms | 191,338 | 241,150 | 317,381 | 486,183 | 583,981 |
| Employees | 223,481 | 286,209 | 485,917 | 780,188 | 951,854 |
| Employees per firm | 1.17 | 1.19 | 1.53 | 1.60 | 1.63 |

Sources: Betriebszählung (1930), i. 3, p. 11; Reithinger (1929), p. 340.

2. Parallel to the development of firms the significance of the immediate supply by means of weekly markets, hucksters and pedlars simultaneously decreased, while the shop as a dominating form of retail trade succeeded. This development, begun in the second third of the 19th century, took a varying course depending on the region and was probably finished in the great cities around 1880/1890. Against this background endeavours to concentrate the food retail trade in market halls failed. A contrary movement and a new form of business on the other hand was formed in the shape of the partly very important street trade with sales stalls.[2]

3. The disappearing significance of direct contact between producer and consumer also resulted from the obvious change in the goods sold. The country products and the colonial goods were joined by a third group of industrially prepared and produced foodstuffs. First these manufactures were semi-products like farinaceous products, oat flakes and soup flours, and from the middle of the 1860s the scale of branded articles ready for use also increased, although the actual breakthrough of these products happened in the Weimar Republic.

4. Apart from the generally growing real income and the increasing size of the urban markets this stock extension was the basis of a specialization that made the creation of a delimitable, shop-bound specialized food trade possible. Within this branch of economy recently unknown specializations on single goods and groups of goods respectively took place: the grocer and shopkeeper respectively were joined by milk-, fat- (butter, eggs, cheese), vegetables-, fruits-, bread-, delicatessen-, tobacco-, wine and liquor shops, to name only the most important ones. The extent of these changes can be demonstrated by the following data from Hamburg:

*Table 2:* Specialization of the food retail trade in Hamburg 1800–1913 (Number of shops)

| Year | 1800 | | 1842 | | 1913 | |
|---|---|---|---|---|---|---|
| Retail trade with | | | | | | |
| agricultural products | 104 | (5,4%) | 282 | (8,5%) | 4,453 | (22,8%) |
| Groceries | 263 | (13,7%) | 369 | (11,8%) | 1,488 | (7,6%) |
| Delicatessen | 22 | (1,2%) | 26 | (0,8%) | 741 | (3,8%) |
| Beer | – | | 1 | (0,0%) | 16 | (0,1%) |
| Wine and liquor | 205 | (10,7%) | 247 | (7,4%) | 280 | (1,4%) |
| Confectioneries | 2 | (0,1%) | 1 | (0,0%) | 233 | (1,2%) |
| Bread and baker's ware | 4 | (0,2%) | – | | 1,820 | (9,3%) |
| Meat and meat products | 29 | (1,5%) | 45 | (1,4%) | 29 | (0,1%) |
| Fish | 4 | (0,2%) | 7 | (0,2%) | 200 | (1,0%) |
| Tobacco | 56 | (2,9%) | 92 | (2,8%) | 2,062 | (10,6%) |
| Total | 689 | (35,9%) | 1.070 | (32,1%) | 11,322 | (58,0%) |

*Source:* Author's evaluations of the Hamburg directories of these years. Percentage from all shops in Hamburg.

5. In spite of these remarkable changes the small neighbourhood shops were constantly criticized by consumers and science. In addition to inadequate food hygiene one attributed to them a price-raising effect, a small enterprise structure, minimal own capital resources, no orderly book-keeping, high outstanding debts because cash-payment was unusual, high labour costs caused by daily opening-times of more than twelve hours, small cold-storage-, storage- and salesrooms, and those were the characteristics of the majority of shops.[3] Nevertheless one should not forget that these shops were the most essential innovation, whose internal rationalisation turned out to be the permanent task until the 1960s.

The great possibilities for rationalisation were first of all used by the so-called 'new' forms of business, which nevertheless all began in the form of small enterprises.

Department stores did not exist in the German Empire until the 1890s, and they started selling food in 1892.[4] Used as a competitor, food had to represent the general cheapness of the business. The department stores created a price pressure by means of a mixed calculation, rationalisation pressure through purchasing power and standardization of goods as well as a pressure for innovation by means of new products like canned vegetables and tomatoes. They included delicatessen and basic foodstuffs into a 'shopping event' and appealed to the senses in the food departments. In terms of business and marketing they worked as attacked models, although they did not rise above 0,25 per cent of the foodstuff turnover in 1913.

Greater significance was gained by the consumer co-operative societies that rose particularly since the middle of the 1880s. Since then endeavours, especially from the side of the workers, were made to combine economic and social-political aims even against the resistance of the trade unions and the Social Democrats. They tried to establish a distributive contra-society that could deliver high-quality products at prime cost and at the same time represent a not-commerzialized but cooperative way of life. By means of large-scale efforts aiming at an own production the usual assortment of goods was extended by baker's ware and fresh meat. The sale was made through a broad network of medium-sized shops, while important sales advantages were achieved through the 'Grosskaufsgesellschaft' founded in 1894, and regional purchasing days respectively. Cash, payment and reimbursement at the end of the year improved the internal liquidity. Despite the great increase only 5 per cent of the total turnover was concentrated in their hands in 1913.

The multiple shop trading, which was founded in the 1870s, formed the private economy, counterpart of the consumer-cooperatives. Purchase, stock-keeping, calculation, advertising and administration were centralized, and only the sale was decentralized. Most chain-stores stayed regionally limited, and only a few specialized chains gained a country-wide significance by means of limited assortments arranged around popular products (coffee, chocolate, tobacco). Chain-stores like Kaiser's Coffee-Shop became well-known through uniform advertising and a uniform shop decoration as well as their own trade marks. Still, their share of the foodstuff turnover in 1913 will only have been about 3–4%.

The specialized retail trade reacted to this strongly noticeable competition in two ways. On the one hand it called for government protection. Since the middle of the 1890s this led to special taxes against all new forms of business, whose further development was at least checked.[5] On the other hand attempts to improve the business situation through 'self-help' turned out to be more important. Two developments have to be pointed out:

In the field of sales the middle-sized firms began a large-scale fight against the costly habit of buying on tick. Since the 1890s they switched to handing out 5 per cent discount tickets in the case of each payment in order to diminish the outstanding debts involving heavy losses and to tie the customers closer to the shops. As the generally increasing costs had to be cushioned somehow, further rationalisation endeavours were inevitable. Since 1902 a country-wide organisation in the 'Union of the German Discount Savings Associations' was established and in 1913 about 40,000 food stores were members of this organisation that turned out to be the most important retail trade organisation before the First World War (Table 3).

*Table 3:* The Union of German Discount Savings Associations 1903–1914

| Year | Members | Turnover (10 Million. M) |
| --- | --- | --- |
| 1903 | 12,000 | 10,939 |
| 1904/05 | 18,789 | 18,789 |
| 1905/06 | 33,691 | 29,648 |
| 1906/07 | 41,741 | 40 |
| 1907/08 | 50,423 | 52 |
| 1908/09 | 54,773 | 62 |
| 1909/10 | 57,597 | 64 |
| 1910/11 | 61,500 | 68 |
| 1911/12 | 65,733 | 70 |
| 1912/13 | 70,400 | 74 |
| 1913/14 | 73,495 | 76 |

*Source:* Schmid (1920), p. 140.

As they did not manage to stop a further advance of the new forms of business, as even the multiple shop traders switched to the discount system, it became clear that the discount savings unions were only part of a necessary broader change. The growing communication within the unions made common purchase seem possible as a second innovation, which had already sporadically been practised in the 1870s. After central purchasing commissions had failed repeatedly, the foundation of the association of German retailer-purchasing co-operatives in 1907 led to a long-term successful establishment of a central purchasing union. Since 1912 this Edeka standardized advertising and in part even the decoration of the shop-front of their membership shops, they centralized big parts of the purchase, put through own trade marks and above all promoted the management knowledge of their members.[6] Following the new forms of business, parts of the specialized trade now switched to direct purchase from the producer and therefore managed ultimately to offer products at much cheaper prices.

At least 15–20% of all food stores were members of the discount savings unions and the retailer-purchasing co-operatives before the First World War. Alongside these efficient middle-class firms there were 1. many single and unorganized shops with only small profits and 2. a great number of avocational retailers which only aimed at supplementing the main income and were led mostly by women. Both types represent the actual problem of further rationalisation.

## From dealer to distributor: The food trade in war and inflation 1914–1923

The First World War and the following hyperinflation stopped the slow but steady rationalisation on its own resources. Until the end of the 1940s a period followed that was only interrupted between 1924 and 1932 and was marked by a decisive break in market economy competition structures by means of governmental and corporate regulatory decrees. While the time before the First World War was marked by an increasing approximation to the standard of performance of the Western industrial states, the interval of more than thirty years represented a special development which was not alleviated until the big jump of the 1950s and most of all the 1960s and was finally overcome.

The First World War itself represented first and foremost a problem of acquisition for the food trade. The increasing difficulties in supplying the civilian population with the bare necessaries of life led to a comprehensive rationing of almost all foodstuffs until 1916. The government bureaucracy cooperated most of all with the larger firms and the associations of the retail trade and thereby indirectly promoted a high organisational structure. They gave fixed quotas of foodstuffs to the retailers, who had to distribute them to fixed consumers at fixed prices and in exchange for vouchers. While the continuance of the retail trade thereby tended to be conserved one simultaneously stopped further growth through strict 'keeping away of untrustworthy persons from the trade'. Still, the disintegration of the distributional system could not be countered. The war-time food policy, which was half-hearted due to political considerations, led to a strong intensification of the direct contact between consumer and producer, and illicit trade became essential. While the food trade had profited from the rising prices first, it has shown average losses since 1916.[7] The retention of products, usury and food adulteration strongly increased. The tax burden obviously increased, and in 1916 a limited, and since 1924 a general turnover tax was introduced. This tax actually hit the medium-sized and larger firms in particular, for one had installed minimum tax limits for social reasons and the efficiency of the revenue authorities often failed in view of the small shops. The introduction of the eight-hour day attending the establishment of the Weimar Republic had relative cost advantages for the small shops in connection with the decreasing opening-times. Nevertheless, the significance of the new forms of business altogether increased until the end of the hyperinflation. While the multiple shops kept their positions during the war and slightly decreased later, the co-operative associations doubled their membership figures up to 1923 to almost 4 millions, but had to pay for their consumer-friendly activities with an extensive exhaustion of their reserves.[8] The strong fixation on the First World War as an economic cut blocks the view of the steadiness of the crisis, though. The nutritional situation remained precarious until 1923, the more so as the rationing system was maintained until 1921/22. The sale of the assortment, constantly changing according to acquisition possibilities, was guaranteed until 1923 and it is therefore not surprising that the number of small firms drastically increased between 1921 and 1923, while the hyperinflation was the end for many of them.[9] At the same time the significance of the street trade clearly grew, which helped many war-disabled persons and unemployed to make a frugal living.

## Partial rationalisation: The short boom of the Weimar Republic 1924–1932

Since 1924 a distinct upward tendency of the food retail trade began. Since then the recordable turnovers rose by more than 50% up to 1929 (Figs. 1–2).

The turnover figures illustrate the greater stability of the food retail trade during the downswing in 1926 and the depression of 1929–1933, which was conditional on structure. Analogous with Engel's law, the rule is obviously applicable that the food retail trade's share of the whole trade turnover is in inverse proportion to the free top consumption figure of a society, a thesis which was also confirmed by the development in the Federal Republic of Germany. The number of firms increased slightly during the Weimar Republic, but without reaching pre-war times (Table 4).

*Table 4:* Number of firms and employees in the food retail trade in Germany 1925–1939

| Year | | 1925 | 1933 | 1939 |
|---|---|---|---|---|
| Firms | – Retail Trade | 768.618 | 843.611 | 833.192 |
| | – Food Sector | 383.213 | 441.664 | 426.885 |
| Employees | – Retail Trade | 1,647.404 | 1,916.863 | 2,226.876 |
| | – Food Sector | 676.859 | 813.559 | 848.902 |
| Employees | – Retail Trade | 2,14 | 2,27 | 2,67 |
| per firm | – Food Sector | 1,77 | 1,84 | 1,99 |

*Sources:* Betriebszählung (1930), pp. 270–271; Ergebnisse (1927), pp. 351–352; Betriebszählung (1937), pp. 93–95; Einzelhandel (1942).

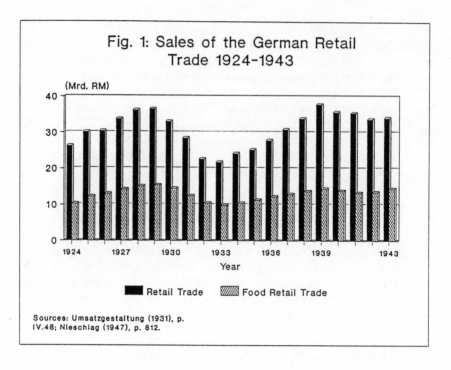

Fig. 1: Sales of the German Retail Trade 1924–1943

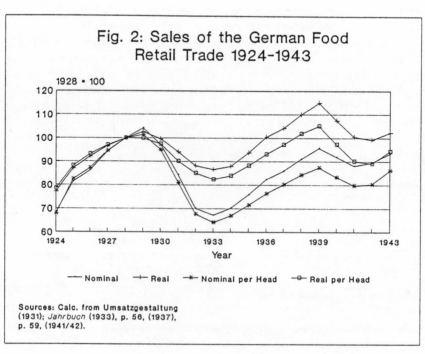

Fig. 2: Sales of the German Food Retail Trade 1924–1943

The business censuses illustrate at the same time the continually rising number of employees per business. They point to far-reaching but altogether only limited internal changes, whose basic significance has been discussed since the middle of the 1920s with the catchword 'rationalisation of trade'. Marketing analysis was to lead to a planned reduction of costs. In view of the consumer's new situation of choice since 1924 the demands concerning choice, packaging, display and quality of the products grew. Rising labour costs as well as a growing tax burden made the cost pressure swell again. The advice of the newly founded retail trade association, especially the 'Hauptgemeinschaft des Deutschen Einzelhandels' founded in 1919, aimed at correct bookkeeping and statistics as well as at a concentration of the purchase. Their effect on the food retail trade stayed small. The stock turnover rate hardly changed until the world depression while the new forms of business could already extend their pre-existing advantages (Table 5).

*Table 5:* Stock turnover rate of the food retail trade in Germany 1924–1931

| Year | Groceries | Edeka | Multiple Shops | Consumer Coop. |
|------|-----------|-------|----------------|----------------|
| 1924 | 4,8 | N.D. | 11 | 18,7 |
| 1925 | 5,2 | N.D. | 11 | 20,2 |
| 1926 | 5,5 | 6,5 | 12 | 22,7 |
| 1927 | 6,6 | 5,8 | 13 | 26 |
| 1928 | 6,7 | 6 | 14 | 25,4 |
| 1929 | 6,5 | 5,9 | 16 | 25,9 |
| 1930 | 7,1 | 7,1 | 17 | 26,3 |
| 1931 | 8,1 | 7,5 | 20 | 27,6 |

*Source:* Benning and Nieschlag (1933), pp. 39–40.

The intensified competition led to a clear intensification of advertising in the retail trade; the costs involved almost doubled compared to pre-war times and lay far above those of the industry.[10] High sums of money were invested in the equipment of shops, shop-windows were installed, the salerooms were decorated with wainscoting and modern lamps.[11] While the surrounding field of the products thereby changed, the assortment stayed relatively unchanged. The share of branded articles clearly rose to 20–30%, and the share of trade marks also increased strongly. On the whole the specialization remained, and only creameries as well as coffee and cocoa shops showed the first signs of integration endeavours. An exception to this rule were the co-operative societies, which more and more gave up the strict separation of groceries and industrial products on one hand and fresh products on the other hand and often offered complete assortments.[12] The small flexibility of the assortment led to a strong growth of the street and huckster trade, which partly determined the fruit and vegetable supply in the big towns by 50% only to increase even more during the world depression.[13]

The forms of sale also hardly changed; the shop counter remained the decisive piece of furniture. Self-service was broadly discussed and had a precursor in the form of the uniform price shops, but was not realized. The Swiss Migros-System was not very successful either. It was based on the sale of packed products at round prices in moving shops.[14] The small purchasing sums and the share of loose and unpacked products, which made up almost a third of all products, supported this structural conservatism.

Small rationalisation efforts were achieved beyond the organisational area. The discount savings unions were ousted through war and inflation, the specialized and central organisations were poorly equipped as far as financial means were concerned and therefore not very efficient. The retailer-purchasing co-operatives were the only positive exception. In 1929 the Edeka linked more than 25,000 shops, the Rewe was the second central retailer-purchasing co-operative to be established and by 1935 it already had 8,000 members. Both associations achieved cost advantages through the purchase of products, but the position they held was still too weak to fasten the industrial production to the rationalisation endeavours of the trade.

The rationalisation of the retail trade only partly succeeded during the Weimar Republic. For one thing it remained confined to the individual business and left consumer and industry almost completely out. Furthermore it took place chiefly in the new forms of business and the senior specialized trade, while the small and smallest shops lost ground dramatically within a few years (Table 6).

*Table 6:* Sales of food of different forms of trade in Germany 1924–1933

| Year | Groceries | General Stores | Department Stores | Consumer Coop. | Multiple Shops |
|------|-----------|----------------|-------------------|----------------|----------------|
| 1924 | 84 | 83 | 94,4 | 61,8 | 85,6 |
| 1925 | 100 | 100 | 100 | 100 | 100 |
| 1926 | 106 | 105 | 127,1 | 121,2 | 109,6 |
| 1927 | 116 | 116 | 156,7 | 143 | 140,1 |
| 1928 | 123 | 124 | 194,8 | 169,7 | 156,5 |
| 1929 | 129 | 128 | 237,1 | 190,1 | 166,6 |
| 1930 | 120 | 124 | 240,2 | 201,3 | 174,4 |
| 1931 | 107 | 108 | 222,3 | 188,5 | 152,5 |
| 1932 | 93,1 | 95,7 | 190,5 | 153,2 | 128,6 |
| 1933 | 90,2 | 94,3 | 155,9 | 115,5 | 91,8 |

*Sources:* *Wirtschaftszahlen* (1932), pp. 6–7; Hasselmann (1971), pp. 707–709; Handel (1933), p. 41; Handel (1934), p. 52.

As a consequence of lacking efficiency the specialized retail trade lost about 10% of its market share while the new forms of business managed to pool almost 24% of the turnover.[15]

## Control through state and corporations: the food trade 1932–1948

The world depression meant a clear economic break for the food retail trade even though the dramatic turnover losses were caused mainly by the strong price decline. The turnover decreased nominally by 35,4% from 1929 till 1933, substantially 'only' by 15,7%. More important was the fact that more and more economic competition was affected by political decisions. The transition to the presidential regime since 1930, the growing significance of the small middle-class parties and the watchwords of the National Socialists orientated by the specialized trade formed the background of a renewed departure from market economic policy, which began in 1930 with a new special tax legislation for large-scale enterprises. The 'take-over' of the coalition of National Socialists and right-wing bourgeoisie in 1933 did not change this policy structurally, but radicalized it clearly.

*Table 7:*  Sales of food of different forms of trade in Germany 1932–1936 (1932 = 100)

| Year | Groceries | General Stores | Department Stores | Consumer Coop. | Multiple Shops |
|------|-----------|----------------|-------------------|----------------|----------------|
| 1932 | 100 | 100 | 100 | 100 | 100 |
| 1933 | 96,8 | 98,5 | 77,8 | 65,6 | 86,5 |
| 1934 | 104,6 | 109,1 | 70,2 | 60 | 80,6 |
| 1935 | 113,6 | 120 | 64,4 | 60 | 84,7 |
| 1936 | 124,7 | 134,5 | 58,2 | 47,8 | 84,3 |

*Sources:*  Calc. from Handel (1934), p. 52, (1935/36), p. 77, (1936/37), pp. 66, 176; Hasselmann (1971), p. 496. 1936 only January-July.

In 1932 an installation prohibition for one-price stores was introduced and extended to all retail trade firms in 1933. The special tax for large-scale enterprises was doubled, clearance sales drastically confined, the granting of discounts through large-scale, especially the consumer, co-operatives, was restrained decisively. The latter were organisationally destroyed and National Socialists took over the leading positions. In 1934 all retail trade enterprises had a general licence liability, the taxes for large-scale businesses were raised again, the sale of vending machines through large-scale firms was prohibited. Jewish owners of department stores were expropriated in exchange for an insufficient indemnification, as happened also to many medium-sized enterprises. The consumer co-operatives received the heaviest blow. They had already had big solvency problems during the world depression because many members had split up their savings accounts and their own food production caused great losses. In 1933 they were exposed to many encroachments and arbitrary apprehensions, and it was considered 'un-german' to buy there. In 1935 the closing down of 82 big co-operatives was decided by law. 40% of the turnover was privatized and transferred to holding companies respectively. In 1941 the NS-State closed the remaining co-operatives. The consequences of this 'competition allevia-tion'[16] were striking: At the beginning of the Second World War the new forms of trade lay below the turnover share they had had in 1913 (Table 7).

On the other hand it is out of the question that the NS-State decidedly pursued a middle-class orientated economic policy. It was rather the aim of the government to establish a broad and decentralized network of indepen-dent and viable single shops. While the smallest businesses were to drop out of the controlled market situation in the long run, the remaining shops were expected to accept fundamental rationalisation efforts. Therefore a trade group 'foodstuffs and luxury foods' was founded in 1935 as a compulsory organisation, which together with the 'Deutsche Arbeitsfront' and the 'Reichsnährstand' formed a corporate network for the realisation of the desired efficiency augmentation. The technical aims were thoroughly com-bined with political aspects, though. Only a rationalised distributional system seemed to 1. make the continuous basic supply possible which was needed for the acceptance of the Regime, 2. make the switch of the foodstuff production conveyable to the consumer and 3. guarantee a trade structure which was close to the consumer and helped in case of a possible expansion of war. To secure a fixed profit various reciprocal trade agree-ments were made between industry, agriculture and trade. Thereby produc-tion, wholesale and retail trade were confined, but firm profit margins granted, which were strengthened by corporately fixed maximum and minimum prices. These measures altogether improved the economic situa-tion of the food trade from 1935, even if the general economic development was surely more significant in this respect. Important basic index numbers rose continually and remarkably. The stock turnover rapidity doubled from 1935 till 1942, the average turnover per employee rose despite the price stop in 1936, substantially by a third.[17] The profitability of the shops improved clearly, and medium-sized firms had the highest profits (Table 8).

*Table 8:* Profits in the groceries retail trade in Germany 1932 and 1937 (% of turnover)

| Turnover (RM) | 1932 | | 1935 | | 1937 | |
|---|---|---|---|---|---|---|
| | at rent | own premises | at rent | own premises | at rent | own premises |
| till 5000 | – | – | 8,8 | 10,7 | 11,6 | 13,6 |
| 5,000–20,000 | 7,0 | 8,5 | 8,1 | 9,6 | 8,9 | 10,1 |
| 20,000–50,000 | 4,3 | 5,5 | 6,7 | 7,7 | 7,5 | 8,4 |
| 50,000–100,000 | 3,2 | 4,1 | 5,5 | 6,1 | 6,2 | 6,9 |
| 100,000–500,000 | 1,3 | 2,1 | 4,6 | 5,2 | 5,1 | 5,9 |
| 500,000–1 Mil. | 1,6 | 1,6 | 3,6 | 4,0 | 4,6 | 5,2 |

*Sources:* *Betriebsstruktur* (1935), pp. 16–17; Umsatz (1937), p. 442; *Betriebsstruktur* (1940), pp. 44–45.

The growing significance of medium-sized firms is also illustrated by the fact that despite the decreasing importance of large-scale enterprises the average number of employees per firm rose by 8,1% till 1939, while the number of businesses decreased by 3,4% despite a distinct population growth. Consolidation was only achieved at the price of increased efficiency. This general development should not obscure the fact that from the middle of the 1930s various supply problems especially of meat, fat and luxury food arose, to which the customary grey and black markets of that time bear witness. The renunciation of the freedom of trade led to an early economy of shades, which is often incorrectly confined by collective remembrance to the time after the Second World War.

The assortment of the food trade grew broader, but lost depth. More and more local products were sold as well as substitutes and surrogates. Because of the high costs packaging was less frequent and loose products became more important.[18] The reciprocal trade contracts provoked clear progress in the field of formation of types and sorts. The shops' phenotype was all the longer more determined by topic- and product-related common advertisements. The shop-windows of the retail trade were a part of the propaganda machinery of the NS-State's strategic direction of consumption. Internal rationalisation, protection of power and preparation of war were combined again. At the same time there was only little progress in the organisation of the retail trade. The strict orientation by the supply chain production-wholesale trade-retail trade restrained the growth of the retailer-purchase co-operatives. And the efforts of some wholesale firms to concentrate the purchase by means of purchase or voluntary groups, where the retailers did not have to give up their independence, were not very successful.

During the war, by which the food trade profited until 1942, the significance of medium-sized shops increased again, and the situation was similar to the First World War. The disintegration did not begin on a large scale until 1944, but was more far-reaching than in 1918.

## Permanent rationalisation in distribution and sale: food retail trade in the Federal Republic of Germany 1949–1991

The situation after the Second World War was similar to that after 1923. After the lapse of various restrictions on freedom of trade from 1948 onwards the sales expanded. From 1949–1991 they rose nominally by more than 15 times, substantially by 6,5 times. At the same time the food sector's relative share of the whole retail trade turnover decreased from 46,8% in 1949 to 35,7% to 27,5% in 1991 (Fig. 3).

The firm figures developed in a different way. While from 1948 till 1952 the number of food stores clearly rose, it then stagnated and continually decreased since the end of the 1950s. Due to the turnover tax statistics, which cannot be compared and had been newly filed in 1962, we cannot

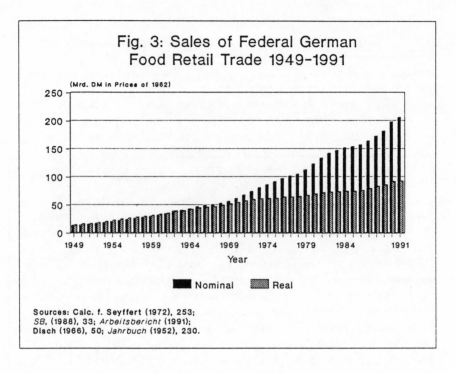

Fig. 3: Sales of Federal German Food Retail Trade 1949-1991

(Mrd. DM in Prices of 1962)

Sources: Calc. f. Seyffert (1972), 253;
*SB*, (1988), 33; *Arbeitsbericht* (1991);
Disch (1966), 50; *Jahrbuch* (1952), 230.

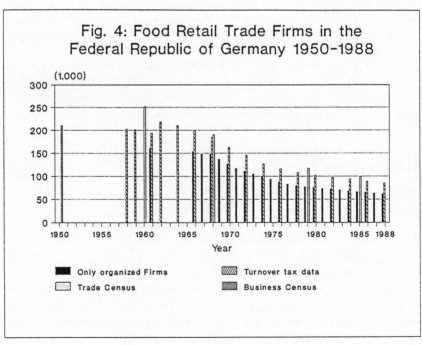

Fig. 4: Food Retail Trade Firms in the Federal Republic of Germany 1950-1988

(1.000)

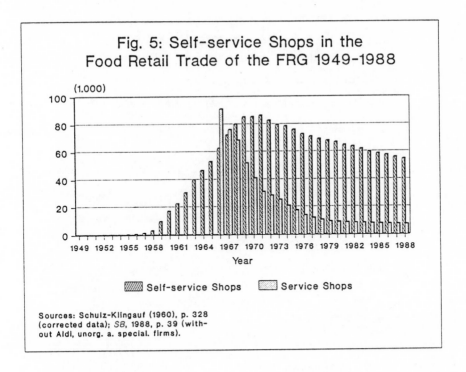

Fig. 5: Self-service Shops in the
Food Retail Trade of the FRG 1949–1988

Sources: Schulz-Klingauf (1960), p. 328
(corrected data); *SB*, 1988, p. 39 (without Aldi, unorg. a. special. firms).

illustrate the change in the 1950s precisely. But it is certain that the decisive decrease happened in the 1960s and the early 1970s, and the number of shops halved between 1962 and 1976 (Fig. 4).

What drove the development were once again the new forms of trade, especially the multiple shop trading and the partly indemnified consumer co-operatives. They were more dependent on the quickly rising labour costs than the medium-sized firms and translated the manifold stimulations from abroad into distribution and sale. Relying on the ability to package products centrally they became the actual pioneers of self-service from 1948, while its general break-through was not before 1957 (Fig. 5). As the acceptance of these shops was small from first, the consumer co-operatives also built up a network of Tempo-shops.

The keeping down of costs could best be achieved through higher turn-overs, therefore the new forms of trade started an aggressive price and advertising policy. Furthermore they clearly increased the share of own trade marks that did not have fixed prices and extended the assortment by fresh products, then frozen foods. Especially fruits, vegetables and meat were freely calculable articles which served as price-political 'drawing cards'.[19] Thereby they increased their turnover share clearly, but could not regain the level of 1932 before the middle of the 1960s (Fig. 6).

There were two reasons for this: on the one hand the consumer co-operatives did not manage to reach their pre-war level, although they were

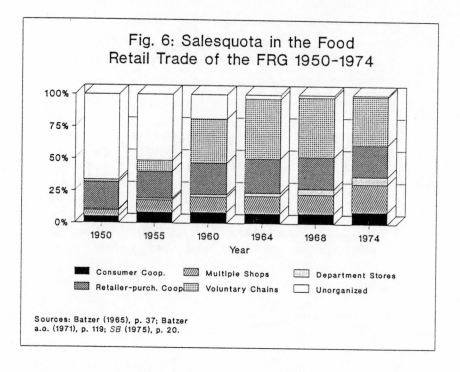

Fig. 6: Salesquota in the Food Retail Trade of the FRG 1950–1974

Sources: Batzer (1965), p. 37; Batzer a.o. (1971), p. 119; *SB* (1975), p. 20.

surely the most innovative form of trade after 1945. The co-operative and discount law in 1954 did not only allow sale to non-members, but confirmed essential elements of the National Socialists' legislation. The reimbursement was confined to 3%, and savings bank functions were not to be practised anymore. Thereby the self-financing of the co-operatives at the moment of comprehensive construction of new larger shops was decisively restrained. Because of the rationalisation of sale activities personal relations with the members broke down. They lacked modernity in the organisational structure and the unprofitable production enterprises enlarged the problems. In 1969 the consumer co-operatives linked together to the Coop-Group, which was changed into a stock corporation in 1974 and thereby actually put an end to the history of the consumer co-operatives.

On the other hand the reaction of the specialized trade was very different from what happened after 1923. Not only the retailer-purchase co-operatives, but also the other specialized dealers accepted – although with a delay – the challenge of the new forms of trade. The wholesale trade, which was hit by the expansion of the large-scale enterprises just as much, tended to form voluntary chains together with the retail traders to centralize purchase from the middle of the 1950s. The cooperation with the international groups like SPAR, VIVO, CENTRA, Végé, TIP, Ifa or A&O became decisive. The headquarters supported similar shop fronts and uniform advertisements, introduced new trade marks and extended the assortments. On the Federal German market since the middle of the 1960s there were only trade groups left which kept their organisations competitive by permanent rationalisation. The strong decrease in the business figures was due to this group rationalisation: a widespread dying-off of single, unorganized shops did not happen in the Federal Republic of Germany, but the small shops rather fell through the grid of self-chosen standards of performance. The heavy price competition led to an increasing significance of the central authorities among voluntary chains and retailer-purchasing co-operatives, while the economic independence of the retailers disappeared quickly. The formation of voluntary groups led to a universalization of multiple shop trading as a dominant form of enterprise in the 1960s. The place of separation according to organisational and purchase structures was more and more taken over by assortment, salerooms, breadth, quality and depth of the supply. The Federal German market was basically saturated at the beginning of the 1960s. One no longer offered scarce commodities but superfluity. The naked price decided imperatively: since the end of the 1950s the discounters set standards for a cheap basic supply and formed the actual quintessence of the prevailing development. Only since the early 1970s can one recognize intensified trading-up endeavours, which aimed at higher profits through more valuable and more expensive products.

At this time the purchasing behaviour had already changed clearly. The cash payment finally succeeded up to the beginning of the 1970s, and the average purchase sums substantially doubled between 1957 and 1989. Packed and conserved products, strict closing-times and the renunciation of weekly labour payments led to an obvious trimming of the full utilization of the food retail trade, which varied according to month and weekday. This general change from customer to consumer led to a comprehensive commercialisation of the relationship of people, products and buyers, who freed themselves from personal elements. This was illustrated mainly by the changes inside the salerooms. Before the counter disappeared due to self-service, especially the new forms of enterprise changed their product presentation from the end of the 1940s. The place of the undiscerning product-hiding shelves and drawers was taken by open shelves. The counter was freed from dominating sets and advertising boards and led back to its serving function. Instead of wood the use of combinations of wood, metal and glass was increased from the beginning of the 1950s. The visual sale began before the self-service. Shop-windows and decorations allowed a look into the shop before it became usual from the end of the 1950s to make special offers prominent by labelling panes. Cash registers and refrigerators as usual equipment now forced their way into the trade, although they had already been used sporadically since the Weimar Republic. The switch to saleable packaging began already before the self-service, although the food industry only contributed decisively from the beginning of the 1960s.

Through self-service the consumer became active and took the place of the shop-assistants. Open shelves, shopping baskets and more and more refrigerators were placed all over the shop, the serving counter only remained as a cash register desk. Since 1957 the statistical floorspace of the average shop increased tenfold, and it trebled in toto. One said good-bye to even prices. The purchase of food seemed to become more self-determined, the assortment visible and tangible. At the same time the assortment was decisively extended. The 1950s and 1960s marked the general transition to a complete assortment, which comprised meat and meat products, fruit and vegetables, bread and baker's ware, dairy products and frozen foods. The specialized enterprises followed this trend or tried trading-up strategies by means of more profound and more valuable assortments. Since then the average structure of the assortment has stayed relatively uniform, only the growing share of convenience products is worth mentioning. The assortments gained in depth, the average number of articles in a supermarket rose from 1,383 in 1954 to 6,620 in 1991.

These changes did not only concern the consumer, but also the industry. The complete assortments supported the emancipation from single trade marks with excellent turnovers, and they were now joined by more and more own trade marks. In 1954 they constituted 9% of the turnover, in 1967 even 25%. Contrary to the branded articles they could be calculated freely and therefore represented the actual spear point in the price competition. At the same time the branded article industry was put under a price-political pressure, the trade groups' growing power of demand forced them to more and more comprehensive super conditions. Since the end of the 1960s there was a power difference in favour of the food trade.

But the history of rationalisation is not only a story of success. More and more the 'economisation of the distribution'[20] came to its own limits. The concentration on questions of assortment formation, the decoration of shops, the power of purchase and making one's mark in contrast to fellow competitors finally led to an education of the consumers to a price-consciousness that did not prevail in other segments of the trade. Services constituted a growing part of the private consumption, in which the food trade decreased relatively. As a consequence the stronger emphasis of shopping events was taken up on a large scale through consumer markets and shopping centres from the beginning of the 1970s. While the supply trade was increasingly marked by the functional discount principle, the larger shops counted on the so-called event-trade. 'Gourmet's Paradises' were created, which offered luxury products and exotic specialities at high prices. This also concerns profitable bio-products. Service and distribution functions were integrated, the offer of prefabricated and consumable products was intensified.

One has to wait and see whether this much-discussed polarisation of the trade will achieve an over-proportional growth. The significance of customer-close sale by means of mobile shops, which has increased since the middle of the 1980s, makes other scenarios seem possible. The concentration on few consumption centres outside the residential areas raises great problems for the basic food supply especially of elderly people who are not mobile. Despite the event trade the satisfaction about the number of retail shops altogether decreases even among urban consumers. In view of the increasing problems of the individual traffic the trade perspectives will perforce connect themselves with an environmentally sensible and forward-looking policy. Modern consumers prefer products with suitable packaging, and deposit systems will get more importance in future. Trading-up strategies will only be successfull, if they consider ecological and hygienic problems caused by new products. If the German food retail trade wants to continue its unique upward trend of the last forty years sucessfully, it has to emphasize not only further economic rationalisation but must also create a new distribution strategy which is close to the life of the customers.

## Notes

1 Batzer (1965), p. 41.
2 Hasse (1892), pp. 101–102; Hasse (1900).
3 Spiekermann (1993).
4 Spiekermann (1994), pp. 29–32.
5 Spiekermann (1994).
6 *Edeka* (1982),pp. 6–14.
7 Lebensmittel-Kleinhandel (1918).
8 Entwicklung (1924); Hasselmann (1971), pp. 706–709.
9 Hirsch (1928), p. 658.
10 *Einzelhandel* (1929), pp. 14–15; Mataja (1929), p. 1241.
11 Keiser/Benning (1933), pp. 141–142.
12 Benning/Nieschlag (1933), pp. 70–71.
13 Weigel (1927), pp. 399–402; Rompe (1933), pp. 400–402.
14 Weghmann (1938), p. 39.
15 Ibid., p. 5; Batzer (1965), p. 36.
16 Förderung (1935), p. 14 ('Milderung des Wettbewerbs').
17 Tiburtius (1949), pp. 26–27, 136.
18 An exception were the self-service shops founded by Eklöh in 1938.
19 Batzer a.o. (1971), pp 123–141.
20 Redwitz (1990), pp. 16–17 ('Ökonomisierung der Distribution').

## Literature

*Arbeitsbericht (12.) der Hauptgemeinschaft des Deutschen Einzelhandels* 1959, (Köln 1960).
*Arbeitsbericht (13.) der Hauptgemeinschaft des Deutschen Einzelhandels* 1959, (Köln 1961).

*Arbeitsbericht (*15.*) der Hauptgemeinschaft des Deutschen Einzelhandels* 1959, (Köln 1963).

*Arbeitsbericht (*34.*) der Hauptgemeinschaft des Deutschen Einzelhandels* 1981, (Köln 1982).

*Arbeitsbericht* 1991 (44.) *der Hauptgemeinschaft des Deutschen Einzelhandels,* (Köln 1992).

*Die nichtlandwirtschaftlichen Arbeitsstätten in der Bundesrepublik Deutschland nach der Zählung vom* 13.9.1950, I. 1, (Stuttgart/Köln 1952).

Barrenstein, Peter F., *Der mittelständische Einzelhandel in der Bundesrepublik Deutschland. Entwicklung, Entwicklungsdeterminanten und gesamtwirtschaftliche Funktionen,* (Frankfurt a.M. 1980).

Batzer, Erich, 'Starker Wandlungsprozess im Lebensmittelhandel'. *Wirtschaftskonjunktur,* 17 (1965), pp. 33–41.

Batzer, Erich, 'Der Strukturwandel im Einzelhandel der Bundesrepublik Deutschland', in Erich Batzer, Laumer, Helmut and Takeshi Suzuki (eds), *Absatzwirtschaft in Japan und Deutschland. Strukturen-Wettbewerb-Politik,* Berlin/München 1992, pp. 37–68.

Batzer, Erich a.o., *Marktstrukturen und Wettbewerbsverhältnisse im Einzelhandel,* (Berlin/München 1971).

Benning, Bernhard and Robert Nieschlag, *Umsatz, Lagerhaltung und Kosten im deutschen Einzelhandel* 1924 *bis* 1932, (Berlin 1933).

*Betriebsstruktur und Besteuerung im Einzelhandel und im Handwerk. Eine Sammlung von Richtzahlen, P.* 1: *Einzelhandel,* (Berlin 1935).

*Betriebsstruktur und Kostengestaltung in wichtigen Gewerbezweigen. Eine Sammlung von Richtzahlen, P. II: Einzelhandel, Gaststätten- und Beherbergungsgewerbe,* (Berlin 1940).

*Gewerbliche Betriebszählung. Die gewerblichen Betriebe und Unternehmungen im Deutschen Reich,* (Berlin 1930) (Statistik des Deutschen Reichs, V. 413).

*Gewerbliche Betriebszählung. Das Gewerbe im Deutschen Reich. Textband,* (Berlin 1937) (Statistik des Deutschen Reichs, V. 466).

Disch, Wolfgang K.A., *Der Gross- und Einzelhandel in der Bundesrepublik,* (Köln/Opladen 1966).

*Edeka. 75 Jahre immer in Aktion* 1907–1982 (s.l. n.d).

*Der Einzelhandel mit Lebensmitteln, Kolonialwaren und Drogen,* Berlin 1929.

'Der Einzelhandel. Ergebnisse der nichtlandwirtschaftlichen Arbeitsstättenzählung 1939'. *Wirtschaft und Statistik,* 22 (1942), pp. 265–271.

'Die Entwicklung des deutschen Einzelhandels 1913 bis 1923'. *Wirtschaft und Statistik,* 4 (1924), pp. 732–733.

'Weitere Ergebnisse der Volks-, Berufs- und Betriebszählung 1925. Das Handelsgewerbe nach den Ergebnissen der gewerblichen Betriebszählung von 1925'. *Wirtschaft und Statistik,* 7 (1927), pp. 350–355.

'Förderung des Mittelstandes'. *Wochenbericht des Instituts für Konjunkturforschung,* 8 (1936), No. f. 16.02., pp. 13–15.

'Handel', *Vierteljahrshefte zur Konjunkturforschung*, 8 (1933), P. B, pp. 40–41.

'Handel', *Vierteljahrshefte zur Konjunkturforschung*, 9 (1934), P. B, pp. 49–52.

'Handel', *Vierteljahrshefte zur Konjunkturforschung*, N.S. 10 (1935/36), pp. 75–78.

'Handel', *Vierteljahrshefte zur Konjunkturforschung*, N.S. 11 (1936/37), pp. 65–67, 176–178.

*Handels- und Gaststättenzählung 1960, I. Einzelhandel*, I. 1, (Stuttgart/Mainz 1965).

*Handels- und Gaststättenzählung 1968, II. Einzelhandel*, I. 1, (Stuttgart/Mainz 1973).

*Handels- und Gaststättenzählung 1979*, I. 2, (Stuttgart/Mainz 1982).

*Handels- und Gaststättenzählung 1985*, I. 1, (Stuttgart/Mainz 1986).

Hasse, E., 'Messen und Märkte', *Statistisches Jahrbuch deutscher Städte*, 2 (1892), pp. 101–116.

Hasse, E., 'Markthallen', *Statistisches Jahrbuch deutscher Städte*, 8 (1900), pp. 337–352.

Hasselmann, Erwin, *Geschichte der deutschen Konsumgenossenschaften*, Frankfurt a.M. 1971.

Hirsch, Julius, 'Entwicklungstendenzen des modernen Handels'. *Magazin der Wirtschaft*, N.S. 2 (1926), pp. 656–660.

Keiser, Günther and Bernhard Benning, *Kapitalbildung und Investitionen in der deutschen Volkswirtschaft 1924 bis 1928*, (Berlin 1931).

'Der Lebensmittel-Kleinhandel im Zeichen der Kriegswirtschaft'. *Deutsche Handelsrundschau* (1918), pp. 259–261.

Mataja, Viktor, 'Die Bedeutung der Reklame'. *Magazin der Wirtschaft*, N.S. 5 (1929), pp. 1241–1243.

Nieschlag, Robert, 'Der Weg des deutschen Binnenhandels. Eine Studie des Deutschen Instituts für Wirtschaftsforschung'. *Europa-Archiv*, 2 (1947), pp. 811–817, 881–886.

Redwitz, Gunter, 'Handelsentwicklung. Wertewandel-Perspektiven für die Handelslandschaft, in Rüdiger Szallies and Günther Wiswede (eds), *Wertewandel und Konsum. Fakten. Perspektiven und Szenarien für Markt und Marketing*, (Landsberg a. Lech 1990), pp. 257–282.

Reithinger, A., 'Vermehrung oder Uebersetzung des Handels?'. *Magazin der Wirtschaft*, N.S. 5 (1929), pp. 339–343.

Rompe, Franz, 'Märkte und Markthallen'. *Statistisches Jahrbuch deutscher Städte*, 28 (1933), pp. 392–418.

*SB in Zahlen. Ausgabe 1974/75*, (Köln 1975).

*SB in Zahlen. Ausgabe 1988*, (Köln 1988).

Schmid, Eugen, *Der deutsche Detailhandel und seine Organisation*, RStwiss. Diss. (Würzburg 1920).

Schulz-Klingauf, Hans-Viktor, *Selbstbedienung. Der neue Weg zum Kunden*, (Düsseldorf 1960).

Seyffert, Rudolf, *Wirtschaftslehre des Handels*, 5th rev. ed., (Opladen 1972).

Spiekermann, Uwe, 'Milchkleinhandel im Wandel. Fallstudie zu München 1840–1913'. *Scripta Mercaturae*, 27 (1993), pp. 91–144.

Spiekermann, Uwe, *Warenhaussteuer in Deutschland. Mittelstandsbewegung, Kapitalismus und Rechtsstaat im späten Kaiserreich*, Frankfurt a.M. 1994.

*Statistisches Jahrbuch für die Bundesrepublik Deutschland* 1952, (Stuttgart/ Köln 1952).

*Statistisches Jahrbuch für das Deutsche Reich*, 52 (1933); 56 (1937); 59 (1941/ 42).

Tiburtius, Joachim, *Lage und Leistungen des deutschen Handels in ihrer Bedeutung für die Gegenwart*, Berlin/München 1949.

'Umsatz, Betriebsausgaben und Gewinn im Einzelhandel mit Nahrungs- und Genumitteln'. *Wirtschaft und Statistik*, 17 (1937), pp. 441–442.

'Die Umsatzgestaltung im Verteilungsgroßhandel und im Einzelhandel Deutschlands in den Jahren 1924 bis 1931', *Vierteljahrshefte zur Statistik des Deutschen Reichs*, 40 (1931), pp. IV. 43-IV.51.

Weghmann, Arnold Maria, *Die Strukturwandlungen des Lebensmittelhandels*, Stwiss. Diss. Halle-Wittenberg, (Stuttgart 1938).

Weigel, Paul, 'Wochenmärkte, Straßen und Hausierhandel, Markthallen'. *Statistisches Jahrbuch deutscher Städte*, 22 (1927), pp. 383–414.

*Wirtschaftszahlen* 1925 bis 1931, (Berlin 1932).

# 17

# FOOD RETAILING, NUTRITION AND HEALTH IN IRELAND, 1839–1989: ONE HUNDRED AND FIFTY YEARS OF EATING

## E. Margaret Crawford

### Introduction

On the eve of the Great Irish Famine two thirds of the population were country dwellers and one half of these were cottiers: i.e. agricultural labourers cultivating the land of tenant farmers. They were rewarded for their services, not by money wages, but by small plots of land on which they cultivated potatoes which grew abundantly in Irish conditions, and when accompanied by buttermilk provided the sole means of subsistence. Some cottiers rented land for which they paid a money rent acquired by selling a pig which was reared on potato scraps. Nevertheless, for more than a third of the population retailing was not part of their lives.

The Great Famine marked a watershed in the economic and social life of Ireland. The population fell from 8.4 million to 6.5 million between 1841 and 1851, and decreased further to 4.5 million by the end of the century. It continued to decline until 1961, after which it increased slightly. The unique post-Famine demographic pattern was the product of falling fertility, static death rates until 1900 and persistent emigration.[1] After the Famine, furthermore, the population became increasingly urbanized. In 1841 13 per cent of the population lived in towns of 2,000 and over. By 1911 the figure had increased to 33.5 per cent and by 1971 to over 50 per cent.[2]

Those who survived the Famine and stayed on the land carved out an existence in ways very different from their fathers. They were now wage-earning agricultural labourers. During the subsistence crisis the number of cottiers and labourers dropped by 40 per cent, and from 1851 to 1911 decreased by a further 40 per cent. The fall in numbers enhanced their value but this was partly offset by a move towards pastoral farming which reduced the demand for labour. While agricultural wage rates remained low between 1840 and 1900 compared with wages in other sectors they increased consistently. Incomes, however, rose less than wages since work was intermittent. In addition, new demands were placed on earnings. Before the

Famine, rent had been the main item of expenditure, but once the market place was entered, food commanded a rising proportion of expenditure. Fortunately the burden of rents fell after the Famine. By contrast, between 1850 and 1870 expenditure on food increased. With the exception of tea and sugar, 'a very large and striking advance'[3] took place in the price of food. Rising money income, nevertheless, made possible a more varied dietary pattern, at first in the east but ultimately throughout the whole country. Imported commodities such as Indian meal (maize meal), wheat flour, tea, and sugar were bought from shops and markets, as also were locally produced goods such as bread, milk and even potatoes.[4] According to one historian 'the most remarkable development of all in the post-Famine era was the greater quantity of shop-purchased food'[5] eaten by all classes.

## Retailing

The history of retailing in Ireland remains to be written, but the fact that shopkeepers and traders constituted 'an increasing proportion of the economically active population'[6] in the second half of the nineteenth century indicates a growing dependence on the distributive trade. Even in rural districts the retailing network extended to meet the developing consumer demand for shop purchased foods.[7]

*Table 1:*  Numbers occupied in food retailing in Ireland 1861–1911

|  | 1861 | 1871 | 1881 | 1891 | 1901 | 1911 |
|---|---|---|---|---|---|---|
| Shopkeepers |  | 24,925 | 24,221 | 27,961 | 30,572 | 24,617 |
| Grocers | 8,726 | 11,321 | 15,406 | 17,106 | 17,140 | 15,407 |
| Butchers | 2,652 | 7,339 | 6,448 | 6,772 | 6,717 | 6,710 |
| Bakers | 9,293 | 9,056 | 9,148 | 9,020 | 8,293 | 7,723 |
| Fishmongers | 1,971 | 2,022 | 2,069 | 2,360 | 1,612 | 1,645 |
| Greengrocers | 967 | 1,909 | 2,864 | 2,611 | 2,039 | 1,614 |
| Milk Sellers |  | 2,758 | 3,717 | 2,219 | 2,317 | 1,968 |
| Cheesemongers | 9 | 2,263 | 1,669 | 440 | – | – |
| TOTAL | 23,618 | 61,593 | 65,542 | 68,489 | 68,690 | 59,684 |
| Grocers/ 10,100 of population | 40 | 100 | 113 | 115 | 115 | 114 |

*Source:*  Census of Ireland 1861; Census of Ireland 1871; Census of Ireland 1881; Census of Ireland 1891; Census of Ireland 1901; Census of Ireland 1911.

Shopkeepers often fulfilled a dual, and in some cases a triple role. They supplied food and also provided credit, so important to labourers' families when earnings were spasmodic.[8] In remote areas they also acted as middlemen or agents, accepting eggs and butter for the local or export market in exchange for Indian meal (maize meal), tea and sugar.[9] The multiple role of the shopkeepers forged insoluble bonds between the shopkeeper and customer which were a source of tension. In a rural society where incomes were low and cash flows small such relationships were inevitable for labourers to live, but the cost of credit was high.

In 1921 Ireland was divided into two political units, the Irish Free State (Eire) and Northern Ireland, which complicates comparison with earlier periods (See Notes 14 & 15). Nevertheless, it is clear that there continued to be a marked growth in retailing until 1936 (see Table 2). During the next decade, however, contraction is evident. The post First World War years were a period of rising prosperity particularly between 1926 and 1931 when real incomes per head rose by 14 per cent in the Irish Free State.[10] In Northern Ireland increases in national income were probably of the same order of magnitude. For although politically divided, living standards in the two countries were similar.[11] After 1931, however, real incomes fell in the Free State as the Great Depression cut deeply into what was still an agriculturally based economy.

*Table 2:*  Numbers occupied in food retailing in Eire 1926–1946

|  | 1926 | 1936 | 1946 |
|---|---|---|---|
| Grocery/Provisions | 14,669 | 17,095 | 16,808 |
| Butchers | 4,547 | 5,246 | 3,350 |
| Vegetable & Fruit | 1,693 | 2,044 | 1,799 |

*Source:*  *Census of Population 1926; Census of Population 1936; Census of Population 1946.* (26 counties)

The 1960s marked the beginning of a 'retail revolution'. The number of independent grocery outlets declined, as large multiple supermarkets increased. Over the thirty year period 1958 to 1988 supermarkets increased 400 fold while grocery shops decreased by just over 60 per cent. The new selling philosophy was 'pile it high, sell it cheap', and this approach resulted in the market share being diverted away from the traditional grocer to the new self service supermarkets, particularly in urban areas. In the 1980s Parker noted that 'multiples' commanded 86 per cent of grocery trade in Dublin but less than one third in the sparsely populated Connaght and Ulster counties'.[12] Toward the end of the 1980s expansion in multiple supermarkets ceased and by 1991 their numbers actually declined.[13]

Irish grocery shops were predominantly family businesses, and in the 1950s almost 75% of them had a turnover of under a £100 per week, while 36.3% brought in less than £20 per week.[16] Of those employed in the grocery business 59 per cent were either proprietors or unpaid members of the owner's family, and only 1.7 per cent belonged to retail chains of 5 units or more. Significantly, though, the retail chains accounted for 13.0 per cent of total grocery sales.[17]

A major disadvantage experienced by family grocers was their inability to compete with the new forms of retailing emerging in 1950s and 1960s. Retail sales which had grown by only 3% per annum in 1950s more than doubled to 7% between 1960 and 1965, consequently encouraging new and larger companies to enter the grocery retail sector. The new stores had bigger turnovers, larger bulk orders and increased rates of discount which in turn were passed to the customers. In an effort to survive, small retail grocers responded by forming collective voluntary groups, to enhance collective bargaining power when dealing with suppliers.[18] Since the late 1980s the 'multiple' market share has fallen by 10 per cent though still has the lion's share at 52 per cent of the market.[19]

*Table 3(a):* Number of Retail Food Outlets in Eire 1956–1988

|  | 1956 | 1966 | 1977 | 1988 | % change (1977–88) |
|---|---|---|---|---|---|
| Grocery Shops | 13,111 | 10,770 | 7,305 | 5,176 | -29.1 |
| Supermarkets |  | 41 | 250 | 433 | 73.2 |
| Grocery & Public House | 3,742 | 3,007 | 1,362 | 921 | -32.4 |
| Fresh Meat | 1,776 | 1,803 | 1,862 | 1,690 | -9.2 |
| Fish & Poultry | 162 | 167 | 141 | 111 | -21.3 |
| Fruit & Vegetables | 546 | 362 | 354 | 327 | -7.6 |
| Bread, Flour & Pastry | 336 | 397 | 270 | 337 | 24.8 |
| Grocery shop/10,000 pop. | 45 | 37 | 25 | 15 |  |

*Source: Censuses of Distribution*[14]

(b) Number of Retail Food Outlets N. Ireland 1965–89

|  | 1965 | 1975 | 1989 |
|---|---|---|---|
| Grocery | 5518 | 2678 | 1471 |
| Other Food |  | 2062 | 1500 |
| Grocery shop/10,000 | 37 | 17 | 9 |

*Sources: Censuses of Distribution (N. Ireland).*[15]
*Retailing in Northern Ireland* (1990).

By 1989 family shopping habits even among the poorer classes had shifted towards supermarket purchasing. Three-quarters of families used major supermarkets at least once a month and 60 per cent at least once a week; two-thirds of households visited local supermarkets at least once a week. On the other hand, small local corner shops were not totally eclipsed. More than half of poor families in Dublin visited local shops and vans two or three times a week and often daily.[20] These outlets continued to provided a service when larder stocks ran dry and credit when needed.

## Diet

Whereas in the past food retailers were merely the purveyors of food, now there is an expectation that their varied stocks should provide high quality and healthy produce.[21] Furthermore, with the advent of shops and later supermarkets eating habits changed.

Dietary surveys help us to chart the development towards more varied fare. The earliest systematic study was carried out in 1839. This was followed by surveys in 1859, 1863, 1903–4, 1948–50, 1988 and 1989.[22] In the late eighteenth century and early decades of the nineteenth century increasing commercialisation of grain and pastoral products left the peasantry with the only two commodities they could not sell, potatoes and buttermilk and these they consumed morning, noon and night. The dietary survey of 1839 by W.H.T. Hawley, a Poor Law Assistant Commissioner in the south west of the country reveals two points: the limited fare, and the large quantities of potatoes consumed. Men on average consumed daily 12 lbs (5.4 kg.) and women 10 lbs (4.5 kg.). This pattern was typical of the whole of Ireland.

During the Famine the potato crop was destroyed in three seasons out of four. Post-Famine dietary surveys in 1859 and 1863 show that changes had already taken place. Potatoes and buttermilk, for all but the poorest, were eaten in smaller quantities, and new foods or items formerly eaten only occasionally, much of which had to be purchased, were added to the menu. One of the enduring legacies of the Famine was the re-introduction into diets of Indian meal.[23] Indian meal had been imported by the government in 1800 as a relief food when potatoes and grain were in short supply. During the Great Famine it was again consumed widely, and it remained part of the daily diet long after the shortage had ceased. Indian meal, more than any other food, introduced the labouring classes to purchased food. Additional items on their shopping list were bread, oatmeal, butter, tea and sugar. Even bacon and meat were now consumed regularly rather than intermittently. Milk, the consumption of which had declined before the Famine, was enjoyed once more, usually in the form of buttermilk or skimmed milk. Writing of the peasantry's eating habits in 1859 C.G. Otway observed the dietary diversification:

> The diet of the labouring classes . . ., has, within the last seven or eight years been much improved both as to quality and variety . . . Before the Famine potatoes with occasional milk was almost the sole diet of the great bulk of the class . . . now, wholemeal wheaten bread, Indian and oatmeal stirabout, and even tea and sugar, as well as milk is used not merely occasionally and as a great luxury, but almost generally.[24]

Once the Irish acquired a taste for tea, they drank it in vast quantities and insisted on the highest quality. Initially tea drinking was concentrated in the east,[25] but during the 1870s and 1880s the habit spread westwards.[26] William Keating of Galway, reported to the Industries Committee (1883–4) that 'the best teas [being] sold anywhere in the United Kingdom are sold in the west of Ireland'.[27] A government official writing from the West in the early 1890s commented that 'tea [was] drunk in excess three times a day by most, and by all once or twice.'[28] Between 1859 and 1903 average daily tea consumption among labourers rose more than ten fold, from 0.03 oz. (0.85 g.) to 0.4 oz.

(11 g.)[29] By the 1950s tea was even more popular, the average intake per head rising to 2.3 oz. (65 g.).[30]

The use of sugar also rose after 1850 in line with tea. Labourers added it liberally to tea and sprinkled it on Indian meal stirabout. Between 1859 and 1904 average sugar consumption among labourers (not including foods rich in sugar) increased ten fold from 8.5 g. to 85 g. per head; during the present century it has risen another ten percent.[31]

White bread was not commonly eaten by labourers until the post-Famine era. W. Hancock noted in 1862 that the importation of cheap and superior flour during the 1860s combined with 'the rise in wages without any rise in [the price of] wheat, . . . brought household bread within the reach of a much larger number of the labouring classes.'[32] During the last quarter of the nineteenth century white bread increased in popularity, particularly in Dublin and other cities. In the countryside it was more common for housewives to buy wheaten flour and bake bread at home. Second, third, or fourth grade flour ceased to satisfy household taste. Keating in the early 1880s observed that 'the poorest of the population of Ireland now . . . will not use even seconds; they buy the finest flour'.[33] Daily bread consumption rose by more than a third in the second half of the nineteenth century. It almost halved, however, during the twentieth century as other foods entered the daily fare.[34]

Despite the importance of butter production in Ireland, it was little eaten by labourers before the Famine. During the second half of the nineteenth century consumption levels remained low, although the average daily intake of butter among the labouring class increased from 0.5 oz (14.2 g.) in 1859 to 1.3 oz. (37 g.) in 1904.[35] During the twentieth century a sharp distinction emerged between the very poor and the better-off labourers. Skilled labourers bought butter in considerable quantities, surpassing the amount consumed by their counterparts elsewhere in the United Kingdom.[36] A high level of butter consumption was maintained through most of the century, though over the past two decades a concerted effort has been made by healthy eating programmes to encourage polyunsaturated spreads instead of butter.

Meat, formerly reserved for festive days, gradually became part of the daily fare, initially in very small quantities. The increase in butchers' shops during the post-Famine decades (see Table 2) reflects the rising demand for meat. Between 1859 and 1904 a six fold rise in average daily consumption in rural areas from 0.05 oz (1.4 g.) to 0.3 oz. (8.5 g.) occurred. During the next five decades consumption rose to just over 2 oz (63 g.) daily and over 3 oz. (90 g.) by 1989.[37] During the inter-war period meat consumption probably rose even higher. The Economic War between Britain and Ireland in the 1930s channelled meat earmarked for the British market into Irish mouths. The war was political in origin, though the battle was waged with economic weapons, in the form of trade duties. Although damaging to the Irish economy, the surplus of meat improved the Irish diet. Between 1926/7 and 1936/7 the number of cattle consumed rose by 79 per cent, and lamb by 37 per cent.[38] Furthermore, following the decision by the Irish Government in 1934 to reduce cattle herds, meat was distributed free to the unemployed for a short period.[39]

By 1900 the transition from subsistence staples to shop purchased food was almost complete. A varied diet was enjoyed by most. The extent to which this process further progressed over the first fifty years of the new century is evident from the Eire national nutrition survey (1948). Compared with the 1904 Board of Trade dietary studies, which listed 17 foods and food groups in the urban study and 11 for the rural, the survey of 1948–50 recorded over 50 foods and food groups. When the household budget survey was carried out in 1987, the list of foods consumed had increased to 125 foods, of which only a very small number were home produced. Table 4 summarises the major changes in food consumption between 1839 and 1989. The data for 1839, 1904, and 1946/8 relate to rural labourers, those for 1989 pertain to urban workers since rural statistics were not available for that date. By the mid twentieth century, however, dietary differences between urban and rural dwellers were not significant.

*Table 4:*  Per capita consumption of major food items in g/ml per day

|                | 1839 | 1904[1] | 1946/8[2] | 1989 |
|----------------|------|---------|-----------|------|
| Potatoes       | 5226 | 795     | 543       | 307  |
| Milk products  | 1647 | 398     | 424       | 513  |
| Eggs           | –    | 17      | 28        | 43   |
| Bread          | –    | 568[3]  | 357[3]    | 231  |
| Butter         | –    | 20      | 28        | 46[4] |
| Meat           | –    | 9       | 63        | 90   |
| Bacon          | –    | 48      | 10        | 55[5] |
| Fish           | –    |         | 6         | 18   |

1 Figures calculated from the rural survey of 1904
2 Figures calculated from survey of Farm Workers' Families and based on their calculation of 'diet-head'.
3 Bread and flour have been aggregated.
4 Butter and margarine have been aggregated.
5 Processed meat.
Sources:  1839 *Sixth Annual Report* (1840).
   1904 *Second Report by Mr Wilson Fox* (1905).
   1946/8 *National Nutrition Survey*, Part V, Dietary Survey of Farm Workers' Families (1950).
   1989 P. Lee & M. Gibney, *Patterns of Food and Nutrient Intake in the Suburb of Dublin* (1989)

This extension of consumer choice was partly the result of developments in agricultural and food processing technology, the establishment of fast transportation networks and improved marketing techniques, as well as a revolution in the kitchen, both in the storage facilities, and cooking methods.

Income strongly determined the type and quantity of foods purchased. In 1859, 80 to 90 per cent of labouring incomes was spent on food. By 1904 this figure had fallen to 60–70 per cent. A further decline to 40 or 50 per cent had occurred by the 1950s. By 1964, despite consumer spending increasing rapidly, the proportion of income spent on food declined to 32.8%.[40] The decline has continued, and in the 1980s the average proportion of total spending allocated to food was 20%,[41] although in manual workers' households the percentage was around 30 per cent.

Prior to the 1950s the link between food purchasing and income was clear cut. The staple foods, potatoes and grains, were essential; it was dairy and meat products which were sensitive to income. A good example of this relationship can be found in the meat and butter consumption of urban working men's families in 1904. See Table 5.

*Table 5:* Average weekly Meat and Butter purchased by Urban Working Men's Families 1904

|  | Meat lbs/kg | | Butter lbs/kg | |
| --- | --- | --- | --- | --- |
| Under 25s | 3.30 | 1.5 | 0.96 | 0.4 |
| 25s to under 30s | 4.32 | 1.9 | 2.13 | 0.9 |
| 30s to under 35s | 8.43 | 3.8 | 2.43 | 1.1 |
| 35s to under 40s | 7.25 | 3.3 | 2.40 | 1.1 |
| 40s and over | 8.62 | 3.9 | 4.04 | 1.8 |

*Source:* *Second Series of Memoranda* (1905)

Expenditure on tea and sugar were notable as highly inelastic.

To-day this linkage is more complex. A wider variety of foods is available at competitive prices. Thus those with small incomes can purchase a good nutritious diet despite limited budgets. A Northern Ireland survey of 1988 demonstrated that among men income levels did not affect the nutritional quality of their diet, whereas for women nutritional standards were influenced by the income of the bread winner.[42]

## Nutrition

Economists usually assume that as income rises, so does well being, including nutritional standards. However, between 1850 and 1900 nutritional standards in Ireland fell; the rise in retailing did little for the health of Ireland's poor. Thereafter, economic improvement and nutritional standards moved in the same direction.

Recent analysis of Irish diets has revealed that in the pre-Famine era, when labourers lived in the most wretched of conditions, their fare was exceptionally nutritious. They consumed daily high levels of protein, carbohydrate, energy value, calcium and iron, and despite their meatless diet the quality as well as the quantity of protein was high.[43] Only the fat content of the diet was low.[44] As consumption of potatoes and milk declined and bread, butter, tea and sugar were widely adopted the nutritional quality deteriorated. Protein, carbohydrate, calcium and energy values fell, and but for the increase in fat the fall in energy value would have been even sharper. It would be misleading, however, to envisage a nation of undernourished people in the post-Famine era. The protein content, for example, in many labourers' diets was more than adequate. For, although in many households only small amounts of meat, bacon, fish and eggs were purchased, amounting to 3/4 to 1 oz (21–28 g.) daily, milk, on the other hand, was drunk in its various forms by almost every family in considerable quantities. But milk, skimmed milk and buttermilk alone did not account for the good protein levels. Potatoes, now eaten in smaller amounts were still important, so too were farinaceous products. Families existing on meatless diets could acquire high protein levels as demonstrated by an example from the 1859 survey in Table 6.

*Table 6:*   A Sample Diet from the 1859 Survey of Labourers' Diets

|  | Quantity per week for family of 7 | Average Daily Protein per Labourer |
| --- | --- | --- |
| Indian meal | 28 lb (12.7 kg) | 38.9 |
| Potatoes | 7 st (44.5 kg) | 20.2 |
| Bread | 1½ lb (682 g) | 1.4 |
| Buttermilk | 21 qt (24 litres) | 2.2 |
| New Milk | 1½ qt (1.7 litres) | 28.5 |
|  |  | 91.2 |

*Source: Thirteenth Annual Report* (1860), p. 72.

By the early years of the twentieth century the protein content had fallen by roughly 25 per cent. Increasing urbanization contributed to the changing pattern of food consumption leading to an overall decline in protein. In towns and cities the shops provided a greater choice of food. Butchers' shops abounded in Dublin; and those in poor districts sold a wide variety of cheap cuts of meat.[45] Nevertheless, the quantities of meat eaten were still very small, and the increase in consumption of protein rich foods – bacon, pork, and eggs – was insufficient to offset the decline in the amount of milk, buttermilk, skimmed milk, and potatoes consumed. Tea replaced milk, bread replaced potatoes, and the increased variety of daily fare reduced dependence on milk, oatmeal, Indian meal and potatoes.

One of the most interesting and significant dietary changes to take place over the period under study is the quite remarkable increase in fat consumption from the 1850s onwards. Prior to the famine diets contained a mere 13 grams of fat which contributed only 3 per cent to the total energy value. A major reason for the low fat content was the dominance of the potato, a food containing only a minuscule of fat. The rise in dietary fat in the post-Famine period, though initially modest, accelerated as butter consumption and the used of animal fats for frying food increased. By the opening years of the twentieth century Irish labouring men consumed about 50 per cent more butter than their English or Scottish counterparts.

Both the quantity and type of fats in the diet have come under scrutiny. The increased consumption of butter and foods fried in animal fat are now causing concern on health grounds. Emphasis is being placed on the substitution of saturated fat by polyunsaturated, consequently the replacing of butter with polyunsaturated spreads is recommended.

To summarise, during the early decades of the twentieth century nutritional standards rose, albeit slowly, so that by the time of the national nutritional survey of 1948–52 a marked change in the balance of the diet was evident. Good protein intakes were maintained, the contribution of carbohydrate foods to the energy value declined, fats increasing their role as an energy provider. Calcium and iron levels too were upheld at a satisfactory level. The change from self-sufficiency in food to purchased food initially marked a deterioration in nutritional standards. The tide turned with improved living standards and healthy eating programmes,[46] instigated to eradicate tuberculosis early in the twentieth century (See Table 7).

*Table 7:* Nutritional Analysis of Irish Labourers' Diets 1839–1959

|  | Protein (g) | Fat (g) | Carbo-hydrate (g) | Energy Value (kcal) | (MJ) | Calcium (mg) | Iron (mg) |
|---|---|---|---|---|---|---|---|
| 1839 | 113 | 13 | 1069 | 4600 | 19 | 1660 | 25.0 |
| 1904 | 83 | 59 | 613 | 3194 | 13 | 754 | 20.0 |
| 1946/8 | 84 | 78 | 428 | 2745 | 12 | 1128 | 17.2 |
| 1989 | 100 | 128 | 409 | 3134 | 13 | 1233 | 13.5 |

Calculated from surveys referred to in Table 4.

## Health

According to George Russell in 1913 the Irish were making the wrong dietary choices to enjoy good health.

There is no doubt that the vitality of the Irish people has seriously diminished, and that the change has come about with a change in the character of the food consumed. When people lived with porridge, brown bread and milk as main ingredients in the diet, the vitality and energy of our people were noticeable, though they were much poorer than they are now. With increasing prosperity . . . we have grown much poorer if our standards are biological and not financial. When one looks at an Irish crowd one could almost tell the diet of most of them. These anaemic girls have tea running in their veins instead of blood. Those weakly looking boys have been fed on white bread. The new is more expensive then the old. We not only pay more for it in cash, but we pay more for it in sickness, in loss of vitality and of pleasures in life, and capacity for work.[47]

Russell's comment on the deleterious effect on the nation's health of the Irish diet was perceptive. The temptations of the highly prized tea, sugar, and baker's bread, enticed the population from the more healthy potatoes and dairy products. Direct indicators of health in the pre-Famine period are few. However, the fact that the Irish achieved high fertility rates before the Famine suggest a healthy population. As nutritional standards fell after 1850 standards of health declined. For example, deaths from tuberculosis increased at the very time when tuberculosis deaths in England and Scotland were declining.

*Table 8:* Deaths registered from Pulmonary Thrombosis in Ireland (1864–1905)

Rate per 100,000 of the population

| 1864 | – | 177 | 1880 | – | 214 | 1895 | – | 212 |
|------|---|-----|------|---|-----|------|---|-----|
| 1870 | – | 185 | 1885 | – | 219 | 1900 | – | 225 |
| 1875 | – | 193 | 1890 | – | 217 | 1905 | – | 206 |

*Source:* *Annual Reports of the Registrar General*, (Ireland)

Both historical and epidemiological evidence supports the clinical view that nutritional status is of importance in tuberculosis,[48] and modern research has demonstrated the decisive role played by nutritional improvements in increasing resistance to all infectious diseases.[49] It is not surprising, therefore, that the mortality rate from tuberculosis rose between 1860 and 1900. Among the urban poor mortality from the disease was exceptionally high. In 1908 mortality in Dublin was 3.4 per 1,000, whereas in rural County Mayo the rate was only 1.4.[50] As T.J. Stafford, Medical Commissioner to the Local Government Board, pointed out 'the poverty which exists in . . . [Dublin and Mayo] is essentially different in its circumstances, but for scantiness of the means of subsistence . . . the inhabitants of County Mayo could scarcely be surpassed.'[51] Stafford, therefore deduced 'that poverty and bad housing, . . . [did] not . . . account for the excessive [death] rate from tuberculoses.'[52] Although poor living conditions prevailed in Mayo, nutritional standards were higher than those of the Dublin poor.[53] Access to more home produced foods in Mayo resulted in superior dietary standard. For example, the mean protein content of rural labourers' diets was almost 20 per cent higher than those consumed by Dublin workers, and 30 per cent greater in energy value.[54]

There are some grounds for believing though, that as Ireland increasingly enjoyed the wealth of its neighbours so it gathered its share of the nutritional ills of affluence. In Ireland today cardiovascular disease is a major killer (see Figures 1a & 1b). While females' death rates started to decline in the 1950s, nevertheless, compared with other developed countries they are still high. Male mortality rates peaked during the 1970s and early 1980s and despite a slow decrease they still rank high by international standards. Furthermore, Northern Ireland is at the top of the world league with a male mortality rate of almost 900/100,000 in the mid 1980s for the 55–64 year olds.[55] A number of risk factors have been identified,[56] in particular a high intake of saturated fat. Has the liking for butter, discernible from 1900, and maintained at a high level throughout the century, left a legacy to the present generation of heart disease? The Irish habit of spreading bread liberally with butter, adding butter to boiled potatoes and other vegetables, and preferring frying to other cooking methods have been identified by nutritionists as particularly injurious to health, increasing the risk of heart disease, and so should be discouraged.[57] One of the objectives, therefore, of health promotion programmes has been to encourage a reduction in fat intake, and recommend the use of polyunsaturated fats.

This paper is merely an overview of the changes in food retailing, food consumption patterns, nutritional standards and health in Ireland over the nineteenth and twentieth centuries. The expansion of grocery shops during the second half of the nineteenth century brought a diversification of diet, but also a decline in nutritional standards and health. In the second half of the twentieth century food retailers, while providing an ever increasing variety of products, have made little contribution to improved nutritional standards. Promotions on healthy eating figure infrequently within their marketing strategy. Research in Northern Ireland has revealed that retailers view healthy eating as being potentially in conflict with their business objectives.[58] There is a danger, therefore, in the late twentieth century, as in the late nineteenth, that nutritional standards could fall again as consumer choice expands, unless health promotion programmes succeed. Lord Trenchard has pointed out 'that people are very conservative about their eating habits, change only very slowly, and mainly for reasons other than either nutritional beliefs or the power of . . . marketing.'[59] The problem is, of course, that 'people do not shop for nutrients, they shop for food'.[60]

## Notes

1  Lee (1973), p. 1.
2  Vaughan and Fitzpatrick (1978).
3  *Report . . . on the Wages* (1870), p. 11.
4  *Thirteenth Annual Report* (1860), p. 60.
5  Clark (1979), pp. 125–6.
6  Kennedy (1978), p. 61; see also, Kennedy (1979), p. 202; Daly (1981), p. 107.
7  Kennedy (1979), p. 202.

Fig. 1(a)  **Deaths from Ischaemic Heart Disease**
Eire 1960–1990

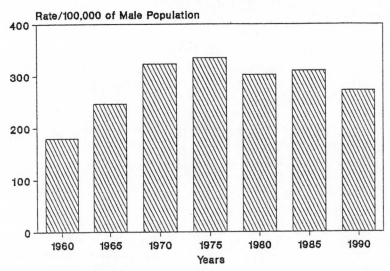

Source: Reports on Vital Statistics

Fig. 1(b)  **Deaths from Ischaemic Heart Disease**
Northern Ireland 1960–1990

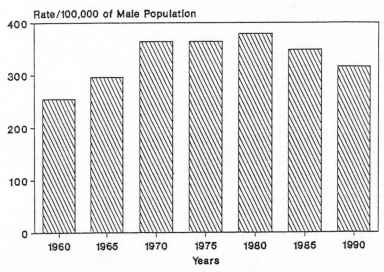

Source: Reports of Registrar General N.I

8  Kennedy (1979), p. 204; Clark (1979), pp. 130–2; Daly (1981), p. 108.

9  Daly (1981), p. 108.

10  Duncan (1939–40), pp. 1–16.

11  Johnson (1985), p. 45.

12  Parker (1989), p. 239.

13  Nutrition Surveillance in Ireland (1993), p 81.

14  *Census of Distribution 1956–9* (1962); *Census of Distribution and Services 1966, 1969, 1970–1*; *Census of Distribution 1971* (1975–7); *Census of Distribution 1977* (1982–3); *Census of Services 1988* (1991).

15  *Report on the Census of Distribution (Northern Ireland)*, 1965 (1969); *Report on the Census of Distribution (Northern Ireland)*, 1975 (1979).

16  O'Rourke and DeLoach (1967), p. 10.

17  O'Rourke and DeLoach (1967), p. 10.

18  O'Rourke and DeLoach (1967), p. 2.

19  Nutrition Surveillance in Ireland (1993), p. 80–1.

20  Lee and Gibney (1989), p. 17.

21  *Research on Nutrition in Northern Ireland* (1993).

22  *Sixth Annual Report* (1840); *Sixth Report of the Medical Officer* (1863); *Thirteenth Annual Report* (1860); *Second Report by Mr Wilson Fox* (1905); *Second Series of Memoranda* (1905); *National Nutrition Survey* (1950); Barker, *et al.* (1988); Lee, and Gibney, (1989).

23  Crawford (1981), pp. 113–131.

24  *Thirteenth Annual Report* (1860), p. 52.

25  *Thirteenth Annual Report* (1860), p. 52.

26  *Royal Commission on Agriculture* (1881), pp. 129–30, Q.3141.

27  *Report . . . on Industries (Ireland)* (1884–5), p. 362. Q. 6612.

28  *Inspectors' Local Reports (Base-line Reports)* (1898), p. 177.

29  Calculated from the *Thirteenth Annual Report* (1860); *Sixth Report of the Medical Officer* (1864); Lumsden (1905); *Royal Commission* (1910): *Second Report by Wilson Fox* (1905).

30  Household Budget Inquiry 1951–2 (1954), p. 113.

31  *Thirteenth Annual Report* (1860); *Sixth Report of the Medical Officer* (1864); Lumsden (1905); *Royal Commission* (1910); *Second Report by Wilson Fox* (1905); *Second Series of Memoranda . . .* (1905); Lee (1989).

32  Hancock (1863), p. 78.

33  *Report . . . on Industries Ireland* (1884–5), p. 362, Q. 6612.

34  *Thirteenth Annual Report* (1860); Lumsden (1905); *Royal Commission* (1910); *Household Budget Survey Eire* (1954); Lee (1989).

35  This calculation is based on the diets of both urban and rural labourers in 1904.

36  *Thirteenth Annual Report* (1860); *Second Series of Memoranda . . .* (1905); *Second Report by Wilson Fox* (1905); Lumsden (1905); *Royal Commission* (1910); *Household Budget Inquiry* (1954).

37  *Thirteenth Annual Report* (1860); *Second Report by Wilson Fox* (1905);

*Second Series of Memoranda* . . . (1905); *Household Budget Survey*
(1954); Lee (1989).
38  Johnson (1985), p. 40.
39  Meenan (1970), p. 101.
40  O'Rourke and DeLoach (1967), p. 2.
41  Halpin and Harrington (1992), p. 43.
42  Barker, *et al.* (1988), p. 61.
43  Crawford (1984), pp 250–252.
44  Crawford (1984), pp 235–6.
45  Cameron (1885), p. 432.
46  Aberdeen (1908).
47  Russell (1913).
48  Dubois (1953) p. 140; Livi-Bacci (1990), p. 38.
49  McKeown (1977), pp. 138–9; Brown, Brown and Record (1972), pp. 355–
357.
50  *Royal Commission* (1910), p. 247.
51  *Royal Commission* (1910), p. 247.
52  *Royal Commission* (1910), p. 247.
53  Crawford (1984), p. 331.
54  Crawford (1984), p. 331.
55  Barker (1988), p 4.
56  *Research on Nutrition in Northern Ireland* (1993).
57  Lee and Gibney (1989), p. 81.
58  *Research on Nutrition in Northern Ireland* (1993), paragraph 6.3.2.
59  Trenchard (1978), p. 225.
60  Lee and Gibney (1989), p. 3.

**Literature**

Aberdeen, Ishbel, ed. *Ireland's Crusade Against Tuberculosis*, 3 vols (Dublin,
1908)
Barker, M.E., S.I. McClean, P.G. McKenna, N.G. Reid, J.J. Strain, K.A.
Thompson, A.P. Williamson, M.E. Wright, *Diet, Lifestyle and Health in
Northern Ireland* (Coleraine, 1988).
Brown, T., and R.G. Brown & R.G. Record, 'An Interpretation of the
Modern Rise of Population in Europe'. *Population Studies*, 26 (1972).
Cameron, Charles 'How the Dublin Poor Live'. *Eastward Ho*, vol. 3 (1885).
*Census of Distribution 1956–9*, Central Statistics Office (Dublin, 1962).
*Census of Distribution 1971*, Central Statistics Office (Dublin 1975–7).
*Census of Distribution 1977*, Central Statistics Office (Dublin 1982–3).
*Census of Distribution and Services 1966*, Central Statistics Office (Dublin,
1969, 1970–1).
*Census of Ireland, 1861*, part iv, British Parliamentary Papers 1863[3204–
III]LIX.

*Census of Ireland, 1871*, part i, vol i, British Parliamentary Papers 1872[C662–I to XIII]LXVII; vol ii, 1873[C873–I to IV]LXXXII; vol iii, 1874[C964–I to X]LXXIV; vol iv, 1874[C1106–I to VII]LXXIV.

*Census of Ireland, 1881*, part i, vol i, British Parliamentary Papers 1881[c3042]XCVII; vol ii, 1882[C3148]1 XXVII, vol iii, 1882[C3204] 1 xxviii; vol iv, 1882[C3268]LXXIX.

*Census of Ireland, 1891*, part i, vol i, British Parliamentary Paper 1890–1[C6515]XCV; vol ii, 1892[C6567]XCI; vol iii, 1892[C6626]XCII; vol iv, 1892[C6685]XCIII.

*Census of Ireland, 1901*, part i, vol i, British Parliamentary Papers 1902[Cd 847]CXXII; vol ii, 1902[Cd 1058]CXXIV; vol iii, 1902[Cd 1123]CXXVI; vol iv, 1902[Cd 1059]CXXVIII.

*Census of Ireland, 1911*, part i, vol i, British Parliamentary Papers 1912–13[Cd 6049]CXIV; vol ii, 1912–13[Cd 6050]CXV; vol iii, 1912–13[Cd 6051]CXV; vol iv, 1912–13[Cd 6052]CXVII.

*Census of Population 1926*, vol ii (Dublin, 1928).

*Census of Population 1936*, vol ii (Dublin, 1938).

*Census of Population 1946*, vol ii (Dublin, 1953).

*Census of Services, 1988*, Central Statistics Office (Dublin, 1991).

Clark, Samuel *Social Origins of the Irish Land War* (Princeton, 1979).

Crawford, E. Margaret, 'Indian Meal and Pellagra in Nineteenth Century Ireland', in J.M. Goldstrom & L.A. Clarkson, eds *Irish Population, Economy and Society*: Essays in Honour of the Late K.H. Connell (Oxford, 1981).

Crawford, E. Margaret, 'Aspects of Irish Diet 1839–1904' Ph.D. Thesis, University of London (1984).

Daly, Mary, *Social and Economic History of Ireland Since 1800* (Dublin, 1981).

Dubois, Rene & Jean, *The White Plague* (London, 1953).

Duncan, G.A. 'The Social Income of the Irish Free State'. *Journal of Statistical & Social Inquiry Society of Ireland* (1939–40).

Halpin P., and E. Harrington, 'The Retail Sector 1980–1991'. *Irish Banking Review*, (1992).

Hancock, W.N., *Report of the Supposed Progressive Decline in Irish Prosperity*, (Dublin, 1863).

*Household Budget Inquiry 1951–2*, Central Statistics Office (Dublin, 1954).

*Inspectors' Local Reports (Base-line Reports) 1892–8*, complied by the Congested Districts Board (Dublin, 1898).

Johnson, David, *The Interwar Economy in Ireland*, (Dublin, 1985).

Kennedy, Liam, 'Retail Markets in Rural Ireland at the End of the Nineteenth Century', *Irish Economic and Social History*, v (1978).

Kennedy, Liam, 'Traders in the Irish Rural Economy, 1880–1914', *Economic History Review*, Second Series, XXXII, No. 2 (1979).

Lee, Joseph, *Modernization of Irish Society* (Dublin 1973).

Lee, Pauline, and M. Gibney, *Patterns of Food and Nutrient Intake in a*

*Suburb of Dublin with Chronically High Unemployment*, Research Report Series, Combat Poverty Series (Dublin, 1989).

Livi-Bacci, M. *Population and Nutrition: An Essay on European Demographic History* (Cambridge, 1990).

Lumsden, J. *An Investigation into the Income and Expenditure of Seventeenth Century Brewery Families and a Study of their Diet* (Edinburgh, 1905).

McKeown, T., *The Modern Rise of Population* (London, 1977).

Meenan, James, *The Irish Economy since 1922* (Liverpool, 1970).

*National Nutrition Survey*, Part I (Dublin, 1948), Parts II-IV (Dublin, 1949), Parts V-VI (Dublin, 1950), Part VII (Dublin, 1952).

*Nutritional Surveillance in Ireland 1993*, National Nutritional Surveillance Centre, University College Galway (Galway, 1993)

O'Rourke. A.D., and D.B. DeLoach, *Survival: Group Action in the Wholesale and Retail Grocery Trade* (Dublin, 1967).

Parker A.J., 'The Changing Nature of Irish Retailing', in R.W.G. Carter and A.J. Parker (eds), *Ireland: A Contemporary Geographical Perspective* (London, 1989).

*Report from Poor Law Inspectors on the Wages of Agricultural Labourers in Ireland*, British Parliamentary Papers 1870 [c.35]XIV.

*Report from the Select Committee on Industries (Ireland)*, British Parliamentary Papers 1884–5 [288] IX.

*Report on the Census of Distribution and Other Services of Northern Ireland*, 1965 (Belfast, 1969).

*Report on the Census of Distribution and Other Services of Northern Ireland, 1975* (Belfast, 1979).

*Research on Nutrition in Northern Ireland*, Health Promotion Agency for Northern Ireland, Agenda Item 6, Paper HPA 3/93 (1993).

*Retailing in Northern Ireland*, – Northern Ireland Economic Council, Report 83 (1990)

*Royal Commission on Agriculture*, British Parliamentary Papers 1881 [c.2778-I] XV.

*Royal Commission on the Poor Laws and Relief of Distress*, British Parliamentary Papers 1910 [Cd 5070] L, Appendix, Volume X, Appendix No. II(D), T.J. Stafford's report is dated 1908 'Notes on the Social Condition of Certain Working Class Families in Dublin'.

Russell, George, [AE], *Irish Homestead*, 20 September 1913.

*Second Report by Mr Wilson Fox on the Wages, Earnings and Conditions of Employment of Agricultural Labourers in the United Kingdom*, British Parliamentary Papers 1905 [Cd. 2376] XCVII, [Rural dietary survey 1904].

*Second Series of Memoranda, Statistical Tables, and Charts prepared in the Board of Trade* which includes 'Consumption and Cost of Food in Workmen's Families in Urban Districts in the United Kingdom' British Parliamentary Papers 1905 [Cd. 2337] LXXXIV, [Urban Dietary Survey 1904].

*Sixth Annual Report of the Poor Law Commissioners*, Appendix (D), No. 22, 'Report on Workhouse Dietaries, British Parliamentary Papers 1840 (245) XVII, [Hawley Survey].

*Sixth Report of the Medical Officer of the Privy Council*, 1863 Appendix No. 6 Food of the Lowest Fed Classes by Dr E. Smith, British Parliamentary Papers 1864 [3416] XXVIII.

*Thirteenth Annual Report of the Commissioners for Administering the Laws for Relief of the Poor in Ireland*, Appendix (A), 'Report on the Subject of Workhouse Dietaries and the Dietary of the Labouring Poor in Ireland', British Parliamentary Papers 1860 (2654) XXXVII.

Trenchard, Lord, 'The Inter-Relationship of marketing and Nutrition' in John Yudkin, *Diet of Man: Needs and Wants* (London, 1978)

Vaughan, W.E. and A.J. Fitzpatrick, [eds], *Irish Historical Statistics, Population 1821–1971* (Dublin, 1978).

# 18

# A RETAIL SYSTEM IN RURAL LORRAINE: ITINERANT FOOD TRADE, 1865–1991

## Claude Thouvenot

The aim of this paper is to give insight into the development of a special retail system, the itinerant food trade. It deals with retailers travelling from one village to another, selling bread, meat and *charcuterie*, dairy products, grocery and non-perishable foodstuffs, fruits and vegetables, fish etc. It is not concerned with the travelling retailers selling their goods on markets in towns or villages.

This food retail system does not only exist in Lorraine. It did exist in the past and still exists in France and Europe. Researchers reported its existence in Germany, Scandinavia and Eastern Europe countries before and after they were ruled by communist regimes. Some emigration and extreme poverty areas in Spain or Italy mountains seem not to have known this retail system.

### The setting up of a new retail system (1865–1914)

The countryside in Lorraine as in other areas has been for centuries a food supply source for more and less rich urban people, lords and other notables living in castles and boroughs. Food collectors sometimes travel great distances to reach the most remote places. Bartering mostly enables people to get some condiments like salt, oil or vinegar. People live on subsistence farming for the other foodstuffs they need[1]. Changes occurred in the nineteenth century: the rising new industry as well as the growing urbanization have consequences for the rural population, especially people living near to towns. The economic system progressively changes and is more and more based on money, while people who did not emigrate are relatively well-off.

One may say rural areas became markets 'to be conquered'. New 'characters', the itinerant food retailers, came forth on a small scale and, at the beginning, for a limited clientele.

From 1865–1870 onward, first near to villages where the new industry sets up, the activity of itinerant retailers intensifies: bakers, butchers on days before feasts; some grocers supplying oil, sugar bars, pepper and coffee; herring sellers as soon as cold weather begins.

Those small-sized retailers are prosperous on a small scale and respected in a town or a borough, sometimes in little villages. The wife keeps up the shop, the husband travels around from village to village to get more money.

From around the 1870s–1880s a round bread is not baked at home in Lorraine country as often as before and the baker's activity increases. He is often at the same time grocer, *café*-owner and even farmer. He goes from village to village, at first carrying a wooden basket on his back or his arm, receives requests from customers and delivers every week ordered foodstuffs. The best customers are farm labourers who have no oven at their disposal, rural artisans and of course notables. As business is expanding, he uses a dog cart, then a horse-drawn cart. Sometimes a person ready to make it for him sells his bread[2, 3].

The butcher's clientele is more limited. Only at the end of the century does he regularly travel to villages and has not many customers. He comes every Friday for those who make 'orders': the *curé*, the *châtelain* ('lord'), the mayor, some notables, sometimes the schoolmaster or any one who has a guest the following Sunday[4]. In most villages the butcher only takes orders on days before the village's feast. He begins to come regularly on Saturdays and Sundays at the end of the century in villages where new activities are set up (coalmines, textile mills, iron works). The butcher, just like the baker does, walks at the beginning with a wooden basket on his back, then he travels on horse back. He buys a horse-drawn cart for travelling to several villages. The meat sold is mostly beef – all pieces at the same price – to prepare *pot-au-feu*, beef soup, more and more eaten by well-off people on Sundays. Towards the 1860s–1870s more humble people are used to eat *pot-au-feu* weddings and religious feasts or family at ceremonies[5].

A long time before 1914 the '*Planteur de Caïffa*' is an excellent example for the itinerant retailer. He travels in other regions than Lorraine, starting from town shops. His little three-wheeler drawn by one or two dogs comes to villages on fixed dates and almost fixed hours. His reputation is mainly due to the excellent coffee he sells. He also sells sardines in tins, noodles, biscuits, chocolate, instant puddings, oil, vinegar, pepper . . . The stock of his one-metre high cart depends on customers' requests, always the same, and he is rarely mistaken. He knows who needs one litre oil within two weeks, who is very keen on coffee or is able to eat three chocolate bars within a week.

The clientele of all those itinerant retailers is regular and foreseeable. As 'Caïffa' does it, the baker plans for example that farmers purchase bread on Sundays as a delicacy.

A food retail system is being set up, meeting wishes and the needs of a clientele, at first scattered and limited, not very hard to please, except for those '*heureux du siècle*' (the rich). The clientele becomes larger with time and is tempted by the new foodstuffs proposed.

## Intensification of Itinerant Food Trade (1920–1960)

The intensification of the itinerant food trade in Lorraine countryside starts after World War I. It is due to two main associated phenomena: retail merchants are travelling by motor car, and some changes occur in the everyday life of many customers.

It is not known how many bakers, butchers or grocers bought vans left by the French and U.S. Armed Forces in our regions located near to the armed conflict or devastated by the war. Those retailers who converted them into delivery vans were able to visit more villages and supply more customers.

The development of the travelling food trade between World War I and World War II is both a cause and a consequence of the progress in rural areas, of changes in farmers' living conditions. Their life style changed, their needs grew and diversified. Their activities consisted at the beginning essentially in mixed farming, but they are now more and more specialized: single-crop farming or setting-up of local industries which gradually reduce subsistence farming. The history of the itinerant food trade between World War I and II is not the same for every commune and several factors give reasons for its presence or absence in a commune, its appearance or disappearance, its growth or decrease.

The itinerant trade activity depends especially on the existence or absence of any local resident shop. The rise or disappearance of any retail merchant in one or another activity may lead to a rise or disappearance of a travelling retail merchant of the same activity. The change in size of the commune is also important. A small country commune which is growing after the setting up of an industry on its territory cannot have only the usual itinerant retail merchants at its disposal. Resident retail merchants set up and replace the former itinerant trade.

The preservation, development or dying out of itinerant trade activity depends also – maybe essentially – on the dynamism of merchants, their know-how and punctuality but also on the population to be supplied, its size, its needs and requests. Several reasons for retail merchants to travel from one village to another exist. First they want to raise their turn-over, but also to replace another retailer or to sell more rapidly perishable goods[6].

A survey made in rural Lorraine in the year 1961 makes it possible to define precisely the itinerant food trade after World War II.

From this time onward the distinction between baker, butcher-*charcutier*, grocer, greengrocer, fishmonger begins to disappear. At the beginning retail merchants were specialized, then they sell more and more foodstuffs offered by other retailers. For example bakers sell pastries, confectionery, some '*petite épicerie*' (grocery) foodstuffs. Butchers sell poultry, rabbits, eggs, canned foods. Greengrocers sell fish and vice-versa, according to the season. But every retailer keeps his main activity so that it is still possible to classify them.

Statistical information has been collected to make maps showing how the various types of itinerant retail merchants 'radiate' in countryside communes of the four Lorraine *départements*: Meurthe-et-Moselle, Meuse, Moselle, and Vosges (map no. 1: North-East France).

Some map examples follow. They do represent areas of trade influence for some types of retailers but no real types of itineraries of these retailers[7].

Bakers and baker-grocers generally set up in little communes travel to two or three villages located near to their shop, every day or every second day or at least three times a week. Some other non-visited villages have no itinerant but only resident bakers (map no. 2).

The key is the same for all maps:

Size of centres (where itinerant retailers start from)

| | |
|---|---|
| ● | less than 250 inh. |
| ■ | from 250 to 500 inh. |
| ○ | from 501 to 1000 inh. |
| □ | from 1001 to 2500 inh. |
| ● | from 2501 to 5000 inh. |
| ■ | from 5001 to 10,000 inh. |
| ⊙ | more than 10,000 inh. |
| ○ | village 'visited' by retailers |

Butchers-*charcutiers* mostly come from boroughs and little towns. They used to come once or twice a week, preferably on Wednesdays, Saturdays, or on Sundays mornings. Sometimes several butchers start from the same place to the same commune. As for bakers, this itinerant trade type is a 'proximity' trade. The retail merchant rarely travels more than 20 kilometres a day (map n°3).

Itineraries of independent grocers (40 per cent) are mostly complicated, showing a strong competition between retail merchants, sometimes four to five, travelling once or twice a week, sometimes four or five times even if the village has one or more resident retail merchants.

'Chain-store' grocers[8] – representing 60 per cent- start from middle-sized communes (700–3000 inhabitants). They have a larger selection of goods than grocers working on their own account, offer prices and free gifts, and pose a serious threat to independent grocers who cannot keep up with them. Maps carried out for independent and chain-stores grocers are not shown in this paper but do exist.

Greengrocers (fruit and vegetables) and fishmongers – mostly in winter – come from the town but are also present in smaller villages. They travel once a week, mostly on Thursdays, and in winter especially on Fridays, to sell seafish. Herring was still the most sold fish in the 1960s in Lorraine country. Mullet and whiting are also sold as well as mussels and oysters, especially for Christmas and New Year's Eve (map no. 4).

MAP Nº 1

LOCATING MAP NORTH-EAST FRANCE

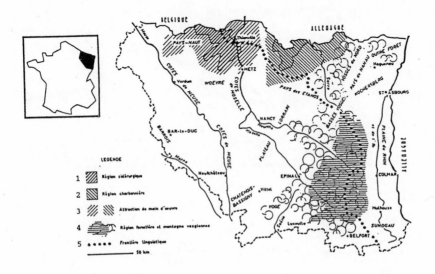

1 - iron and steel industry area

2 - coal industry area

3 - labour attraction area

4 - Vosges forest and mountain area

5 - linguistic boundary

MAP N° 2

BAKERS RADIATING FROM SEVERAL COMMUNES
in Bar-le-Duc area (Meuse)

1961

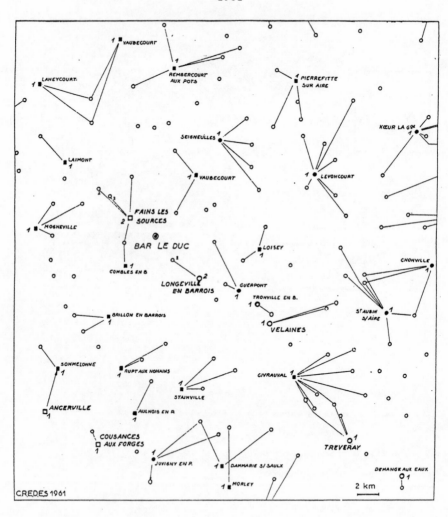

CREDES 1961

2 km

244

MAP N° 3

BUTCHERS - *CHARCUTIERS* RADIATING FROM SEVERAL
COMMUNES
in Stenay-Montmedy area (Meuse)

1961

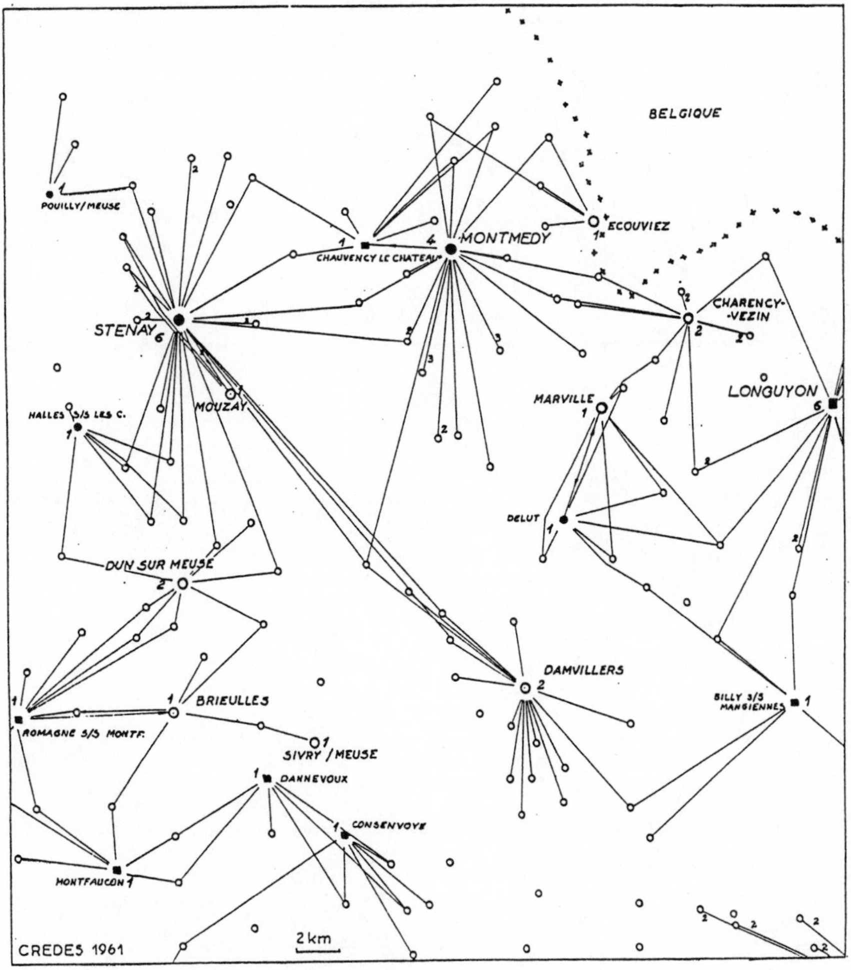

MAP Nº 4

FISHMONGERS RADIATING FROM SEVERAL COMMUNES
in Vaucouleurs area (Meuse)

1961

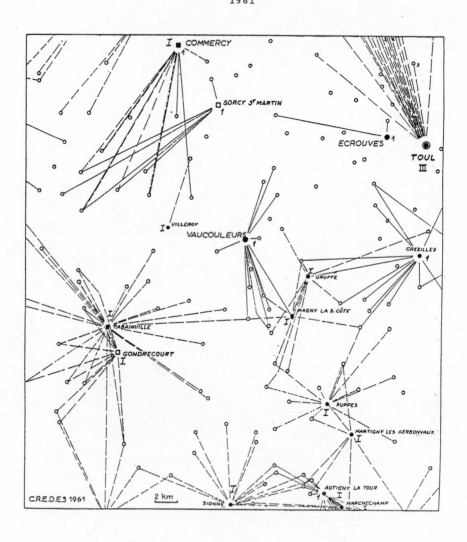

246

Grocers, greengrocers and fishmongers cover greater distances, sometimes up to 50 kilometres a day, and even more.

The clientele essentially consists of farmers and workers. The demand is well defined and regular: bread, meat, grocery foodstuffs, fruit and vegetables (especially early fruits and vegetables) because seasonal subsistence farming is still alive, except for a few oranges and bananas, symbols of a recent exoticism.

This clientele changes as the standard of living improves and people wish a better existence after hard war deprivations. It is now more hard to please as far as quality is concerned. Nevertheless the clientele does not question very much, and is compelled to buy the foodstuffs offered by the only retailer travelling to their village. In the next period the situation is going to change completely.

## Decline and disappearance of traditional retail merchants (1961–1991)

A survey carried out in 1991 in the Lorraine département, 'Meuse', which remains for the most part a rural area, enables us to show the changes that occurred since the beginning of the 1960s.

Bakers who sell not only bread but also pastries, 'general food' foodstuffs (former grocery products) are travelling more and more, as resident bakers closed their shops. Map no. 5 carried out in 1991 looks like the one made in 1961 (see map no. 2).

In fact business is not as financially viable as before. Modern vehicles are expensive, the employment of a person costs much money. The selling of pastries, especially on Sundays, partly balances the costs but it takes time to travel from one village to another and the profit is low. Competition with factory-baked and deep-frozen bread is not very hard, at least in 1991 and in a region which remains very rural.

Butchers-*charcutiers* are still travelling, and even more than in 1961 in some areas (see map no 3). They are declining if compared with the times when the quantity of regular customers was more important. Only elderly people buy regularly, and young people are mostly occasional customers on Sundays, when they have some guests and want high-quality meat. The quantity of customers decreases sometimes down to only three or four regular customers in each village, and the butcher is compelled to travel in a greater number of villages as he sells less meat; a butcher who sold two 'animals' ten years ago sells now only one half.

Seafishmongers are still travelling. They are spreading out to the same extent as in 1961. A great number of customers want to eat fresh fish and sea food. Fishmongers sell fresh products and they come on Wednesdays and Fridays (survival from the past of an almost forgotten religious practice), they are in a good position to compete with new stores or suppliers of 'chain-stores' for deep-frozen fish.

MAP Nº 5

BAKERS RADIATING FROM SEVERAL VILLAGES
in Bar-le-Duc area

1991

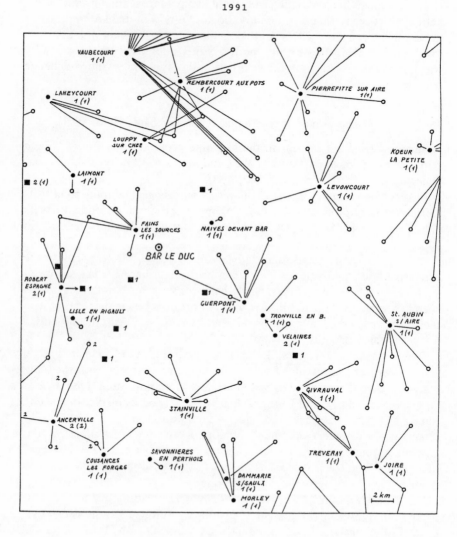

MAP N° 6

FISHMONGERS RADIATING FROM SEVERAL COMMUNES
in Stenay-Brandeville area (Meuse)

1991

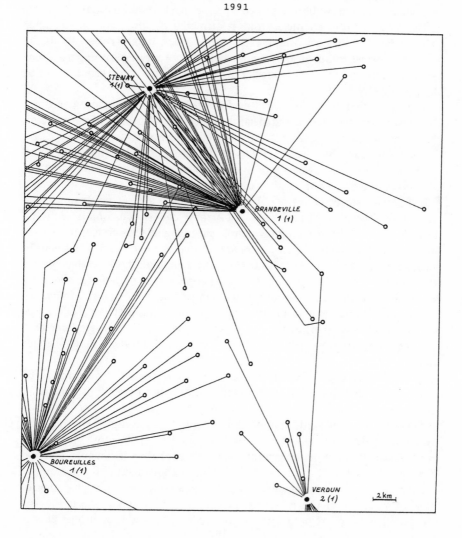

As in the past, some itinerant retail merchants sell, from the beginning of May to mid-August, fruit and vegetables instead of sea products. Others sell only fish, or both during summer months as the cooling equipment makes it possible (see map no 6).

The travelling trade of independent grocers nearly totally disappears. 'Chain-store' grocers who triumphed once over small country grocers thirty years ago, almost disappear, sometimes very suddenly after the 'collapse' of parent companies which have been replaced by supermarkets and hypermarkets.

The main country clientele today is attracted by itinerant long-distance modern retail modes for deep-frozen and non-perishable grocery foods for various reasons: frequent and regular delivery, orders on catalogues, competitive prices, advertisment, special offers . . . Where is the grocer's van of the former days?

The new living conditions existing from the years 1965–1970 onward are the reason for the decline and disappearance of traditional itinerant retail merchants a hundred years after their first appearance in Lorraine.

The motor car which was useful to retail merchants between the First and the Second World Wars develops in the country and leads a greater number of people, especially young people, to travel.

Self-service stores (*supermarchés, hypermarchés*) are set up around 1965 and change the purchasing habits of Lorraine country customers. Between 1970 and 1980 in France country people shopping in self-service stores rises from 10 to 30 per cent. These stores are located at the outskirts of towns in huge shopping centres. Whereas town retail merchants came to the country at the beginning of the century, the rural people are now going for shopping to the outskirts of towns. No countryman in Lorraine or elsewhere in France has to travel more than 30 kilometres to go for shopping to the self-service stores. He may go on his own or be driven by someone for enjoying immense diversity, attractive prices, animation. Even coach services to self-service stores exist . . .[9]

In the last ten years, TV brings rural areas even closer to 'town lights', by means of advertising. It changes, often without that being conscious of it, their needs and wishes.

The itinerant food trade, a more or less compulsory complement to a local 'resident' trade, is dying out or is even totally dead. It has lost much of its importance in the Lorraine rural area and probably the whole of rural France. The new food retail systems seriously challenge the former ones.

Both causes and consequences of new living conditions: the customer of itinerant retail merchants is not the same as sixty years ago. It was in the past regular, it is now irregular, even evanescent. Only the fourth age, elderly people, who cannot go for shopping to these stores see the itinerant retailer as a 'company and a security'. He services those who usually go for shopping outside, such as young farmers, and new countrymen who have left the town. The itinerant merchant also services a more and more growing number of pensioners, people having a second home or coming for week-ends or even holidays, holiday-makers eager for walks, calm, greenery and sometimes good 'farmhouse' products and dishes . . .

The successors of these retail merchants who started the conquest of the rural food market a hundred years ago are now pessimistic, resigned, even angry. Most women are sullen and give up first[10].

Retail merchants lost most of their former clientele and seem to lead a kind of 'rearguard fighting'. The market is not fast-expanding any more. They have lost the status and the role they had in the past in rural communities opening to the 'market'. They feel it in a confused way and some of them say it straight out. Their trade patrimony, both 'resident' and 'itinerant', which they have been working a life time for, has no value any more. It is going to die with them and they will not hand it over to their children, who do not want it any more. This situation is probably the hardest one for some French minds.

## Notes

1  Thouvenot (1975) pp. 378–387.
2  Thouvenot (1969) pp. 16–19.
3  Thouvenot (1987) pp. 23–35.
4  Cressot (1952) pp. 45–50.
5  Thouvenot (1971) pp. 289–300.
6  Clerc-Péchiné (1963) pp. 15–31.
7  Clerc-Péchiné (1963) pp. 121–130. Three types of real itineraries do exist:

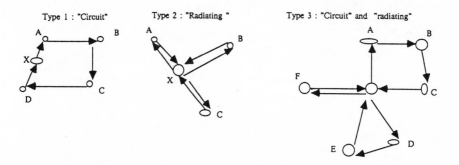

8  Clerc-Péchiné (1963) pp. 64–70. 'Chain-store' grocers: i.e. managers of independent stores owned by cooperative or non-cooperative chain-stores were well-known in Lorraine and even in France after the Second World War: *Coopérateur de Lorraine, Sanal, Eco, Familistère*, etc.
9  Pottier (1974) pp. 36–38.
10  Gérard (1991) pp. 7–9.

## Literature

Clerc-Pechiné, Nicole, *Essai sur le rayonnement commercial. Les tournées de commerçants en Lorraine*, Faculté de Droit et des Sciences Economiques, CREDES, (Nancy, *1963*).

Cressot, Joseph, *Le pain au lièvre, Souvenirs d'enfance*, Le Républicain Lorrain, (Metz, 1952).

Gérard, Claude, 'L'inéluctable (et douloureuse) évolution du commerce au village' *Villages Lorrains*, no. 54, (Nancy, 1991), pp. 3–9.

Ministère du Commerce, de l'Artisanat et des Services, in '*Le commerce en milieu rural 1976–1985, dix années d'intervention des pouvoirs public*', Direction du Commerce intérieur, (Paris, 1987).

Pottier, Micheline, 'Présentation d'une série d'enquêtes sur les magasins à grande surface en Lorraine'. *Bulletin de l'Association des Géographes Français*, no 413–414, (Paris, 1974), pp. 36–45.

Thouvenot, Claude, 'Le pain paysan dans la France rurale de l'Est'. *Cahiers de Nutrition et de Diététique*, IV, 4, (Paris, 1969), pp. 16–23 and VI, 1, (Paris, 1970), pp. 18–20.

Thouvenot, Claude, 'La viande dans les campagnes lorraines'. *Annales de Géographie*, May-June 1971, (Paris, 1971), pp. 288–327.

Thouvenot, Claude. *Les consommations et les habitudes alimentaires dans la France du Nord-Est. Essai de géographie sociale*, Thèse de Doctorat d'Etat, (Paris, 1975).

Thouvenot, Claude. *Le pain d'autrefois, Chroniques alimentaires d'un monde qui s'en va*, Editions Leson (Paris, 1977), new edition: Presses Universitaires de Nancy, (Nancy, 1987).

# 19

# THE DEVELOPMENT OF PUBLIC DISTRUST OF MODERN FOOD TECHNOLOGY IN THE NETHERLANDS. PROFESSIONALS, LAYMEN AND THE CONSUMERS' UNION

*Anneke H. van Otterloo*

'Bad news for cannibals. Human meat is so polluted that one must be advised against its consumption[1]'.

The quotation above refers to a blood-curdling message from 1985 on the amount of CFCs found in the fat tissue of the average Dutch population. The DDT-rate among these substances is, the message continues, twice as high as is officially permitted for animal fat destined for human consumption. This type of information belongs to a multitude of similar communications which are a characteristic part of the contemporary news coverage in the media. Obviously the attention of the consumer public is regularly focused on information about alien substances in food that are deemed harmful. Producers, food experts or authorities of all kinds seem able to resort to appealing to this belief.

Public sensitivity and anxiety about the possibly detrimental consequences of the consumption of certain foodstuffs has probably increased considerably over recent years. These negative feelings do not primarily refer to those delicacies forbidden because of fears of becoming fat, though this is an important contemporary trend as well. Rather, food is blamed for allergic reactions, behavioural disturbances, cancer, poisoning and other life-endangering illnesses. This public distrust is intimately connected with a suspicion of the poor quality of the foodstuffs that are produced by modern technological methods. In view of a great many recently held symposia and newly issued publications, one can agree to the current existence of a fundamental and sometimes conflict-ridden societal debate on the topic of food safety[2].

From a historical and sociological point of view several questions can be posed. Which issues and parties are involved? Since when and how did this public worry rise and develop into its contemporary dimensions? How can one account for the peculiar fact that the lay public and professional experts differ sharply in the estimation of the dangers involved? A closer look at the socio-historical context of this phenomenon may offer some insights into the questions posed. In this article I will make a modest start with this project, considering present problems as a phase in a long-term process.

The theme of public distrust and food scares belongs to the category of lay belief systems about food and health. As such it has much ground in common with experiences and beliefs in the field of alternatively growing and eating, ideas of pregnant mothers about cravings and aversions and the views of vegetarians. Detailed historical and sociological studies on such lay outlooks until now are not abundant[3]. This is a reason to focus here on this subject by means of an analysis of the consumers' movement view in matters of food safety, on which more will be explained in a moment. Although the data presented will be largely restricted to the Netherlands, it is suggested that the phenomenon dealt with is common in other countries possessing advanced food industries, especially in Europe, the United States and Australia[4]. First the parties and opinions involved in the present debates on food quality are considered, following the trail back to comparable issues in the past. Next a study of a consumers' magazine will be discussed.

### The quality of food: a century of debates (1890–1990)

Nutritionists and other food experts have recently gained an important societal position in the Netherlands. They succeeded in initiating a state food policy of which the basic principles are embodied in a government memorandum issued in 1983, about a decade ago. This note, which is considered as an important document from a public health point of view, sets a framework for government measures concerning 1) provisions for a sound supply of foodstuffs, and 2) promotion of sound eating habits[5]. Instruments of policy consist of advice and consultation with the public in the second case and in the maintenance, extension and legislation regulating the production and distribution of foods in the first. The emergence of this document on food and nutrition policy or *Voedingsnota* is an indication of the rise of a societal discourse about food and of both the state's and the (food) scientists' involvement in it. Other examples are to be found in the present proliferation of multi-action committees and other lay organizations, dealing with the quality of food[6]. Food professionals in universities, business and trade or government institutions, have criticized lay views in the eighties and early nineties. Consumers' organizations in their turn have attacked both food industry and government. And an obvious fifth important party in the debate on food quality is the press[7].

According to many scientists present food problems mainly consist in the wrong estimation of the relative health-endangering risks of food choices and food safety by the consumer public. In their opinion, the Dutch simply eat too many fats, sweets and salts. The ordinary eater, however, is afraid first of all of alien substances in foodstuffs, for none of these escapes the grasp of technology today. In their eyes the production of food has been reduced to a frightening process of 'chemicalisation'[8]. For the experts in food safety, one has to distinguish the following substances: additives, chemical and microbial contaminants and natural toxicants. The distrust of the general public has recently been directed at additives, a cover concept for a great many substances used in the industrial production and processing of food. Among these are colourings, flavourings, preservatives and processing aids (emulsifiers, thickeners).

Toxicologists do not understand fears about this type of substances, because additives in particular are thoroughly tested before use. Moreover, the quantities present are so small that nowhere they do exceed anything like the margins of safety. Professionals maintain that the same is true for chemical contaminants for instance, consisting of residues in foods or ingredients, coming from different sources. The most important are: environmental pollution; pesticides, veterinary medicines or other aids in the production processes of agro-business or bio-industry; packaging materials; nuclear pollution. National and international standards are being developed for a harmonizing of rules and legislation on the acceptable daily intake (ADI) of additives and other alien substances. In the eyes of toxicologists, however, microbial contaminants are not at all safe. Frequently caused by a lack of hygiene in the preparation of foods in the kitchen, they lead to food poisoning and gastric disorders up to an estimated rate of a few hundreds of thousands of cases a year. The effects of natural toxicants, finally, are not yet all very well known and need more study[9].

Research among the consumer public in the late eighties in fact reveals the existence of widespread worries about food among which the fear of pesticides, additives and veterinary medicines scores highest and hygiene in the kitchen at home or during transport lowest. Consumers are of the opinion that, though some additives are perhaps indispensable, their use should be limited and the information clearer. Food worries appear to be linked with an extreme lack of knowledge on processes of food production, but -interestingly enough- not in a consistent way[10]. Food experts have pointed to several societal forces as a cause for the much regretted public opinion. These are: the media, the trade and industrial style of food-advertising, extolling the absence of additives, the information by organized consumer's unions and a gigantic lack of knowledge among the lay public about food production techniques and their 'real' risks. During a conference on 'additives and product-information' held in 1990 the leader of an important government research institution even asserted that consumers are 'deceived' by their organizations 'who want to incite the public and the government to action in compliance with their wish by means of alarming publications on additives'[11]. In his opinion the problem of additives is principally 'a problem of communication.' The remedy can be found in

enlightment of the public so that the consumer can make his own independent choice.

These assertions in particular prompted me to focus in this paper mainly
on the role of the consumer's organizations as a factor in the development of
public distrust. Consumer movements in western countries have increased
considerably in societal power since World War II. Issues of food quality
currently make up an important part of their activities[12]. As it is impossible
to take into account the full range of organizations (which differ in socio-
political stance) I confine myself to consideration of the *Consumentenbond*,
the most sizable Dutch consumers' union. The section below presents a
tentative impression of the news about food which this organization has
spread over the last forty years via its periodical. The next few paragraphs,
though, are devoted to the points about food quality in a more distant past.

Industrialization in the Netherlands emerged sluggishly. Full economic
growth was barely underway before 1890. In the developing food industry
Jurgen's margarine factory, established in 1871, took an important position.
This is true both for its role as the first producer of an essential synthetic type
of fat, and as a booming business expanding into a large-scale world-
concern. The history of the Unilever enterprise forms an excellent example
of the processes of growth, differentiation and specialization, which have
been characteristic of industrialization in general and of the industrial
production of foodstuffs in particular. The crucial role of science and
technology in this development, already important in the nineteenth century, cannot be stressed strongly enough. Foodstuffs, originally produced
and processed in a completely different way, have become liable to the same
processes of mechanization and 'chemicalisation' at successive points in
time[13]. The rise of the food industry has been one of the most important
factors in overcoming recurrent food shortages and hunger, that were usual
for people living only a few generations ago[14].

The problems of quality in the nineteenth century were at least as serious
as those of quantity, perhaps even more. During this whole period food
adulteration was widely practised, mainly because of a lack (or complete
ineffectiveness) of government legislation and control. Individuals and
groups concerned for that ordinary consumer of foodstuffs were not only
to be found among the 'hygienists', doctors and other scientists interested in
public health. Cookery teachers attached to the schools of household
economics, established during the 1890s, circulated knowledge on buying
food economically and safely, and lectured on preparing nutritious meals.
They taught housewives to identify signs of food adulteration and warned
mothers not to give their children 'sickly coloured sweets consisting largely of
chalk'[15]. Other women of about the same social position, i.e. the well-
educated middle-class, initiated the establishment of an association to
promote the 'professional' interests of housewives after the turn of the
century. One of their tasks consisted of both advice and criticicism of the

manufacturers of the goods needed in their profession, such as kitchen utensils and food packages. This housewives' union can, in a way, be viewed as a predecessor of the future consumer's organizations, as can the co-operative societies dating from the interbellum[16].

A Food Act finally became operative after World War I in 1919. This had only been possible by a shift in the structure of political power positions of relevant societal groups. Representatives of the incipient disciplines of nutrition, toxicology and social medicine kept insisting on the need for legislative public health measures, while food producers' interest groups, for instance butchers, defended the freedom of their trades as long as possible. Liberal political influences at the local and central level made parliamentary and government agencies slow to take responsibility. The final issuing of government rules on the composition and safety of food opened up possibilities for the protection of consumers, especially the poor, the sick and the ignorant; food safety became a task in the care of the state[17].

## Food quality mirrored in the Consumer's Guide (1953–1993)

De *Nederlandse Consumentenbond* (Dutch Consumers' Union) starts in the spring of 1953 with a few dozen people striving to protect the interests of the consumer in opposition to the strong position of producers and distributors of commodities. The Union aims to realize this goal by means of consumer research, advice and consultation. The definition of the then novel word 'consumer' as 'a spender of income in the most profitable way to himself'[18] is conspicuous for its simplicity. One may assert that the task of 'wise spending' has been extricated from a complex of duties, which only recently belonged to the job of housewifery; after the war apparently, this particular duty lost its feminity. Foreshadowing the coming affluence, the consumer's movement arises incidentally a year after the abolition of the rationing of coffee, a last remnant of wartime food scarcity. A decade later, membership has increased from 1010 (end 1953) to 25,000 and in 1970 to 275,000. By that time, as the magazine records, the Union and the interests it represents are taken seriously by the authorities, trade and business and other consultative partners. The *Consumer's Guide* is referred to as an influential source of information for questions, posed in the Lower Chamber of Parliament[19]. Food items are found in every volume of this journal[20].

### The frugal fifties

From an inspection of the tiny first volume of the *Consumer's Guide* one gets the impression that the Union's claims about consumer's difficulties in choosing from 'the variety of products', is much overdone. The Guide reflects no such thing for it mainly covers the basics of material existence: food and fuel. Prices and qualities of milk, meat, margarine, eggs, coffee and tea are critically appraised, and the Union consultations with other responsible parties in the field of food (state, trade and business) are reported. Nonetheless, one may conclude that the consumer as an eater has been explicitly represented by the Union right from the start. Coverage of 'the expensive book', figures in the next volume as the first non-food or basic-necessity topic. Besides the basics, the results are presented of consumer research on ready-made peasoup; preserved and ready-made foods (especially snacks) will continue to receive attention in future Guides as well.

Another message (1954) catches the eye: 'Danger of poisoning in agriculture'. The author comments on a report from the Provincial Agricultural Association Zeeland, dealing with the issue of spraying as follows: 'the progress in counteracting plant diseases and insects has opened up the possibility of the mass production of crops to the advantage of producers and consumers.' However, the Guide continues, there are disadvantages as well: for the market gardener, who uses insecticides, and for the consumer, who gets these poisonous substances on his table. The report advises against the consumption of unpeeled fruits; the gardeners' assertion on the timely exhaustion of the poison is deemed not very reassuring by the Guide. The comment ends with the conclusion that only unharmful substances are acceptable: 'a check must be put on the indiscriminate spraying of vegetables and fruits'. The hope is expressed that the work of two committees established by the authorities to study this problem 'will end in measures which put conditions on the application of pesticides in order to protect the health of the consumer'[21]. To the observer this communication, dating from six years before Rachel Carson's book *Silent spring* came out (1962), is alarming enough. The Guide's tone however is not; on the contrary, the news is phrased in a rather neutral way.

The last two volumes of this decade witness the take-off of Dutch consumer society. There is already critical comment on slimming pills (1958: 18); fatness and its deceptive cures will be a recurring theme in the years to come. This also applies to a warning about the lack of hygiene in the kitchen, ending up in 'summer diarrhoea'. The number of communications on food decreases in proportion to the number on non-food items, such as records, TVs, cameras, refrigerators and ball-points[22].

*The sixties; the expansion of consumer society*

The decrease in quantity of the articles on food relative to those on industrial products like body-odour sprays, kitchen utensils and do-it-yourself equipment, reflects the changing way in which consumers spend their rising incomes. Yet the food section continues to claim a substantial proportion of readers of the Guide's attention. The news on basic necessities like bread, milk, peanut-butter and tinned meals never misses. Some topics catch the eye because they belong to a pluperfect: school-milk and cod liver oil. Other themes, touching on food and health, are always factual: means of weight-control; the relative advantages of vegetable as opposed to animal fats; vitamins; sweeteners; bio-dynamically cultivated fruits; 'caffeine' and nicotine. Food safety issues are already present in various and unexpected forms: an untested emulsifier, food 'irradiation', the use of hormones in the raising of chickens, food poisoning from salmonella.

In the 1960 volume one comes across the notorious Planta-affair. The consumption of Planta, a vegetable margarine produced by the Unilever concern, is blamed for the rather large-scale incidence of skin-irritations. The margarine appears to contain an insufficiently tested emulsifier which may have caused the reported health problems. The Guide's rather restrained commentary consists of the establishment view that 'it apparently has been possible to use a substance in the production of a generally consumed foodstuff of which the harmlessness is not guaranteed.' The magazine concludes that 'legislation is necessary, even for the most reputable companies (. . .)'; the Union is not opposed to the use of emulsifiers as such, but rather opposes the insufficient degree of examination'[23]. In the next issue the Guide reports on the Union's action on the occasion of the use of hormones in the poultry-industry, in co-operation with other consumer organizations: the minister of agriculture responsible is asked to enact an 'absolute prohibition of the use of substances which are not proved to be totally non-noxious.' To those belong, it is explained, 'besides the infamous Planta-emulsifier, hormone-preparations, antibiotics and other substances'[24]. The Guide's tone remains polite, but now appears a little sterner.

The end of the sixties in the Guide is marked by much information on cars and travelling. Soft drinks, pudding-powders, meals ready for use and the hygiene of packages are subjects of consumer research, just like rolled oats, peas, beans, mustard and vacuum packaged sausage. Health comes into the picture several times when, once more, it concerns smoking and the use of sweeteners in coffee or tea. A novel food, soya-meat, is considered cheap, nutritious, but tasteless. Finally attention is drawn to the rights of the consumer, among which *safety* (protection against the marketing of commodities which are dangerous for health or life) is the first and foremost.[25].

## The seventies: the awakening of environmental consciousness

An important change in political and cultural climate in the context of economic crisis and environmental pollution, sets up favourable conditions for the realization of a range of ecologically orientated experiments, critical of the social structure. The Union's activities in watchdogging the achievements of producers and distributors of foodstuffs and those of the authorities in controlling them, had already been strengthened by the trade unions' consumer's organization, from the second half of the fifties. Yet now suddenly a whole set of newly founded or reactivated radical movements and action groups springs up around the production and consumption of food. They do not primarily watch food business' and government's every step, but offer alternative ways of growing, selling and preparing foods which are ecologically sound[26]. What is the Consumers' Union point of view in these changed circumstances? As to the issue of environmental protection the Union sees the authorities as responsible in the first place, but it wants to back up this goal proceeding from its own (research) field, by freely paying attention to aspects of pollution control. The Union recalls that it has already done this for years: 'if we examine food we have to bear in mind chemical additives and residues of pesticides, in the case of lawn mowers we have to think of noise and in the case of exhaust fumes we attend to toxicity'.[27] This is presented in the same volume as a report on a phosphate-free detergent. An important food theme in the seventies is the need for a revision of the Food Act, by then fifty years old. Straight away in the February 1970 issue an extended article is found on the history and merits of this Act which always has been supported, the Guide explains, by two pillars: 1) control and inspection of foodstuffs, to enforce the rule that they must not be harmful (to health) or unreliable and 2) honest names in order to prevent fraud. In the Union's view, protection for the consumer has been considerable, but recently a revolution in the production and distribution of ingredients and foods has taken place, which leads to new problems. It is concluded that 'the rapid development of technology and industry urges the adaptation of (. . .) the Food Act'. Package-labelling is especially needed, while the increasing use of additives (of which a great many are not yet sufficiently tested) 'must be restricted'. Public health, honesty in trade and the consumer's rights on safety and information are already under discussion. In a later issue the same point is made, now dealing with the international developments concerning the Codex Alimentarium: Dutch legislation is lagging behind.[28]

This explicit call for the need for restrictions to control the ever growing industrial use of additives and other substances, differs from the Union's position and tone with regard to the Planta-Affair in 1960. Then it asked for thorough testing, not restriction. In the same volume the issue of food irradiation is discussed once more. Is there any risk to public health? The Guide tells the reader this is highly probably not so and explains in a rather neutral way the pros and cons of this method of preservation. Other topics in this decade include: the drop in bread consumption and its nutritional consequences, the soya bean and the products made out of it (which are praised), minced-meat hot dogs and soft drinks (which are disapproved of) both from a health point of view. In 1979 the Guide resumes its stance on the Act and expresses the expectation that the new bill will soon be passed.[29]

*The eighties: going into the details of 'food pollution'*

An extensive article on the new legislative requirements for the composition and labelling of jams opens the 1980 volume, whose size has now expanded to 608 pages. A consequence of this space is a notable increase in the length of articles on food (as well as on other commodities), which opens up the possibility of going into much greater detail. The usual buyer's information is adapted to the demands of the time: bran bread, free-range eggs, but also frozen French fries and alcoholic beverages. The mysteries of the new proliferation of dairy products are revealed by information on the composition, nutritional value and other quality aspects of the different varieties of butter and cheese. Several communications are found on the increasing use of vitamins, which in most cases is deemed unnecessary.[30] Two years later the low-fat and low-sugar trend is ridiculed: in the opinion of the Union this type of product induces the consumer to spread twice as much on his bread. Its down-to-earth judgement is simple: those who want to slim should avoid fats, sugar, alcohol and snacks. In this type of 'Good Food' communication the Union's advice appears to resemble the recommendations of the Nutrition Council.

A similar matter-of-fact attitude is expressed concerning the 'alternative' food trend. As is noted in the Guide, 'alternative' eating in all its diversity has much increased in popularity, but how much quality do you get for the often higher prices? The Union's examination of organically grown products reveals, the Guide continues, that there is a lower sort of contamination with nitrates, but some other commodities come out no better than regular ones. As legislative control, commodity control and consumer research of these products are lacking, 'the consumer is left with no more than the unstable base of trust.' It is concluded, that positive points can be indicated, but consumer research is much needed; the Guide plans to pay more attention to products of conservationist enterprises in the future. There is a final, striking communication in this volume: a call for members to be present at a Symposium organized in co-operation with other consumers' and ecological groups on the delay in the enactment of the new Food Act.[31]

It appears towards the end of the decade that, in addition to shopper's news, the trend toward presenting broad and very detailed information on food quality is consolidated. This trend is backed up by research performed on the Union's own account. A conspicuous example is represented by a twelve-page article on the different aspects of fat. Not a single dimension of this particular food topic seems to be left out. The following matters are raised in succession; the consumption of too many fats (a specimen of nutritional enlightenment), shopper's information on 'light' products and very fat snacks, advice in slimming and, last but not least, the property of fats that function as a storage of contaminants in food. The last subject in particular offers the Union the opportunity simultaneously to display its chemical knowledge (PCB, PCE, DDT, HCH, dioxine and so on) and its point of view in 'the continuing story of food pollution.' The Guide explains the different types and sources of this pollution, expressing its expectation that (because of the advanced technologies of both food production and detection of contaminations) more 'food scandals' will follow in the future. The Union is furious about the government's policy of secrecy in some of these affairs and condemns the paternalistic attitude of the authorities, while simultaneously showing its research capacities. In the cases of food pollution (olive oil, fat fish, mother's milk) standardized rules and legislation are also necessary. Health risks are possible in the case of a one-sided diet, the Guide maintains. As to pesticides the opinion is expressed that non-biodegradable substances should be prohibited.[32]

*The nineties: towards European and environmental standards*

At the start of the nineties the Guide continues to expose a series of 'food scandals' in an extensive and well-documented mode. Titles like 'Consumers' Union advises against the consumption of meat from Belgium' and 'Imported vegetables and fruits bring poisonous residues on your plate' point to a shift in the scope of food issues to the international level. Official rules, prescriptions and prohibitions in agri-business and bio-industry appear to differ between the Netherlands and importing countries. Standards of acceptability and control in the use of pesticides and other aids in food production differ as well. An example is found in the use of hormone-based veterinary medicines combined with antibiotics in order to speed up the fattening of animals for slaughtering or to alter the quality of meat. These practices, the Guide explains, have been forbidden in the European Community for two years; however, watertight controls are not established everywhere, as appears in the case of Belgium. Residues of these substances are found in imported beef, which for health reasons must not be eaten. The story about poison in imported vegetables and fruit is of a similar tenor and content. It is concluded that insecurity exists about the acceptable daily intake; experts are not all of the same opinion. What is needed is the following: better control, cleaner production and the prohibition of very poisonous substances. [33]

Inspection of the last volumes of the Consumer's Guide leaves the observer with two impressions about its dealing with the issues of food quality. A continuation of the more radical style of reporting on food, adopted in the eighties, and at the same time a more subtle and restrained way of informing the consumers. The problem of nitrates and other potentially poisonous substances in vegetables and potatoes is tackled in the first way as follows. As a result of testing, it is advised to abstain from certain regular products, such as potatoes, and to try the ecologically grown alternatives: they are environment-friendly. Yet the issues of food irradiation and the allegedly carcinogenic influence of additives are dealt with in the second mode. In the case of irradiation (a topic once more on the agenda) it harks back to a very critical communication dating from 1990: 'Food irradiation forced through (. . .) the experiences until now are far from reassuring.' The relative harmlessness of this method of preservation is amplified and the present improvement in legislation is applauded. Moreover, in an article on cancer and its prevention readers are told not to be worried about the consumption of additives (colourings, preservatives) in this respect.[34]

### Concluding remarks

The quality of food has been an important issue right from the start of the Consumers' Union's existence as an organization. Both continuity and change in dealing with the many aspects of food have been observable on examination of its most important mouthpiece, the Consumer's Guide. Much earlier than expected contaminants and additives in food are noted; these alien substances remain sources of worry, particularly the first-mentioned type. Continuity too is to be found in the attention to the aspects of price and quality, yet this last concept has changed into a broad complex of dimensions. In the Union's view it now covers: reliability plus clarity (in the labelling of packages), safety regarding health plus harmlessness to the environment, nutritiousness plus taste. Food safety issues have increased in importance; 'food pollution' in particular must be counteracted by 'clean' production and sound control.

The fundamental changes in the technology of food production have turned the Union's activities as watchdog of the industrial and government accomplishments concerning food quality into a gigantic task. The realization of this job has apparently not been possible without the aid of science and research. The impressive growth in the Union's membership during the past forty years has provided the funds for an independent examination of the composition of foods and the detection of the presence of alien substances. Armed with this knowledge and backed up by the common consumers whom it represents, the Union has become strong enough to raise its voice in the debate on food safety.

Though the tone of this voice has recently become more alarmist and the demands for the issuing of rules have increased in strictness and radicality, there is no solid base for seeing these changes as deceiving the consumer public. The Union sets itself up as an expert in the midst of other experts, who by virtue of their knowledge are allowed an independent interpretation of the results of scientific research and its margins of insecurity. These margins are open for discussion and may provoke different conclusions by professionals, also depending on the dissimilar societal contexts and positions they are involved in. The Union's expertise, however, raises the question of the contrast between lay and professional beliefs and knowledge in matters of food safety already touched on in this chapter. It appears that the view of the Consumers'

Union can barely be reckoned any more to represent the category of lay beliefs about food and health. The access to the sources of scientific knowledge the Union has acquired may imply a rapprochement with the already established science-supported parties in the debate and at the same time a drifting apart from the consumers represented. Yet one may expect the Union to be an important opinion leader among the 'organized' and perhaps even 'unorganized' ordinary eaters; another type of study is needed to find out to what extent this is the case.

Among the many paradoxes of modern technological societies those around food form an interesting example. The early successes of food science and – industry in western countries in overcoming the ever lurking danger of famines and shortages in the recent past have been forgotten. Nowadays, a hundred years later, their victory seems to have changed into the opposite, at least in some respects. Food riots have disappeared in our part of the world, but a broad public distrust of the quality of modern technological food has taken its place. Consumers and their organizations have to say a lot in the food safety debate with professionals, authorities and the food business. The participation of consumers is an indication of a shift in the social structure of power between the different parties interested in questions of food. Looking back into history, especially concerning the long-lasting and painful establishment of the Food Act of 1919, a process of democratization of scientific knowledge about food (necessary for determining criteria of safety) is discernible. Consumers now have access to their own independent sources of information in order to decide for themselves. If and how they do this, is another point.

## Notes

1  *De Kleine Aarde* (1985) no 52, p. 15.
2  Stigt Thans (1988); Stasse-Wolthuis and Hautvast (1989). See also 'Additievenprobleem vooral communicatieprobleem' [The problem of additives is mainly a problem of communication], in *Voedingsmiddelentechnologie* no 13, 28 June 1990 and the reports on the 'Day of Agriculture', in *Landbouwkundig Tijdschrift* (1991) no. 8.
3  Mennell et al. (1992), pp. 45–47.
4  Farrer (1983); Massart and others (1980); Millstone (1986); Packard (1976); Pyke (1972).
5  *Nota Voedingsbeleid* 1983–1984 (*Food and Nutrition Policy in the Netherlands*), pp. 3–4.
6  Huis in 't Veld (1983) pp. 347–348; Reijnders and Sijmons et al. (1973).
7  See for a comparable case Belasco (1990) pp. 154–186.
8  See for this label Van Otterloo (1990) pp. 52–52 and Mennell et al. (1992), pp. 71–74.
9  Feron (1989); Van der Heijden (1989); van Kasteren (1988); Schuddeboom (1988); Rombouts (1989).

10 Feenstra and Hamstra (1989) pp. 76–78. See also Feenstra (1989), pp. 6–7 and Feenstra (1991) pp. 13–15.

11 See Van der Heijden in: 'Additievenprobleem vooral een communicatieprobleem', in *Voedingsmiddelentechnologie* no 13, 28 june 1990 and Van Kasteren (1988) p. 201.

12 Meulenberg (1992), p. 215, van Nieuwland (1992), p. 257.

13 See Van Otterloo (1990) pp. 52–89; Mennell et al. (1992), pp. 68–75; see for England Burnett (1968) pp. 127–144.

14 Teuteberg (1972), pp. 70–73.

15 Van Otterloo (1990), p. 138.

16 Jonker (1987), pp. 67–87.

17 Den Hartog 1982, pp. 79–81, see also Van Otterloo (1990) pp. 101–106 and De Swaan (1988).

18 See *Consumentengids* (1953), p. 1.

19. *Consumentengids* (1970), pp. 212–214, p. 411. See also idem (1978) p. 157, for a retrospective look at the past 25 years; in the early nineties the membership is about 640,000.

20. The selection of volumes for content-analysis is focused on the years at the start and at the end of a decade: 1953–54 and 1958–59; 1960–61–62 and 1968–69; 1970–71–72 and 1978–79; 1980, 1982, 1988; 1990, 1991, 1992. The number of pages per volume in four decades has increased from 4 to about 60.

21 *Consumentengids* (1954) p. 2.

22 *Consumentengids* (1958) p. 18. In 1953–54 the number of food-communications exceeds the news on non-food products (ratio about 3:2, information on services not included); in 1959 the ratio food – non-food has become 1:4. The number of food entries per volume remains more or less constant, while those on non-food products or services in the future will always increase.

23 *Consumentengids* (1960) pp. 139–140.

24 *Consumentengids* (1960) p. 164.

25 *Consumentengids* (1962) p. 47, p. 80, (1968) pp. 139–140, p. 158, (1969) p. 283.

26 Meulenberg (1992) p. 222; Van Otterloo (1990) pp. 184–210.

27 *Consumentengids* (1970) p. 219.

28 *Consumentengids* (1970) pp. 46–49, p. 298.

29 *Consumentengids* (1978) pp. 82–85, p. 149, (1979) pp. 516–617.

30 *Consumentengids* (1980) pp. 34–37, pp. 430–435, pp. 444–448.

31 *Consumentengids* (1982) pp. 196–199, pp. 388–392. Actually an 'Alternative Consumers' Union' has been established in the same year, see *Voeding en Milieu* (1992) p. 3. A revised Food Act finally became operative in 1988.

32 *Consumentengids* (1988) pp. 450–462.

33 *Consumentengids* (1990) pp. 150–158, pp. 450–461.

34 *Consumentengids* (1990) p. 569, (1992) p. 367, pp. 568–569, pp. 688–691.

## Literature

Belasco, Warren, J., *Appetite for Change. How the Counterculture took on the Food Industry (1966–1988)* (New York, 1990).

Burnett, John, *Plenty and Want. A Social History of Diet in England from 1815* to the Present Day (Harmondsworth, Middlesex, 1968).

Carson, R., *Silent Spring* (Boston, 1962).

Farrer, K.T.H., *Fancy eating that! A closer look at food additives and contaminants* (Melbourne, 1983).

Feenstra, Marijke. Hamstra, A., *Veilig voedsel: de consument een zorg?* [Safe food, a consumer's concern?] (Den Haag, 1989).

Feenstra, Marijke, Hamstra, A., 'Veilig voedsel: eten zonder zorgen' [Safe food, eating without anxiety], in Marian Stasse-Wolthuis and Joseph G.A.J. Hautvast (eds.), *Voedselveiligheid van teelt tot consument*, (Alphen aan de Rijn/Brussel, 1989), pp. 70–81.

Feenstra, Marijke, 'Voedselveiligheid: zorg voor of van de consument?' [Food safety, care or concern of the consumer?], *Landbouwkundig Tijdschrift* (1991), no 8, pp. 13–15.

Feron (1989), V.J., 'Toxicologie van ons voedsel: additieven veiliger dan te veel en te eenzijdig eten.' [Toxicology of our food], in Marian Stasse-Wolthuis and Joseph G.A.J. Hautvast (eds.), *Voedselveiligheid van teelt tot consument* (Alphen aan de Rijn/Brussel, 1989), pp. 6–19.

Hartog, Adel, P. den (ed.), *Voeding als maatschappelijk verschijnsel* [Food as a social phenomenon] (Utrecht/Antwerpen, 1982).

Heijden, C.A. van der, 'Toxicologische beoordeling en norm stelling van voedseltoevoegingen, contaminanten en residuen op nationaal en EG-niveau'. [Toxicological norms for food-additives at the national and EC level], in Marian Stasse-Wolthuis and Joseph G.A.J. Hautvast (eds), *Voedselveiligheid van teelt tot consument* (Alphen aan de Rijn/Brussel, 1989), pp. 64–55.

Huis in 't Veld, G. (red.), *Voedsel. Produktie, samenstelling, afzet, consumentenbelang.* [Foods: production, composition, consumer's interest] (Amsterdam, 1983).

Jonker, I., *Huisvrouwenvakwerk.* 75 jaar Nederlandse Vereniging voor Huisvrouwen (Baarn, 1987).

Kasteren, J. van, 'Onrust over voedsel te wijten aan vervreemding'. [Anxiety about food caused by alienation]. *Voeding* 49 (1988), pp. 200–202.

Massart, D.L., H. Deelstra, Apr. G. Hoogewijs, *Vreemde stoffen in onze voeding. Soorten, effecten, normen.* [Alien substances in our food] (Antwerpen, 1980).

Mennell, Stephen, Anne Murcott and Anneke van Otterloo, *The Sociology of Food: Eating, Diet and Culture* (London/New Delhi, 1992).

Meulenberg, M.T.G., 'Consumentisme – in het bijzonder in relatie tot de consumptie van voedings- en genotmiddelen'. [Consumerism relative to food], in *Voedingsmiddelen en Consument* (Utrecht, 1992), pp. 213–229.

Millstone, Erik, *Food additives. Taking the lid off what we really eat* (Harmondsworth, Middlesex, 1986).

Nieuwland, L. van, 'Voedingsbeleid en consumentenorganisaties'. [Food policy and consumer's organisations], in *Voedingsmiddelen en consument* (Utrecht, 1992).

*Nota Voedingsbeleid* 1983–1984. [Food and Nutrition Policy in the Netherlands] (Den Haag/Rijswijk, 1984).

Otterloo, Anneke, H. van, *Eten en eetlust in Nederland (1840–1990)* Een historisch-sociologische studie [Eating and Appetite in the Netherlands *1840–1990*] (Amsterdam, 1990).

Packard Jr., Vernal S., *Processed Foods and the Consumer. Additives, Labelling, Standards and Nutrition* (Minneapolis, 1976).

Pyke, Magnus. *Technological Eating, or Where does the Fishfinger Point?* (London and Southampton, 1972).

Rombouts, F.M. et al., 'Microbiële risico's van de voeding' [Microbial risks in food], in Marian Stasse-Wolthuis and Joseph G.A.J. Hautvast (eds), *Voedselveiligheid van teelt tot concument* (Alphen aan de Rijn/Brussel, 1989), pp. 19–32.

Reijnders, Lucas and Rob Sijmons et al., *Voedsel in Nederland Gezondheid, bedrog en vergif* [Food in the Netherlands. Health, deceit and poison] (Amsterdam, 1973).

Schuddeboom, L.J., 'Kwaliteitsperceptie door de consument' [Consumer's perception of quality]. *Voedingsmiddelentechnologie* 18–2 (1988) no. 4, pp. 11–15.

Stigt Thans, M.J. van, *Hoe veilig is ons voedsel?* [How safe is our food?] (Amsterdam, 1988).

Swaan, Abram de, *In Care of the State. Health Care, Education and Welfare in Europe and the US in the Modern Era* (New York, 1988).

Teuteberg, Hans J., Günter Wiegelmann, *Der Wandel der Nahrungsgewohnheiten unter dem Einfluss der Industrialisierung* [Changes in food habits and industrialisation] (Göttingen, 1972).

# 20

# THE ROLE OF NUTRITION IN FOOD ADVERTISEMENTS: THE CASE OF THE NETHERLANDS

## Adel P. den Hartog

### Introduction

The growth of the modern food industry is closely connected with developments in food technology, food science and nutrition.[1] From the end of the 19th century, the food industry has made use of nutritional knowledge and concepts in advertisements. This was incorporated in their efforts to convince consumers to buy certain food products. For more than a hundred years the food industry has disseminated nutritional information among the general public. Possible long lasting effects of food advertisements on nutritional knowledge and food habits are difficult to measure, if not impossible.[2] However, it is possible and useful to analyse what kind of information on nutrition has been directed towards the general public.

### Aim

The aim of the paper is to give insight on how the food industry tried to spread knowledge on nutrition among consumers as part of their food advertisements, taking the Netherlands as an example.

It is focused on the following three issues:

- in what way did the food industry make use of nutritional knowledge and new developments of the nutritional sciences
- the nutritional message of food advertising and changes in the course of time
- reactions from nutritionists and the medical profession to food advertising.

The paper relates to the general consumer, but does not cover advertisements for infant foods, nor special diets for people suffering from a particular disease such as diabetes.

The core of the paper is based on a content analysis of nutrition information in Dutch family and women's magazines in the period 1900–1985.[3] In total 4203 food advertisements have been analysed. Needless to say, the objective of advertising is to persuade consumers to buy a certain product and not promote health or nutrition. However, nutrition is just one of the many persuaders used in advertising. Certain products, due to their very nature, are more likely to have a nutrition component in the advertisement than others. Classical examples are baby and infant foods, condensed milk products in tins, tinned foods in general and margarine.

### Diffusion of knowledge of nutrition among the population

Nutritional knowledge has two dimensions, traditional knowledge and scientifically based nutritional knowledge. The traditional knowledge of nutrition, or food ethnology of what is good to eat or not to eat and with whom, is handed on from mother to daughter. In the industrialized countries the traditional knowledge on nutrition is to a large extent superseded by a scientifically based nutritional knowledge. This, however, does not mean that present consumers act according to the ideas of the nutritional sciences!

At the end of the 19th century nutrition emerged as a new discipline, giving scientifically based evidence of the relation between food and health.[4] In the Netherlands nutritional knowledge has been diffused from the beginning of the 20th century by the following agencies of change:

- advertisements of the food industry in newspapers and magazines, informative brochures and booklets.
- child care centres, of which the first was established in 1901. From the 1920s a vast network of child care centres spread over the country
- the Bureau of Nutrition Education from 1941 onwards.

Apart from the above mentioned agencies, nutritional knowledge on cooking has been part of the curriculum of vocational training for girls, in particular in the years 1920–1970.[5] In the 1930s programmes of nutrition education were implemented in rural and urban areas.[6] One may say that the food industry among all these agencies of change has the longest record of being involved in bringing nutritional knowledge to the general public. This gives a good reason to single out food advertising and to analyse food advertisers' activities.

### Food advertising

Food advertising is closely linked with the development of a wider circulation of newspapers and magazines and the emergence of brand names of food products and food in the latter part of the 19th century. In the Netherlands proprietary claims of brands were for the first time regulated in 1893 by law. This took place during the rise of mass production of consumer goods in small packaging.[7] Influenced by English and American advertising and marketing practices, the foundation of modern advertising was laid in the years 1914–1929.[8] This meant among other things, that advertisements became more target orientated, with a balance between illustration and text, and the introduction of marketing research.

A pioneer in the development of brand names and large scale advertising is the margarine industry. As a substitute for butter, an 'ersatz', there was a necessity to profile the new food.[9] Coffee and tea firms have also played an important role in the development of brand names and food advertising in various European countries.[10]

The food industry had an early interest in using nutrition and nutrition related items in their advertising activities. This included health, hygiene and recipes. In the 1920s and 1930s some firms asked home economists to prepare booklets on new cooking techniques and recipes. Well-known booklets were among others the recipe booklet of the cooking oil firm of Calvé.[11] Also classics in the Netherlands are the baking booklets of the German firm of Oetker.

A clear example is the firm of Liga, the manufacturer of well-known nutritious children's biscuits.[12] The Liga biscuit could be used by the mother for the young child as a healthy snack or by soaking it in milk as a porridge. The firm informed consumers in the 1930s of the nutritional aspects of the biscuits by means of:

- food advertisements in newspapers and women's magazines
- the publication of nutrition information in leaflets and booklets
- information on the packaging.

When discussing food advertisements it is of importance to realize that they are focused on women. Despite changes in gender roles, most food purchasing is still done by women. However, the image of women in advertisements has changed considerably from housewives to independent professional women.[13]

### Food advertisements in women's magazines

The analysis of food advertisements in the Dutch women's magazines covers the period 1900–1985.[14] The nutritional information has been analysed according to three main aspects:

- relation with health
- composition of the food product in terms of nutrients as well as ingredients
- utilization of the food product.

The women's magazines studied are not trendsetters, but follow trends, directed at ordinary women with their families.

### From informative to modern food advertising (1900–1939)

Characteristic for the early food advertisements was their informative nature. Information was, however, limited. The name of the product, the brand name and the food quality were mentioned and that was it. Nutritional knowledge and health claims were little used. In the beginning of 1900, the concept of the nutritional sciences was still that for good nutrition, proteins, carbohydrates and fats could suffice.[15] Growth of children could according to advertisements be stimulated by the use of protein rich foods, consumption of gingerbread,

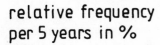

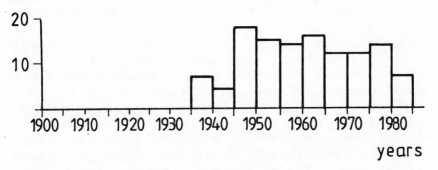

Figure 1.  Relative frequency of the mention of vitamins in food advertisements in Dutch women's magazines, 1900–85.
Source: Bos et al.

chocolate and porridge. Even eating sweets could be appetizing. A range of different products was mentioned as healthy, alcoholic beverages such as Geneva (the Dutch gin), sweet snacks and dairy products.

The doctrine of the contagious diseases, which dominated so much medical thinking in the second part of the 19th century, was also reflected in advertisements for coffee, tea, cocoa, margarine and butter. For all these products it was mentioned that they had been hygienically processed and packaged.

In the period 1920–1930 the character of advertisements changed. The advertised food products often appealed to a level of prosperity which was out of reach of the common man. Informative aspects still remained of importance. Despite the rather spectacular progress made in nutrition research on the existence and role of vitamins, food advertisements only sporadically referred to them. The term vitamin for the first time regularly appeared in advertisements during the economic crisis of the 1930s and in particular in the years 1935–1939 (Fig. 1). It concerned mainly processed foods and porridges. These products were called healthy, of importance for growth of children, the building up of resistance against diseases and the development of bones (Table 1). In the same period the relative frequency of the mentioning of health in food advertisements increased from 6% in the years before to 21% in the period 1935–1939 (Fig. 2).

It is of importance to note that in the same period health authorities were much concerned with a decrease in the quality of nutrition among unemployed households. Several nutrition surveys were initiated on the health situation of the unemployed.[16] Another striking phenomenon is the depiction of slimness and American-style ideas of beauty. It is clearly a break with the concept of fatness as a sign of prosperity and health. Needless to say, these ideas were inspired by the American film industry and to a lesser extent by the nutritional sciences. On the whole, in the period 1930–1939 nothing directly referred to the economic crisis, nor to the threat of a coming war.

During the Second World War food advertising continued. In advertising a shift took place from healthy to nutritious food. In a period of increasing food scarcity the saturational aspects of food became of importance. Also new were the advertisements for substitute products.

In the years after the war, the health of the vulnerable groups, children and pregnant women, has a central place in food advertising. A whole range of products is recommended to mothers for their children and even their unborn children. To vitamins, nearly magical properties were attributed (Fig. 2). An example from a margarine advertisement in 1948 read:

'. . . And the nutritional value? Look at these stout, healthy children, eating Blue Band. It is made from exquisite natural fats and besides it contains the "sunshine" vitamins A and D. Those vitamins construct the osseous system and increases our resistance against disease.[7]' In later years vitamins B and C received attention. They were good for growth, resistance, appetizing, blood stimulation and lessening of digestive problems. Various manufacturers started to vitaminize all sorts of products. In 1949 the vitaminizing of food products was regulated by law. Fat was strongly associated with the digestibility of food and was valued in a positive way. On the other hand attention to a slim figure continued. The term 'calorie' appeared for the first time in advertising in the beginning of the 1950s (Fig. 3).

**Healthy, pleasant and tasty**

In the years 1963–1975 the tone of advertising is changing. Attention is still given to nutrients, but they are less emphasized than in the period just after

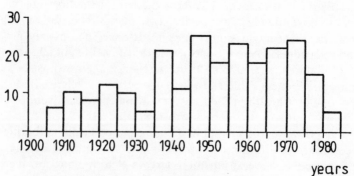

Figure 2.   Relative frequency of the mention of the notion "healthy" in food advertisements in Dutch women's magazines, 1900–85.
Source: Bos et al.

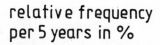

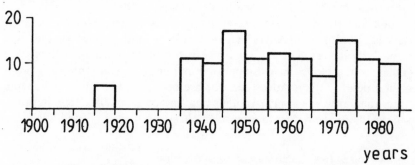

Figure 3.  Relative frequency of the mention of energy and related subjects in food
advertisements in Dutch women's magazines, 1900–85.
Source: Bos et al.

the Second World War. Social aspects of nutrition are now put forward, such
as pleasant and tasty. The word 'healthy' is now indiscriminately used. The
claim 'good for your figure' is mentioned in 12% of all food advertisements.
In this period of an unprecedented prosperity for nearly all categories of
society, two foodstuffs received a less favourable attention: fats and sugar.

The results of nutrition research on cardiovascular diseases were reflected in
food advertising. In advertisements, particularly of the margarine industry,
consumers are warned against the development of overnutrition and cardiovascular diseases. Polyunsaturated fats are recommended for better health.

Carbohydrates are less mentioned, and when mentioned, in a rather negative
way: 'contains less sugar', 'free of sugar', or: 'not sweetened and for that reason
good for your figure.' Gradually consumers become suspicious of food
additives. Advertising, flexible as it is, starts to mention what a product does
not contain such as: no additives, preservatives, colourants or emulsifiers.

It is of interest to note that at the beginning of the 1970s a start has been
made with a new phenomenon, a male presence in the kitchen. In the middle
of the 1970s the number of advertisements in magazines diminished food and
non food. This was due to an increase in TV and radio commercials. At the
same time, however, the share of food advertisements increased.

## A Healthy Nutrition

A healthy nutrition becomes a central theme in food advertising in the period
1976–1985. In the 1970s health claims were made in more than 35% of all
advertised food products. After 1980 the food act forbids the mentioning of the
term 'healthy' or 'good for your health' in advertisements.[18] In a very suggestive
way the food industry got round this problem by depicting a concept of health in

the form of healthy looking slim persons. Increasing attention is now given to what a product does not contain. It goes along with chemophobic tendencies among consumers. The claim that food products are made from pure or natural ingredients is more frequently made than before.

Food advertisements are mainly targeted at women. Women were for years depicted as housewives or in the role of mother (Fig. 4). This was particularly the case in the years between 1950–1965. After 1980 pictures of women as housewives have disappeared, but not altogether those of women in the role of mother. Advertisements are now aimed at adults in general, rather than at women only. Another trend becomes manifest, less information on the food product and more emphasis on the sphere and image.

### Critical voices from nutrition and health circles

Advertisements have always received critical receptions from various sections of the society. In the 1920s there was a strong move in society against

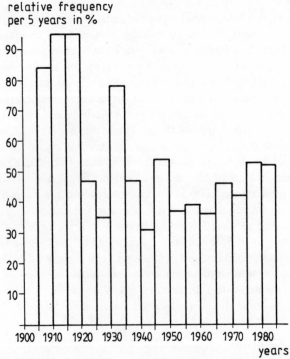

Figure 4.  Relative frequency of the mention or depiction of women in the role of housewife[1] or mother in food advertisements specifically directed to women in Dutch women's magazines, 1900–85.
Source: Bos et al.
[1] includes male servants till the 1930s.

advertising, in particular against advertisement boards dotted all around towns and along roads. Advertising was considered as clamorous, obtrusive and damaging to esthetic values.[19] The criticism of advertising increased after the Second World War with the rise of consumerism.[20] Likewise, the medical profession and nutritionists were often suspicious of food advertising.

In America, the cradle of modern advertising, the food chemist Alfred W. McCann, a former employee of the food industry, stated in 1918: 'The advertising manager can not state the whole truth in a food advertising campaign . . . their advertisements center about the talking points that will sell their products, always clear of controversy'.[21] In the 1920s and 1930s food advertisements were mainly criticised for ways in which they dealt with aspects of the quality and hygiene of food. Nutritional aspects were hardly taken into account by critically minded health professionals.[22]

The Nutrition Council, created in 1940, played an important role in getting food advertising regulated in such a way that it would not be in conflict with direct public health interests and scientific evidence. Thanks to the work of the Nutrition Council, vitaminizing of food products was regulated by the Food Act in 1949.[23] As a result less emphasis in food advertising was given to vitamins. In the UK the Advertising Association prepared on a voluntary basis a code of conduct on how to deal with vitamins in advertising. This was a clear attempt to avoid discrediting food advertising. A summary appeared in 1958 in the Netherlands Nutrition Journal.[24] In the Netherlands the regulation of food advertisements happened later than in the UK, in 1964 and likewise on a voluntary basis.[25]

The Nutrition Council has on several occasions forwarded complaints to the Advertising Code Commission (and the Advertising Council for TV and radio). A major conflict developed on the use of health claims. Nutritionists and consumer organizations alike become very concerned about the abuse of health claims in food advertisements. They were of the opinion that health claims were misleading, such as: healthy bread, healthy margarine, good for your health, good for your cardiovascular system, and fresh is healthy. In 1977 the Nutrition Council advised the government on the handling of health claims in advertising.[26] After 1980 health claims are permitted no longer.

In the 1970s the consumption and frequency of consumption of sugar and sugar-containing snacks came under attack by nutritionists and dentists. Caries, in particular of young children, became a public health issue. Advertisements like, 'sugar makes you slim', caused irritation. In the United Kingdom the nutritionist John Yudkin (1972) fiercely attacked the sugar industry with his book entitled 'Pure, white and deadly, the problem of sugar'.[27] This provocative publication, with a mix of scientific evidence and speculation, had likewise in the Netherlands a negative impact on the attitude towards sugar. Because of these developments against sugar, the Advertising Code Foundation prepared a code on sugar-containing snacks in 1980. Important points were: less emphasis on children below the age of 14 years, no suggestion that a sugar-containing snack may replace a meal or eating a snack just before going to bed.[28]

In the years after 1980 one may observe a kind of rapprochement between the nutritionists and the food industry. It reflected a change in culture which gradually took place in Dutch society. Flower power and provocative public happenings were important elements of public life in the 1960s and 1970s. After 1980 a trend appeared towards more harmonious and individualistic approaches. Nutritionists and the food industry are now more prepared to listen to each other's arguments. Major food firms now take the nutritional dimensions of their food products seriously into account in their advertisements and other ways in reaching the consumer. They have employed nutritionists on their staff in order to avoid conflicting situations and to tie in with new developments in the field of nutrition.

This does not mean, of course, that the conflict of interests has ended between the nutritional sciences and the food industry. It has, however, made an end to sterile antagonistic approaches.

### A discussion on food advertising and nutrition

Looking at the food advertisements studied for the period 1900–1985, we can conclude that food advertisements in general provide limited information with a nutritional scientific undertone. Other arguments such as tasty, pleasant and distinctive are dominant. Nevertheless, nutritional terms and concepts from the nutritional sciences have frequently been used in food advertising, for a very long period. The length of time between new scientific knowledge and application in food advertisements becomes shorter. In 1912 in London Casimir Funk introduced the term 'vitamin', which appeared more than 10 years later in Dutch women's magazines[29].

The margarine industry played an important role in providing scientific evidence in its advertisements. The relation between cholesterol and health was more rapidly picked up in food advertising. It concerns scientific knowledge on nutrients that may be a threat to health. Of interest also is the introduction of nutrition information in a rather negative way in the 1980s, such as no additives, no sugar or low in fat.

What has been the long lasting impact of food advertisements on the nutritional knowledge of consumers? This is very hard, if not impossible, to measure. On the other hand one may assume that the food industry in the course of time has contributed much to a greater familiarity with nutritional terms such as vitamins, proteins, calories, cholesterol, linoleic acid and the problems of cardiovascular diseases. Advertisers make use of those parts of scientific information only that may promote the sale of their products. This coincides often with current research themes.

*Table 1:* Nutritional concepts and terminology utilized in food advertisements in Dutch women's magazines 1900–1985

| Nutritional concepts and terminology | Appearance in magazines first time years | most frequent | Share of total no. of advertisements percentage | Trend |
|---|---|---|---|---|
| Energy (total) | 1915–19 | 1946–50 | 18% | fluctuates after 1935 approx. 10% |
| Nutritious | 1910–14 | 1946–50 | 16% | around 1940–45 |
| Protein | 1905–09 | 1971–75 | 7% | after 1956 approx. 5% |
| Fat | 1910–14 | 1956–60 | 12% | after 1940 approx. 70%, absent in 1961–65 |
| Linoleic acid | 1960–64 | 1976–80 | 5% | stable approx. 5% |
| Carbohydrates (general) | 1900–04 | 1981–85 | 10% | approx. 5% |
| * sugar | 1900–04 | | | |
| * less sugar, free of sugar | 1935–39 | | | |
| * starch | 1920–24 | | | |
| * nutritional fibre | 1976–80 | | | |
| Vitamins (general) | 1935–39 | 1961–65 | 13% | increasing till 1961, after that decreasing |
| Vitamin A and D | 1935–39 | 1946–50 | 8% | only in 1946–6 |
| Vitamin B and C | 1935–39 | 1976–80 | 5% | fluctuates approx. 3% |
| Minerals (total) | 1900–04 | 1940–45 | 16% | before 1940 approx. 4% after 1945 approx. 10% |
| Calcium | 1920–24 | 1946–50 | 7% | around 1940–45 |
| * salt | 1910–14 | | | |
| * low in salt | 1960–65 | | | |
| * iron | 1920–24 | | | |
| Additives (general) | 1905–09 | 1981–85 | 20% | highest in 1935 (13%) lower in 1956 (64%) |
| Contains no additives | 1905–09 | 1981–85 | 7% | before 1981 sporadic |
| * contains additives | 1905–09 | | | |
| * contains artificial sweeteners | 1946–50 | | | |
| Pure ingredients | 1900–04 | 1981–85 | 11% | low between top years 1940 (9%) 1981 (11%) |
| Pure vegetable food | 1951–60 | 1976–80 | 6% | after 1961 approx. 4% |

*Source:* den Hartog, et al. 1989.

**Notes**

1  See e.g. Pyke (1968) as far as the U.K. is concerned and for the Netherlands, Lintsen (1992).

2  It is, however, possible to measure short term effects of food advertisements on the nutritional knowledge of consumers as was done by Vermeersch and Swenerton (1972, 1980) in California, U.S.A.

3  A study of 85 years of food advertising in the Netherlands has been carried out by G.J. Bos, P.A. Flach and N.G.A. van Solingen as part of a project on the development of the modern Dutch diet. Some of the results have been published in Dutch by Bos et al. (1987) and den Hartog et al. (1989). Much assistance has been received from Sioekie Kroes in preparing this chapter.

4  Pyke (1968), pp.1–2.

5  den Hartog (1992), p. 311, Jobse-van Putten (1987), van Otterloo (1985).

6  den Hartog (1983), p. 37.

7  Nijhof (1986), p. 33.

8  Nijhof (1986), pp. 8–10, Schreurs (1989), pp. 85–86.

9  van Stuijvenberg, 1969, p. 248. The studies of Charles Wilson on the history of Unilever (1954, 1968) give a good insight into the role of food advertising in the development of the modern food industry.

10  Bantje (1981), pp. 180–191, Teuteberg (1989).

11  Jobse-van Putten (1985), p. 7.

12  A study by the Department of Human Nutrition, Wageningen Agricultural University, is in progress on the nutritional concepts of the firm of Liga, covering the period 1920–1992.

13  van Lieshout (1980), p. 49–57.

14  The data presented in the following paragraphs on food advertisements are mainly from unpublished material of the study carried out by Bos et al. (1987).

15  McCollum (1957), pp. 201–2.

16  den Hartog (1983), pp. 34–5.

17  den Hartog et al (1989), p. 227.

18  de Bekker (1980).

19  Schreurs (1989), pp. 73–83.

20  Schreurs (1989), pp. 166–9.

21  McCann (1919), p.v.

22  When searching the volumes of the educational journal on nutrition and hygiene (1920–1935) published under the auspices of the Netherlands Institute of Public Nutrition (Nederlands Instituut voor Volksvoeding) hardly any references were found to the nutritional message of food advertisements. Likewise the National Health Council was not concerned with matters related to nutrition and food advertising in the period 1902–1940. The advisory work of the Council as far as nutrition was concerned, dealt with food hygiene and health, and the quality of food in general (Rigters, 1992, pp. 94–97, 157–159).

23  den Hartog, C. (1980) pp. 94–95.
24  Nutrition (1958), p. 72, Voeding (1958), pp. 740–1.
25  Since 1964 advertising is, on a voluntary basis, regulated by the Advertising Code Foundation (Stichting Reclame Code). It deals with advertisements in newspapers, magazines and other printed media and those of the cinema. The implementation of the Code is entrusted to the Advertising Code Commission (Reclame Code Commissie). Advertising by television and radio, for the first time allowed by law in 1967, is supervised by the Advertising Council (Reclame Raad), but that lies beyond the scope of this paper.
26  de Bekker (1981) p. 8, Rijneveld-van Dijk (1982), pp. 250–1.
27  Yudkin (1972), a revised version appeared in 1986.
28  Voeding (1980), p. 443.
29  McCollum (1957), p. 217, Todhunter (1976), p. 361.

## Literature

Bantje, H.F.W., *Twee eeuwen met de weduwe. Geschiedenis van de Erven de Wed. J. van Nelle N.V..* [The history of the coffee and tea firm van Nelle] (Rotterdam, Van Nelle, 1981).

Bos, Gerda, J., Flach, P.A., Solingen, N.G.A. van, Hartog, A.P. van. '85 Jaar voedingsmiddelen advertenties in Nederlandse tijdschriften'. [85 years of food advertisements in Dutch magazines], in Annemarie de Knecht-van Eekelen and Marian Stasse-Wolthuis (eds), *Voeding in onze samenleving, een cultuurhistorisch perspectief* (Alphen a.d. Rijn/Brussel, Samsom Stafleu, 1987), pp. 135–159.

Bekker, George J.P.M. de, 'Voeding, reclame en gezondheidsclaims'. [Nutrition, advertisements and health claims]. *Voeding*, 41 (1980), pp. 138–142.

Hartog, Adel P. den, 'Dietary change and industrialization: the making of the modern Dutch diet'. *Ecology of Food and Nutrition*, 27 (1992), pp. 307–318.

Hartog, Adel P. den, 'Food habits in a situation of crisis: the unemployed and their food in the years 1930–1939 in the Netherlands'. *Ernährungs-Umschau*, 30 (1983), supplement, pp. 33–6.

Hartog, Adel P. den, Flach, P.A., Bos, G.J., Solingen, N.G.A. van. 'Voedingsinformatie in reclame, een analyse van 85 jaar voedingsmiddelenadvertenties'. [Nutrition information in advertising, an analysis of 85 years of food advertisements]. *Voeding*, 50 (1989), pp. 224–9.

Hartog, Cornelis den, 'Perioden in de ontdekking en waardering van vitamines'. [Periods in the discovery and appreciation of vitamins]. *Voeding*, 41 (1980), pp. 89–95.

Jobse-van Putten, Jozien, 'Met nieuwen tijd, komt nieuw (w)eten. Invloed van het voedingsonderricht op de Nederlandse voedingsgewoonten, ca 1880–1940'. [Influence of nutrition training on Dutch food habits]. *Volkskundig Bulletin*, 13 (1987), pp. 1–29.

Lieshout, Jan van, *Het kan wel op al is het lekker! Het dagelijks leven van kleine man tot Jan Modaal, zichtbaar gemaakt in 50 jaar reclame.* [Daily life of the man in the street visualized in 50 years of advertising] (Bussum, Unieboek, 1980).

Lintsen, H.W. (ed), *Geschiedenis van de techniek in Nederland*, Deel I *Techniek en modernisering, Landbouw en voeding.* [History of technology in the Netherlands, Part I Technology and modernization, agriculture and nutrition] (Zutphen, Walburg Pers, 1992).

McCann, Alfred W., *The Science of Eating* (London, Evans Brothers, 1919).

McCollum, Elmer V., *A History of Nutrition, The Sequence of Ideas in Nutrition Investigations* (Boston, Mass., Houghton Mifflin, 1957).

Nijhof, P., *Emaille reclame borden in Nederland* [Enamel advertising posters in the Netherlands] (Amsterdam, van Soeren, 1986).

Nutrition, 'Advertising of vitamin products.' *Nutrition* 12 (1958), p. 72.

Otterloo, Anneke H. van, 'Voedzaam, smakelijk en gezond. Kookleraressen en pogingen tot verbetering van eetgewoonten tussen 1880 en 1940'. [Cookery teachers and efforts to improve dietary habits between 1880 and 1940]. *Sociologisch Tijdschrift*, 12 (1985), pp. 495–542.

Pyke, Magnus, Food and Society (London, John Murray, 1968).

Rigter, René B.M., *Met Raad en Daad. De Geschiedenis van de Gezondheids-raad 1902–1985.* [By word and deed. The History of the Health Council] (Rotterdam, Erasmus Publishers, 1992).

Schreurs, Wilbert, *Geschiedenis van de reclame in Nederland.* [History of advertising in the Netherlands] (Utrecht, Spectrum, 1989).

Stuijvenberg, J.H. van (ed), *100 jaar margarine.* [100 years of margarine] ('s-Gravenhage, Martinus Nijhoff, 1969).

Teuteberg, Hans, 'Entwicklung und Funktionen der Lebensmittelwerbung'. *Ernährungs-Umschau*, 36(1989), pp. 17–31.

Todhunter, E. Neige, 'Chronology of some events in the development and application of the science of nutrition'. *Nutrition Reviews*, 34(1976), pp. 353–365.

Vermeersch, J.A., Swenerton, H., 'Consumer response to nutrition claims in food advertisements'. *Journal of Nutrition Education*, 11(1979), pp. 22–6.

Vermeersch, J.A., Swenerton, H., 'Interpretations of nutrition claims in food advertisements by low-income consumers'. *Journal of Nutrition Education*, 12(1980), pp. 19–25.

Voeding, 'Het adverteren van vitamineprodukten'. [Advertising of vitamin products]. *Voeding*, 19(1958), pp. 740–1.

Voeding, 'Nieuwe gedragscode voor suikerhoudend snoepgoed'. [New code of conduct for sugar containing sweets]. *Voeding*, 41(1980), p. 443.

Wilson, Charles, *The History of Unilever*, 3 Vols (London, Cassell, 1954, 1968).

Yudkin, John, *Pure, White and Deadly: the Problem of Sugar* (London, Davis Poynter, 1972).

# INDEX